Oxford Handbook of
Cancer Nursing

PUBLISHED AND FORTHCOMING OXFORD HANDBOOKS IN NURSING

Oxford Handbook of
Cancer
Nursing

Edited by

Mike Tadman
Oxford Brookes University, Oxford, UK

Dave Roberts
Oxford Brookes University, Oxford, UK

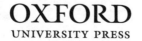

OXFORD
UNIVERSITY PRESS

OXFORD
UNIVERSITY PRESS

Great Clarendon Street, Oxford OX2 6DP

Oxford University Press is a department of the University of Oxford.
It furthers the University's objective of excellence in research, scholarship,
and education by publishing worldwide in

Oxford New York

Auckland Cape Town Dar es Salaam Hong Kong Karachi
Kuala Lumpur Madrid Melbourne Mexico City Nairobi
New Delhi Shanghai Taipei Toronto

With offices in

Argentina Austria Brazil Chile Czech Republic France Greece
Guatemala Hungary Italy Japan Poland Portugal Singapore
South Korea Switzerland Thailand Turkey Ukraine Vietnam

Oxford is a registered trade mark of Oxford University Press
in the UK and in certain other countries

Published in the United States
by Oxford University Press, Inc., New York

© Oxford University Press, 2007

The moral rights of the authors have been asserted
Database right Oxford University Press (maker)

First published 2007

British Library Cataloguing in Publication Data
Data available

Library of Congress Cataloging in Publication Data

Data available

Typeset by Newgen Imaging Systems (P) Ltd., Chennai, India
Printed in Italy
on acid-free paper by LegoPrint S.p.A.

ISBN 978–0–19–856924–4 (Flexicover:alk.paper)

10 9 8 7 6 5 4 3 2 1

Foreword

These are exciting, but testing, times for cancer nursing. As treatment regimes become more complex, targeted therapies introduce new challenges in administration and symptom management, and patterns of care delivery change, cancer nurses need to expand their knowledge and adapt to new ways of working whilst ensuring that the unique contribution they make to the care of people with cancer remains intact.

That unique contribution depends on a genuine understanding of the emotional and physical impact of cancer and its treatment, an ability to assess (with sensitivity and timeliness) how the person is dealing with that impact and a high degree of skill in anticipating (and preventing if possible) the problems that might be waiting around the corner. Cancer nursing, perhaps more than any other specialty, encapsulates the art and science of caring – combining emotional support, information and education with an intensive level of personal and physical care throughout treatment as well as rehabilitative support and care once treatment is over.

This excellent handbook manages to communicate both the art and the science of cancer nursing by paying equal attention to the physiological basis of cancer and the complexities of managing the disease as well as to the personal and social experience of cancer and its psychological sequelae. The handbook comprehensively deals with a huge range of obvious and not so obvious topics, providing crucial information, up to date and balanced arguments, and sensible advice for cancer nurses working in all areas of practice. Its accessible style will appeal to cancer nurses of all levels, and it deserves to live up to its name as a book which is kept close at hand, rather than on the shelf.

Mary Wells
Clinical Research Fellow in
Cancer Nursing
University of Dundee
October 2006
Dundee, Scotland

Preface

When given the opportunity to write this handbook, we were aware of the lack of a concise, instant reference book for cancer nurses in the UK. Several exist, though they are mainly North American and these are not always useful within a UK context. Larger textbooks, of which there are several, are impractical to have at hand within everyday practice. We therefore wanted to create a handbook that would be sufficiently detailed but easily accessible to support a wide range of practice situations that nurses may encounter.

Our first problem was how to decide what to leave in, what to leave out and how much depth on each particular topic to cover? Several sessions working on various outlines and considering available cancer curricula led us to an initial format, which was eventually distilled down to this final version.

Some topics easily fitted the format of one page per topic, for example a quick reference on how to manage a particular emergency or side effect. To achieve this we have given concise and up to date, practice-focused and evidence-based information throughout. However, other areas did not fit this format so comfortably. How can you reduce the complexity of communication skills down to a few key points? To help readers deal with these more subtle and complex practice issues, we have included reflection points. These provide an opportunity to draw on personal practice knowledge, and consider how practice might be improved or developed. There are also a number of blank pages where readers can make notes and add further information from their own experience or additional reading.

We knew that with the continuously changing face of cancer care it was important to cover recent developments in understanding of cancer biology and current developments in treatment modalities. However, we have aimed to put the patient, their family, and the experience of cancer, at the heart of this book. Insights are provided, in the form of direct patient quotes, into what it is like to have cancer, how individuals and families cope, and how to support them. There is a strong psychosocial focus, with a consideration of the social context within which cancer takes place, and how it affects every aspect of a patient's life.

We hope that we have got the balance right and covered the essential topics at an appropriate level. We know, however, that in such a concise book some readers will be disappointed at the lack of depth on topics of particular interest to them. We hope therefore that this handbook will complement larger, more detailed texts and encourage and inspire practitioners to further explore areas of interest.

Repetition does exist at times within the book, but this is intentional in an effort to keep appropriate material together for the purpose of the book.

We believe that this book is a valuable aid to clinical practice and fulfils its role as a practical handbook, remaining in a uniform pocket or practitioner's briefcase rather than on a shelf at home.

We would welcome any feedback on this first edition to help improve and develop any future editions.

Acknowledgements

We must firstly acknowledge the silent contribution of the many patients and their families we have worked with over the years. It has been our privilege to work with them, and we are grateful for the ways in which they have shared some of the most difficult days of their lives.

This book is a distillation of many years of wisdom, compassion and expertise, acquired through working alongside professional colleagues. We thank them all.

Specific mention must be made of:

Hazel Robertshaw, who was involved from the beginning, but whose destiny took her elsewhere.

The staff at OUP; Catherine Barnes who supported us through the initial development of the project, Nic Ulyatt who helped in such a positive way to keep it on target, and to Helen Hill for her final support in bringing the book to press.

Our colleagues at the School of Health and Social Care, Oxford Brookes University: Jane Appleton, Dorothy Bean, Helen Bennett, Gillian Chowns, Lorraine Dixon, Sue Duke, and Kay Leedham.

We thank all of those who have contributed to writing, editing and reviewing sections of the book and ensuring that it remained true to its original intent of being a practical aid to clinical practice.

Mike: to my long-suffering wife and children who have been neglected too often throughout this project and yet managed to keep me sane (and well fed) throughout.

Dave: my thanks to all of my family and friends, but particularly James and Mary, for their love and support.

Acknowledgements

Contents

Detailed contents

Contributors

Jane Appleton
Oxford Brookes University,
Oxford

Angela Avis
Oxford Brookes University,
Oxford

Helen Bennett
Oxford Brookes University,
Oxford

Graham Collins
John Radcliffe Hospital,
Oxford

Lorraine Dixon
Oxford Brookes University,
Oxford

Sarah Durrell
Churchill Hospital, Oxford

Gail Eva
Sir Michael Sobell House,
Oxford

Andrew Fishburn
Lancashire Teaching Hospitals
NHS Trust, Preston

Mark Foulkes
Royal Berkshire Hospital, Reading

Maggie Grundy
The Robert Gordon University,
Aberdeen

Mandy Harbottle
University of West of England,
Bristol

Helen Jeffries
Nuffield Orthopaedic Centre,
Oxford

Meinir Krishnasamy
Hospice in the Weald, Tunbridge
Wells

Sian Lewis
Velindre Cancer Centre, Cardiff

Shelley Orton
Churchill Hospital, Oxford

Joan Palmer
Royal Berkshire Hospital, Reading

Nicola Stoner
Cancer Research UK Medical
Oncology Unit, Oxford

Gilly Tomsett
Royal Berkshire Hospital, Reading

Sandy Wellman
Churchill Hospital, Oxford

Linda Whitehead
Littlemore Hospital, Oxford

Annie Young
University of Birmingham,
Birmingham

Reviewers

Sue Atkins
Oxford Brookes University

Nick Bates
Churchill hospital, Oxford

Dorothy Bean
Northampton General Hospital,
Northampton

Sue Duke
University of Southampton,
Southampton

Megan Edwards
Leeds General Infirmary, Leeds

Sara Faithfull
University of Surrey, Guildford

Nicky Haynes
Churchill Hospital, Oxford

Sandy Hayes
John Radcliffe Hospital, Oxford

Kay Leedham
Oxford Brookes University,
Oxford

Ruth Moxon
Royal Berkshire Hospital,
Reading

Lisa Peck
Gloucestershire Royal Hospital,
Gloucester

Nicky Sillwood
Royal Berkshire Hospital,
Reading

Bridget Taylor
Oxford Brookes University,
Oxford

Jacqui Warden
Churchill Hospital, Oxford

Mary Woolliams
Oxford Brookes University,
Oxford

Sue Ziebland
DIPEx Research Group, Oxford

Abbreviations

5FU	5-fluorouracil
AFP	alpha-feroprotein
AHP	allied health professional
AI	aromatase inhibitor
AM	intramuscular
AML	acute myeloid leukaemia
BCC	basal cell carcinoma
BCG	bacillus calmette guerin
CBT	cognitive behavioural therapy
CEA	carcinoembryonic antigen
CIN	cervical intraepithelial neoplasia
CML	chronic myeloid leukaemia
CNS	clinical nurse specialist or central nervous system
CT	computed tomography
CTZ	chemoreceptor trigger zone
CXR	chest X-ray
DCIS	ductal carcinoma *in situ*
DiPEx	Directory of Personal Experiences of Health and Illness
DNA	deoxyribonucleic acid
DVT	deep venous thrombosis
ECM	extracellular matric
ER	(o)estrogen receptor
FBC	full blood count
FNA	fine needle aspiration
G-CSF	granulocyte colony stimulating factor
GI	gastrointestinal
GM-CSF	granulocyte macrophage colony stimulating factor
GU	genitourinary
GvHD	graft versus host disease
Hb	haemoglobin
H&N	head and neck
HCG	human chorionic gonadotrophin
HIV	human immunodeficiency virus
HPV	human papilloma virus
HSCT	haematopoietic stem cell transplant

ICP	inter cranial pressure
IT	intrathecal
IV	intravenous
IVU	intravenous urography
LCIS	lobular carcinoma in situ
LDH	lactate dehydrogenase
LFTs	liver function tests
LHRH	luetinising hormone releasing hormone
MA	malignant ascites
MDT	multidisciplinary team
MPM	malignant pleural mesothelioma
MRI	magnetic resonance imaging
NHS	National Health Service (UK)
NICE	National Institute for Health and Clinical Excellence
NMSC	non-melanoma skin cancer
NSAID	non-steroidal anti-inflammatory drug
NSCLC	non-small cell lung cancer
NSGT	nonseminomatous germ cell tumour
OGJ	oesophago–gastric junction
OM	oral musositis
PET	positron emission tomography
PR	progesterone receptor
PSA	prostate specific antigen
RINV	radiotherapy induced nausea and vomiting
SC	subcutaneous
SCC	squamous cell carcinoma
SCLC	small cell lung cancer
SSRI	selective serotonin reuptake inhibitor
SVCO	superior vena cava obstruction
TCC	transitional cell carcinoma
TLS	tumour lysis syndrome
TME	total mesorectal excision
TNF	tumour necrosis factor
TNM	tumour node metastasis
TRALI	transfusion related acute lung injury
TSG	tumour suppressor gene
TURP	trans urethral resection of prostate
US	ultrasound
UTI	urinary tract infection
VC	vomiting centre
WHO	World Health Organization

Dedications

MT: This book is dedicated to Nic, Morgan and Finlay
who inspire me continuously and who make everything
in my life worthwhile.

DR: I dedicate this book to the memory of my parents,
Irene Roberts and Griffith Davies Roberts.

Section 1

Introduction

Introduction

Scientific advances

Oncology and cancer nursing are both rapidly developing specialties. Major breakthroughs in science within the last two decades are having a major influence on practice in a number of different ways.

Advances in our understanding of cancer biology have enabled the development of more accurate screening methods, improved preventative strategies and improved diagnostic and prognostic indicators. The development of a range of new biological treatments that target specific changes in cancer cells, offers greater hope and choice to many individuals with cancer. It also creates new challenges for practitioners, supporting patients with difficult treatment choices and complex symptom management.

Technological advances have also enabled quicker and more targeted radiotherapy planning and treatment. This has led to more intensive treatment regimes in a number of cancer sites. There have also been developments of new chemotherapy drugs and new combinations of treatments for many cancers, for example an increased use of concurrent chemotherapy and radiation and the addition of biological therapies to standard chemotherapy regimes.

These changes have occurred in the context of extended life expectancy, leading to increasing rates of cancer. More people are now living with cancer in the community. Improved access to information has led to higher patient expectations about treatment choices and support. In the UK there has also been public criticism of poor cancer survival rates, compared to other developed world countries.

Future scientific breakthroughs will ensure that these remain exciting and hopeful times for all those working within the cancer nursing specialty. However, the pressure of expensive new drug treatments, an ageing population, and increased patient expectations all create their own difficulties for the health services resources, which are already under pressure.

Policy initiatives

England and Wales

The Calman-Hine report (1995)[1] 'A Policy Framework for Commissioning Cancer Services' highlighted variations in care, a lack of national standards, out-dated demarcations between staff, barriers between services, and a lack of clear incentives to improve performance in cancer care. Since then cancer policy has aimed to improve services and reduce inequality across patient groups and geographical regions. The NHS Cancer Plan (2000)[2] set out the government strategy to tackle cancer, linking prevention, diagnosis, treatment, care, and research. This overall strategy has been actioned through the setting up of the 34 Cancer Networks in England and Wales. Specific quality standards of care have been outlined in the Manual of Cancer Services[3] (2004) that are assessed through a process of Peer Review.

These policy initiatives have led to:
• Key waiting times initiatives, reducing the time for individuals between initial suspicions of cancer, to diagnosis and onwards to treatment
• An increase in the number of site-specific clinical nurse specialists and nurse practitioners
• A demand for greater involvement of primary care
• An increasing emphasis on the role of palliative care at all stages of the care pathway.

The National Assembly for Wales, Health and Social Services Committee is currently undertaking a review of cancer services for people in Wales. The terms of reference are to review equality of provision and equity of access to services and to identify the barriers to good service and measures to overcome them. This report should be completed in March 2007.

Cancer Policy Scotland

In Scotland the Scottish Executive Health Department set out the Scottish cancer strategy for improving cancer services in, Cancer in Scotland: Action for Change (SEHD 2001). The Scottish Cancer Group is responsible for overseeing the implementation of this strategy and regional Cancer Advisory Groups monitor its progress. Cancer in Scotland: Sustaining Change (SEHD 2004a) looks at more recent progress and future steps required for further effective development.

Specific clinical guidelines are issued by Scottish Intercollegiate Guidelines Network (SIGN), through its umbrella organisation NHS Quality Improvement Scotland (NHSQIS). This mirrors the role of The National Institute for Health and Clinical Excellence (NICE), in England and Wales. The implications of NICE guidelines for Scotland are considered by SIGN.

1 Department of Health (1995). Policy Framework for commissioning cancer services: A report by the Expert Advisory Group on Cancer to the Chief Medical Officers for England and Wales. (Known as Calman–Hine Report.) London: DoH.
2 Department of Health (2000). The NHS Cancer Plan: a plan for investment, a plan for reform. London: DoH.
3 Department of Health (2004). Manual For Cancer Services. London: DoH.

A strategy framework for nursing people with cancer in Scotland (SEHD 2004b) was also published in 2004.

These and other useful cancer publications can be found at the *Cancer in Scotland* website, http://www.cancerinscotland.scot.nhs.uk/

Clinical implications

The clinical implications of these advances and policy initiatives have been many:

- An increase in survival rates in some major cancers, e.g. breast cancer
- An increasing number of individuals being actively treated including older patients and those with lower performance status, who are more susceptible to major side-effects
- Increasingly specialized cancer treatment and support
- The development of cancer multidisciplinary teams
- An increasing move from in-patient care to ambulatory care, which has had major consequences for resources in outpatients and primary care
- Escalating cost of cancer treatments having major implications on resources, both in hospital and in the community
- Inpatient units may be particularly busy with mainly acutely unwell patients. This has the potential knock-on effect of increasing staff stress.

These changes offer nurses many opportunities to develop new knowledge, skills and career opportunities, for example running nurse-led clinics, for both patient follow-up and diagnosis. However, as nurses take on a range of different tasks and roles the blurring of professional boundaries, particularly with junior doctors, is also a potential area for conflict.

New treatments add another layer of complexity to decisions that patients and health care professionals must face. It can be difficult managing the patients' expectations of new treatments, which may in reality offer only limited advantages. Nurses have a major role to play in providing informational and psychological support for these patients.

The move to more out patient treatment may improve quality of life for many patients and their families. However, patients now have less time to be fully assessed, informed and supported by health professionals. Many more patients face potential acute episodes such as neutropaenic sepsis whilst at home. There will also be an increased need for specially trained and experienced primary care practitioners to offer safe and effective care to these individuals.

These changes are taking place within the context of a health service that faces financial pressures, shortages of specialist nurses and an increasingly ageing nursing workforce. Cancer nurses will be expected to find ever more efficient and flexible ways of working within their current resources, whilst specialist nurses may face increasing caseloads of patients to support. Other demands include the need for continuing professional and educational development, at a time when study leave is also under pressure.

Cancer care and cancer nursing will continue to be an area of constant change and development in the near future. Though some of the developments can be predicted and therefore planned for, e.g. the continuing increase in cancer prevalence, others are less certain. For example who would have predicted 10 years ago that the most successful treatment for chronic myeloid leukaemia would be an oral drug, with limited side-effects? It is this unpredictability that makes this area such an exciting specialty to be involved in.

Specialist nursing roles

Clinical Nurse Specialists

One of the most significant developments in cancer nursing has been the recent development of a number of specialist nurse posts. Many of these are site-specific clinical nurse specialists, nurses who have responsibility for the care of a particular cancer site. Examples are found in breast cancer, head and neck cancer, lung cancer, neuro-oncology, gynae-oncology, haematology, palliative care and many others.

The clinical nurse specialist roles allow patients and their families to receive a comprehensive and holistic approach to care from a single professional who will often remain their key worker throughout their cancer journey. With their in-depth knowledge of individual patients, clinical nurse specialists are well placed to facilitate continuity of care within multidisciplinary teams, and across the boundaries of primary, secondary and tertiary care.

Clinical nurse specialists require a high level of specialist skills and knowledge. This includes expertise in the care of a specific cancer site, and also broader communication, consultation, educational, managerial and research skills. These enable them to effectively support patients and their families, and also to support non-specialist staff in working directly with cancer patients.

Clinical nurse specialists often play a key role in developing and improving patient services. Examples include developing and improving patient pathways, reducing delays in diagnostic clinics and providing patient and family centred follow up.

However, many nurse specialists have ever more complex roles, with continuously increasing caseloads, as new treatment options are developed. They will face increasing demands on their time.

Nurse-led clinics

Another important recent development has been the increasing number of nurse-led clinics. These often provide follow-up for patients after treatment, and offer specific therapeutic interventions for groups of people with cancer, or with specific cancer-related symptoms and problems. Examples include breathlessness clinics, relaxation, massage and psychological support services and oral chemotherapy support clinics. There is a growing evidence base for the effectiveness of many of these clinics, in terms of safety, job satisfaction and for their popularity with patients.

Other nursing roles

As policy continues to demand a flexible workforce to meet the changing needs of the population, new nursing roles continue to develop. Nurse Practitioners carry out a number of highly specialized investigative and treatment procedures within cancer care, for example nurse-led cystoscopy, intravesical chemotherapy and proctoscopy services. Nurse consultants, alongside consultants from allied health professions (AHPs), contribute a higher level of expertise, leadership and practice development. Greater clarity of the nature of higher-level practice, and its registration, will hopefully consolidate these roles, and ensure that they have a substantial future in the development of cancer services.

The role of the patient in cancer care

One of the most radical shifts in our understanding of cancer care in recent years has been the enhanced profile of the patient. This is in part due to the actions of patients themselves, making their voices heard in a variety of ways, including writing their own accounts in newspaper articles, autobiographical accounts or in blogs. The subjective patient experience is now also supported by a significant body of research. The accounts that have emerged are illuminating for the professional and they also help patients and carers to feel less isolated by putting their experiences into a broader social context.

There are also a number of ways in which we as professionals have begun to rethink the patient's and carer's place in the health care system. Cancer is best understood as a chronic disease, one that people may live with for many years. Patients therefore need help to manage their own lives, as well as deal with the process of treatment, and whatever outcome it has for them. Resources need to be targeted on supporting patients, their families and carers, as well as on treating the cancer. No one is better placed to identify the needs of people with cancer than the patient themselves, especially with the improvements that have taken place in accessing information about cancer and treatment options.

There are other political trends that support the centrality of patient experience. Consumerist ideas have now been active within the British health care system for over a decade, and these ascribe rights to the user or consumer of services. For any improvements to be made to cancer services, the voice of the patient must be heard, recognised, and responded to. There are a number of ways in which this is taking place. Individuals and user groups are frequently involved in or consulted on decisions about the allocation of resources. Services aim to work in partnership with service users, and they are sometimes employed as advisers. However, people with cancer do not always wait to be asked for their view. The debate over the availability of Herceptin as a treatment for breast cancer has shown just how powerful the patient voice has become.

Various new labels have arisen to represent the recipient of cancer services, e.g. 'service user', 'consumer'. Although these terms have a role in redefining our views of people with cancer, the term 'patient' remains popular with the public and professionals alike, and is the term used mostly in this book.

The multidisciplinary team (MDT)

The Multidisciplinary Team (MDT) is established as a feature of the effective management of cancer within the UK National Health Service. It usually involves a number of medical, nursing and AHP specialists, and focuses on a specific cancer site. The size of the population served will depend on the incidence of the cancer. Regular meetings ensure that information is pooled, expertise is shared and the complexity of the patient's needs can be dealt with. This creates a managed network and care pathway for the patients with a particular cancer.

Within each MDT, each patient should have a key worker, negotiated with the patient, who provides a clear point of contact, and manages the continuity of their care. This person will often be the site specific clinical nurse specialist, who is well placed to fulfill this particular role.

The contribution made by clinical nurse specialists to decision-making in the MDT are very important. Patients are often more open with nurses about particular problems that they may be facing, or their wishes concerning treatment and palliative care options. The nurse input into the MDT can enable a more patient centred approach to be maintained, with a focus on the needs of the patient and their family.

National guidelines aimed at cancer services, eg Improving Outcomes Guidance issued by The National Institute for Health and Clinical Excellence, highlight the importance of effective MDT work and recommend the overall makeup of different MDTs for specific cancers.

The National Institute for Health and Clinical Excellence (NICE)

The National Institute for Health and Clinical Excellence (NICE) is an independent organization, which provides national guidance for the National Health Service. It does this through,

Public Health Guidance: guidance on the promotion of health and prevention of ill health.

Health Technology Appraisals. These offer guidance on the use of new and existing medicines, treatments and procedures for cancer within the NHS.

Cancer Service Guidance. These offer advice on the appropriate treatment and care of people with cancer within the NHS.

Cancer networks throughout England and Wales are expected to take NICE guidance fully into account when planning services and treatments for individuals with cancer. In Scotland specific clinical guidelines are issued by Scottish Intercollegiate Guidelines Network (SIGN), which considers the implications of NICE guidelines for Scotland.

With the high cost of many new cancer treatments the role of NICE will become increasingly important in ensuring equitable access to treatment throughout the UK.

NICE and this handbook

The suggested approaches to treatment laid out in the *Major Cancers* and *Symptom Management* sections of this handbook are based on the most up-to-date national guidance at the time of writing.

However, treatment guidelines are changing frequently in the light of new research, particularly via the NICE service guidance and health technology appraisals.

Note: It is important that you check the latest guidance via the *National Institute for Health and Clinical Excellence* website, at www.nice.org.uk. You can also check for local guidelines from your Cancer Network. Practice in individual centers may vary and may change as new guidelines are updated and published.

For the latest Scottish guidance, please go to the Scottish Intercollegiate Guidelines Network (SIGN) website at: www.sign.ac.uk

References and further reading

Department of Health (1995) Policy Framework for commissioning cancer services: A report by the Expert Advisory Group on Cancer to the Chief Medical Officers for England and Wales. Known as Calman Hine Report. London: DoH.

Grundy M (2006) Cancer care and cancer nursing. In: Kearney N, Richardson A (eds). *Nursing Patients with Cancer. Principles and Practice.* London: Elsevier Churchill Livingstone.

Department of Health (2000) *The NHS Cancer Plan: a Plan for Investment, a Plan for Reform.* London: DoH.

Department of Health (2004) *Manual For Cancer Services*. London: DoH.
Scottish Executive Health Department (2001). *Cancer in Scotland: Action for Change*. Edinburgh: The Scottish Executive.
Scottish Executive Health Department (2004a). *Cancer in Scotland: Sustaining Change*. Edinburgh: The Scottish Executive.
Scottish Executive Health Department (2004b). *Nursing People with Cancer in Scotland: a Framework*. Edinburgh: The Scottish Executive.

Websites

Cancer in Scotland website: http://www.cancerinscotland.scot.nhs.uk/
Department of Health website: http://www.dh.gov.uk/Home/fs/en

Section 2

The cancer problem

Chapter 2

Cancer epidemiology

cancer problem

ch year 10.9 million people worldwide are diagnosed with cancer, and ..7 million die from the disease. This equates to around 12% of annual deaths worldwide.

The proportion of all deaths caused by cancer varies, from 4% in Africa to 23% in Northern America. As cancer is mainly a disease of older age, much of this difference is explained by differences in the age of the population in regions of the world. Currently 10% of people in the world are aged 60 and above. In developed regions, 20% of the population are over 60, compared with 8% in the less developed regions. By 2050, it is expected that 20% of the world population will be over 60 years old. This increase will lead to more cases of cancer.

The most common cancers world-wide are lung, breast, bowel and stomach (see Fig. 2.1). Lung cancer now accounts for 12% of all cancer worldwide and its incidence has doubled since 1975. The rate of lung cancer is predicted to increase in the next 20 years in areas of the world where smoking prevalence has risen—such as Eastern Africa, Central America, and South East Asia.

There are wide regional variations in the most common cancers. In Europe, breast, bowel, prostate, and lung account for 50% of cancer incidence. This reflects the ageing population, and lifestyle factors such as high fat diets and levels of smoking. In Eastern Africa, Kaposi's sarcoma, and cervical cancer account for nearly 30% of the cancer incidence, reflecting the AIDS epidemic and high rates of sexually transmitted infections.

Survival rates vary from region to region. In resource-poor countries there may be limited access to screening programmes, diagnostic procedures, and many of the drug treatments that may improve survival rates. The stigma associated with cancer and the burden of the cost of treatment may delay diagnosis and treatment.

The World Health Organization (WHO) is encouraging a public health approach to reduce the causes and consequences of cancer, focusing on:
- Developing and strengthening national cancer control programmes.
- Early detection of cervical and breast cancer.
- Developing guidelines on disease management.
- Support for low-cost approaches to respond to global needs for pain relief and palliative care.

The regional differences in incidence rates highlight the need for specifically targeted public health measures in each world region.

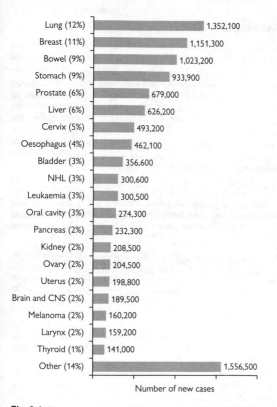

Lung (12%)	1,352,100
Breast (11%)	1,151,300
Bowel (9%)	1,023,200
Stomach (9%)	933,900
Prostate (6%)	679,000
Liver (6%)	626,200
Cervix (5%)	493,200
Oesophagus (4%)	462,100
Bladder (3%)	356,600
NHL (3%)	300,600
Leukaemia (3%)	300,500
Oral cavity (3%)	274,300
Pancreas (2%)	232,300
Kidney (2%)	208,500
Ovary (2%)	204,500
Uterus (2%)	198,800
Brain and CNS (2%)	189,500
Melanoma (2%)	160,200
Larynx (2%)	159,200
Thyroid (1%)	141,000
Other (14%)	1,556,500

Number of new cases

Fig. 2.1 The most commonly diagnosed cancers* worldwide, 2002 estimates.

* Contributing more than 1% of total number of cases and excluding non-melanoma skin cancer.
Statistics used by courtesy of Cancer Research UK.

UK situation

Incidence

This is the number of new cancer cases arising in a specified period of time, normally over a period of one year. In 2002* more than 275,000 people were diagnosed with cancer in the UK. The biggest risk factor for cancer is increasing age, with 64% of cancer diagnosed in people age 65 and over (see Fig. 2.2, age at diagnosis). The ageing population in the UK means that the incidence of cancer will continue to increase in the near future.

Although there are more than 200 different types of cancer, just four types; breast, lung, bowel and prostate cancer account for over 50% of cancer diagnosed each year in the UK (see Fig. 2.3).

Prevalence

This is the number of people who have received a diagnosis of cancer and who are alive at any given time. This reflects both the incidence of cancer and its associated survival pattern.

Risk

An individual's risk of developing cancer depends on many factors, including their smoking behaviour, diet, and genetic inheritance. It is estimated that in the UK around half of all cancers could be prevented through changes to lifestyle such as stopping smoking, limiting alcohol intake, eating healthily, and protection from sun exposure. (📖 Aetiology).

UK males

Prostate cancer is now the most commonly diagnosed cancer (in males), in the UK. It has recently overtaken lung cancer, with almost 32,000 cases diagnosed in 2002.

In the last ten years the incidence of prostate cancer has increased by around 60%, mainly due to increased TURP and PSA screening. Lung cancer incidence dropped by 28% during the same period, relating to a decrease in smoking amongst males. Bowel cancer is the third most common and these three cancers account for over 50% of male cancer incidence.

UK females

Over 41,700 women were diagnosed with breast cancer in 2002, accounting for 31% of female cancer. The next most common cancer is bowel cancer, (12%), followed by lung cancer at 11% of cases. Rates of lung cancer have remained quite steady over the past 10 years, reflecting the stabilization of smoking rates amongst women.

---

* The UK cancer registries do not release cancer statistics right up to the current year. There is normally a 4-year time lag with incidence statistics and a 2-year time lag with mortality statistics.
Cancer Research UK Website: http://info.cancerresearchuk.org/cancerstats/
This is an excellent resource for UK cancer statistical information.

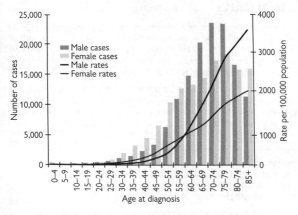

Fig. 2.2 Numbers of new cases and age-specific incidence rates by sex, all neoplasms (excluding NMSC), UK 2002. *Statistics used by courtesy of Cancer Research UK.*

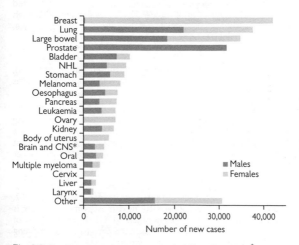

Fig. 2.3 The 20 most common cancers in the UK-incidence 2002[*]. *Statistics used by courtesy of Cancer Research UK.*

[*] Non-melanoma skin cancer (NMSC) is omitted from the CRUK statistics shown here. It is a very common condition but is virtually always curable. Registration is known to be incomplete and up to 100,000 cases might be diagnosed each year in the UK.

UK mortality

Cancer is the cause of 28% of all deaths in the UK. In 2004 over 152,000 individuals were registered as having died from cancer. Over one fifth of all cancer deaths are from lung cancer. The next three most common cancers are of the bowel, breast, and prostate cancer. 48% of all cancer deaths can be attributed to these four cancers (see Fig. 2.4).

The difference between incidence and survival statistics for particular diseases reflects the wide variation in 5- and 10-year survival statistics for each disease, with some cancers often being very successfully treated and others having a very poor overall prognosis. (See following topic, Survival).

The overall rate of mortality from all cancers has fallen by 11% in the last 10 years, though there are large variations in this trend between different cancers (see Fig. 2.5). The main reasons for the decrease in mortality are:
• Primary prevention of cancer, for example a reduction in smoking.
• Earlier detection due to screening programmes.
• Better treatment, for example new drugs to treat breast cancer.

Despite the fall in lung cancer mortality, it is still by far the most common cause of death from cancer in UK men, causing a quarter of all male cancer deaths. Over 80% of lung cancer deaths are linked to tobacco smoking.

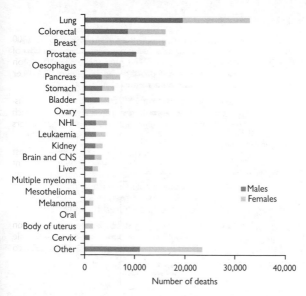

Fig. 2.4 The 20 most common causes of death from cancer (UK, 2004). *Statistics used by courtesy of Cancer Research UK.*

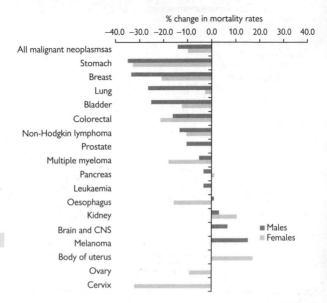

Fig. 2.5 Percentage change in European age-standardized mortality rates, major cancers, by sex (UK 1995–2004). *Statistics used by courtesy of Cancer Research UK.*

The UK cancer registries do not release cancer statistics right up to the current year. There is normally a 4-year time lag with incidence statistics and a 2-year time lag with mortality statistics.

Survival

Cancer survival has improved for most cancers in the last 20 years. However, survival rates between different cancers vary dramatically and are very dependent on the stage of disease at diagnosis.

Site and gender

The variation in survival between disease sites is highlighted by testicular and pancreatic cancer. The UK 5-year survival rate for testicular cancer is around 95%, whereas for pancreatic cancer it is around 2% (although recent changes in treatment may improve this last figure in the next few years). For most types of cancer women have a small survival advantage over men. Fig. 2.6 shows the survival rates for the most common cancers in males and females.

Age

Survival decreases with increasing age for most cancers. This may be due to less aggressive treatment in the elderly, later diagnosis, and several cancers being more chemotherapy sensitive in younger patients. Exceptions to this rule are breast and prostate cancer, which tend to be more aggressive diseases in the youngest age group.

Deprivation

There is lower survival in a range of cancers in more deprived groups, including prostate, colorectal, and breast cancer. Reasons for this could include:
- Later diagnosis e.g. difference in access to PSA testing.
- Treatment delays, poorer access, and lower compliance.
- Worse general health.

Though differences due to deprivation are small in percentage terms, the large overall number of diagnosed cancers in the UK means that deprivation could account for several thousand avoidable cancer deaths each year.

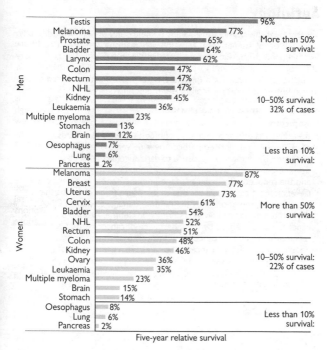

Fig. 2.6 Five year age standardized relative survival (%), adults diagnosed 1996–1999, England and Wales by sex and site. *Statistics used by courtesy of Cancer Research UK.*

Aetiology

The study of the causes of cancer is complex and fraught with difficulty. Epidemiological studies look at whole populations and try to correlate risk factors with specific cancers. Problems occur due to the complexity of factors such as diet and various chemicals. Confounding variables are a problem, e.g. is it obesity, a high-fat diet, or lack of activity which plays a role in bowel cancer, or is it all three to differing degrees?

Key factors in cancer causation

Host factors

- *Age:* cancer is primarily a disease of older age with two-thirds of cancer being diagnosed in those over 65 years of age. This can be explained by increasing exposure to carcinogens, the fact that cancer development requires multiple genetic mutations (□ Cancer biology) and the reduced effectiveness of the immune system in older people.
- *Genetics:* most cancer occurs due to exposure to carcinogens that cause genetic mutations plus the random damage to human DNA that occurs during cell division during our lifetime. Around 5% of cancers may be caused by the inheritance of cancer-related genetic mutations. Hereditary cancers tend to occur at an earlier age, and people with an altered cancer gene can have a greater risk of developing other cancers (□ Cancer biology). More cancer related genes are being discovered each year as research into the cellular causes of cancer continues.

Likely risk factors for cancer causation (UK)[1]

Causes	% in 1998
Tobacco	29–31
Diet	29–31
Medicines	<1
Infective causes	10–20
Ionizing and UV light	5–7
Occupation	2–4
Pollution: air, water, food	1–5
Physical inactivity	1–2

Some inherited cancer genes and their related cancers

Implicated gene	Related cancer (and syndrome)
BRCA1, BRCA2	Breast and ovarian cancer
WT1, WT2	Wilms' tumour
RB1	Retinoblastoma
APC	Adenomatous polyposis coli; bowel cancer
MLH1, MSH2	Hereditary non-polyposis coli: bowel cancer
RET	Thyroid cancer
P53	Li Fraumeni syndrome; multiple types of cancer
XPA	Xeroderma pigmentosum: skin cancer

Carcinogen

A carcinogen is any substance or agent that promotes cancer development. Carcinogens generally cause genetic mutations, i.e. they damage DNA in cells, therefore interfering with normal biological processes.

Environmental factors

Exposure to a range of *environmental* carcinogens increases the risk of developing cancer. This is supported by changes in cancer incidence found in migration studies and varying rates of cancer in different socio-economic groups.

Note: 'environmental' refers to the physical environment in which we live as well as lifestyle factors such as diet and smoking habits.

---

1 Doll R (1998). Epidemiological evidence of the effects of behaviour and the environment on the risk of human cancer. *Recent Results in Cancer Research*, **154**: 3–21.

There are thousands of known carcinogens, but epidemiological studies suggest that radiation, pollution, and occupational exposure account for less than 10% of known cancer risk. Tobacco and diet are easily the most important known risk factors.

- *Tobacco:* this is the most important known carcinogen and a well-established risk factor in many cancers, including lung, head and neck cancers, oesophageal, and stomach cancer. The number of cigarettes smoked and the number of years that a person has smoked are risk factors. Smoking cessation programmes should have a major role to play in reducing the risk of cancer.
- *Alcohol:* the main effect of alcohol is its combined effect with tobacco smoking in head and neck cancers and cancers of the oesophagus. Alcohol by itself is implicated in liver cancer and may contribute to some cancers of the breast and bowel.
- *Diet:* according to a range of epidemiological studies, diet may be the most important cancer risk factor. However, it is difficult to measure a person's diet over time, and we need to know what people ate in the past to explore links to cancer. Diets high in fat and low in fruit and vegetables have been implicated in bowel cancer. Diets high in fruit and vegetables seem to have a protective effect against a number of cancers, including stomach, oesophageal, and larynx cancer. There is no clear role for any one vegetable, though some evidence suggests that brassicas, e.g. cauliflowers, cabbages, Brussel sprouts, may have specific preventative properties. High levels of salt have been linked to stomach cancer. Contamination of food by aflatoxins increases the risk of liver cancer. Other areas linked to diet are physical activity and obesity. Physical inactivity is now related as a risk factor to cancers of the colon, breast, and prostate.
- *Infections:* these account for between 10–20% of worldwide cancer incidence, although in many developing regions of the world this figure is far higher. A range of viruses are implicated in cancer incidence. HPV may account for between 80–90% of cervical cancers and hepatitis B and C are linked to 80% of liver cancer. The AIDS epidemic (HIV infection) has seen a huge increase in Kaposi's sarcoma and lymphomas. Other important infections relating to cancer incidence are Epstein–Barr virus (lymphoma) and the bacterium *Helicobacter pylori*, which is an important risk factor in stomach cancer.
- *Sun exposure:* there is fair evidence that reducing exposure to ultraviolet radiation (sun exposure) reduces the incidence of non-melanoma skin cancer. Increasing exposures of UV light over a lifetime increase the risk of basal cell and squamous cell carcinoma.

Melanoma risk also appears to have a clear link to UV exposure. The most important risk factors are intensity of and age of exposure (high risk from childhood exposure). Skin type plays a part with fair and redheaded people at highest risk.

Further reading

▣ Cancer Research UK Website: http://info.cancerresearchuk.org/cancerstats/ Excellent resource for UK cancer statistical information.

Mckinnell R G, Parchment R E, Perantoni A O, et al. (2006). *The biological basis of cancer.* 2nd edn. Cambridge: Cambridge University Press.

Yarbro C H, Frogge M H, Goodman M (eds) (2005). *Cancer Nursing, Principles and practice.* 6th edn. Massachusetts: Jones and Bartlett.

Cancer biology

Introduction

Knowledge of cancer biology has leapt forward in the last 20 years. This has improved understanding of the disease process of cancer and has opened up the opportunity for targeted treatments and methods of screening.

Cancer is not one disease but many; although there are some striking similarities in how all cancers develop. Cancer is a monoclonal disease, i.e. all the cells in a tumour come from only one ancestral cell. The transformation of a normal cell into its malignant counterpart is an accumulative, multistage process of gene mutation. As each mutation occurs, the cell's DNA becomes less stable. The genes involved control the process of cell division (cell cycle).

It may take many years for multiple mutations of a single cell to occur. This explains the increasing risk of cancer as we get older.

Cell cycle

The sequence of stages through which a cell passes between one division and another is known as the cell cycle (see Fig. 3.1). Chemotherapy drugs target different phases of the cell cycle, some are cell cycle dependent whilst others are cycle independent ($\square$ Chemotherapy). Therefore a working knowledge of the cell cycle is important in order to understand treatment.

At any one stage most cells in the human body are not dividing, and are in an inactive phase called G_0. Growth factors can stimulate cells to move into the cell cycle and divide. For example when the skin is cut, growth factors released by platelets at the site of an injury stimulate skin cells to divide and close the wound.

The four stages of the cell cycle are: gap phases G_1 and G_2, where the cell builds up the energy required for division (see Fig. 3.1), S (synthesis) phase where replication of DNA occurs. and M (mitosis) phase, where doubled DNA splits and two identical daughter cells are created.

A set of proteins (cyclins), and their associated enzymes called cyclin dependent kinases (CDKs), control the cell cycle. The concentrations of these rise and fall during cell division. As the cell moves through the cycle, a series of controlling checkpoints have to be passed. These check the integrity of the DNA and ensure safe and accurate cell division.

The genes that code for the proteins that regulate the cell cycle are known as oncogenes and tumour suppressor genes ($\square$ Oncogenes and tumour suppressor genes). Damage to these genes can knock out the controlling aspect of cell division, driving division forward. This allows cells to ignore checkpoints and damaged DNA to be replicated, leading to out of control cell replication. Cancer can therefore be seen as a disease of the cell cycle.

Key genes that regulate the cell cycle include *p53* and *Retinoblastoma* (Rb), which are implicated in a large number of different cancers.

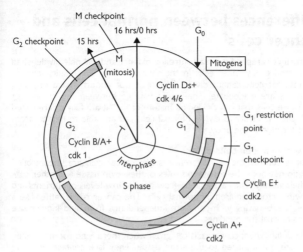

Fig. 3.1 The cell cycle and its checkpoints. Taken from Pecorino L (2005). *Molecular biology of cancer: mechanisms, targets, and therapeutics.* Reproduced with permission of Oxford University Press.

Differences between normal cells and cancer cells

Normal cells reproduce in a controlled manner and will only divide when instructed to by other cells in their vicinity. This 'community' control means that cells cannot divide if there is not enough space or when nutrients are inadequate. There is a balance between the number of immature cells that can divide and mature cells that are fully differentiated and lose the ability to divide. Normal cells are not able to migrate from their location in the body.

How do cancer cells differ?

Lack of control: the key difference is that cancer cells are uncontrolled and do not obey the signals and rules of their own tissue and other cells in their vicinity. They are able to grow despite low levels of nutrients and growth factors required by normal cells. The cancer cell is rather like a renegade, behaving with complete independence from, and indifference to, its normal surroundings.

Growth inhibition: cancer cells can grow when there is no room or when they are not attached to the same tissue. They lack contact inhibition (which will prevent normal cells from growing when there is no room) and anchorage dependence (the need to be attached to other cells of the same tissue, known as 'cell–cell adhesion').

Differentiation: this is the process by which young, immature (unspecialized) cells take on individual characteristics and reach their mature (specialized) form and function. Cancer cells do not fully differentiate and therefore maintain the ability to divide. This lack of differentiation also means that cancer cells do not function as effectively as the normal cell counterparts of their original tissue. The lack of proper differentiation varies amongst cancer cells. The least differentiated cancers tend to be more aggressive and more likely to metastasise.

Metastatic spread: cancer cells can develop the ability to invade other tissue space and grow at other sites. This is the most dangerous aspect of cancer, and is the reason for a majority of cancer deaths (metastasis).

Angiogenesis: once a tumour reaches a size of around $1–2cm^3$ its oxygen supply and nutrients are insufficient for further growth, unless it can establish its own blood supply. Cancer cells do this by sending out angiogenic factors, which stimulate new capillaries to grow towards the tumour from nearby blood vessels. The new blood vessels not only provide oxygen and nutrients for the tumour but also create a route for metastatic colonisation. Angiogenesis is not unique to cancer cells. However, in cancer the process lacks effective controls.

Cell surface changes: numerous changes take place on the surface of cancer cells. These lead to changes in behaviour, including a lack of proper cell–cell adhesion, promotion of metastasis and increased response to growth factors.

Oncogenes and tumour suppressor genes (TSGs)

Of the 30,000 human genes there are now over 100 known oncogenes and tumour suppressor genes. Each has a role in regulating growth. These genes code for a series of molecules, which transmit growth signals from the extracellular environment into the cell and on to the nucleus (see Table 3.1).

Oncogenes

These are genes that drive cell division (akin to an accelerator). These genes produce proteins that include growth factors, growth factor receptors, signal transducers, and nucleus transcription factors. When mutated, they can produce the wrong protein or too much protein, which can drive cell division inappropriately. An example of this is aberrant Erb-B2 receptors, now targeted in treatment by the drug Herceptin®.

TSGs

These provide the negative feedback (or brakes) required in cell division. They can block growth signals at any point in the overall chain, from the surface to the nucleus. When mutated, their function is lost, and cell division cannot be stopped.

Other key mechanisms

Other aspects of cell growth control are important in cancer development.

Apoptosis (programmed cell death): cells normally have a protective mechanism to stop damaged DNA being replicated. If a cell is found to have damaged DNA it is either repaired or the cell self-destructs. Key genes in this process include BcL2 genes and also p53, known as the guardian of the genome, which is mutated in over 50% of cancers. If this gene is not functioning properly, then the accumulation of errors in DNA is speeded up, leading to a greater risk of developing cancer.

Immortal growth: most cells can only divide a finite number of times. After each division the tips of their chromosomes (telomeres) shorten. When these get too short, the chromosomes unravel and cannot divide. Some cancer cells can produce telomerase, an enzyme that maintains the length of these tips during division, therefore extending the number of potential divisions indefinitely.

Tumour heterogeneity: as cancer develops, the inherent genetic instability leads to different cell populations within a single tumour. This can cause difficulty in treating tumours, as some cell populations within a tumour may be resistant to cytotoxic drugs and radiotherapy. This lack of uniformity makes it difficult to eradicate all cells in a tumour with systemic treatments.

Table 3.1 Common TSGs and oncogenes

TSG	Cancers linked with gene damage
APC (adenomatous polyposis coli)	Familial adenomatous and noninherited colorectal cancers
BRCA1, 2 (breast cancer 1 & 2)	Inherited breast cancers; ovarian cancers
DCC (deleted in colon cancer)	Colorectal cancers
p53	Over 50% of human cancers, including bladder, breast, colorectal, oesophageal, liver, lung
Rb (retinoblastoma)	Retinoblastoma, sarcomas; bladder, breast, oesophageal, prostate, and lung cancers
Oncogenes	
abl/bcr	Chronic myloid and acute lymphoblastic leukaemias
HER2/neu	Breast and cervical
ras	Many cancers including pancreas (90%), colon (50%), lung (30%), thyroid (50%)
myc	Lymphoma, leukaemia, lung cancer
Src	Breast, colon, small cell lung

Tumour growth

In normal tissue, homeostasis is maintained by the balance of cell replication, apoptosis (cell death), and differentiation. Fully differentiated cells tend to lose the ability to divide. Within a cancerous tumour there is an imbalance. Tumour cells are not fully differentiated and maintain the ability to divide. The apoptosis programme is not fully functional and due to telomerase (📖 Apoptosis), many cells can go on dividing indefinitely.

Note: it is this imbalance that causes tumour development.

Cancer growth is normally described in terms of doubling time—the time taken for the number of cells in a tumour to double. This may vary from hours to months (the average is 2–3 months).

Doubling time:
• Burkitt's lymphoma: 2–5 days.
• Testicular cancer: 3 weeks.
• Colon cancer: 3 months.

From initial cancer development 30 doublings will produce a tumour of about 1cm in diameter (approximately a billion cells).

▶ Slower growing tumours may therefore be many years old before being discovered.

Several mechanisms impact on the rate of tumour doubling time:
• *Average cell cycle time:* this is usually 1–5 days.
• *Growth fraction:* this is the fraction of cells within a tumour that are actively dividing at any one time. It is often well under 50%.
• *Cell loss:* the main reason that volume doubling times are so much longer than the average cell cycle time, is the high percentage of cell loss in tumours. This is mainly due to cell death, through necrosis and apoptosis, but also includes loss due to metastatic spread.

Implications for treatment

Dividing cells are more sensitive to cytotoxic chemotherapy and radiotherapy than non-dividing cells. Tumours with a high growth fraction are therefore more susceptible to these treatments than those with a low growth fraction.

Many cancers seem to grow faster after starting treatment; so it is important not to have gaps between treatments (📖 Radiotherapy: principles and uses).

Metastasis (spread of secondary tumour)

Metastatic spread is one of the unique characteristics of malignant disease and is the main reason for treatment failure and the eventual death of cancer patients. Approximately 60% of cancer patients with solid tumours have metastatic disease at diagnosis, although only around a half of these will be clinically detectable at that time. Not all cells within a tumour will have the ability to metastasize. This ability will develop in some cell populations if there are further mutations in their DNA.

Routes of spread

Blood and lymph circulation accounts for two-thirds of metastatic spread. Other methods of spread include direct extension along tissue, seeding in cavities such as the peritoneum and spread via the CNS.

Where do cells metastasize to and why?

Most metastatic spread can be explained by anatomical closeness (for example ovarian cancer extending along the fallopian tubes) and also by blood circulation. Cancer cells will get trapped in the first capillary bed they encounter, often in the lungs as part of general circulation, e.g. in breast cancer, or in the liver via the portal blood system, e.g. in colon cancer. Cancer may metastasize to areas such as bone because of changes to cancer cell surface molecules allowing them to interact favourably with tissue or growth factors in specific new sites (see Table 3.2).

The metastatic cascade

Metastatic spread is known to be a complex process requiring each of the following steps.

Angiogenesis (neovascularization): development by a cancer of its own blood supply. The degree of vascularization of a tumour correlates poorly with survival as it offers a perfect route for metastatic spread.

Intravasation: changes in surface molecules (cell adhesion molecules) allow cancer cells to detach from the primary tumour and the extracellular matrix (ECM). They then invade the ECM by secreting digesting enzymes (proteases) and producing motility factors that assist their movement. By gaining access to local blood vessels they can enter the circulation and be transported around the body.

Note: this ability to invade tissue is similar to certain white blood cells, but in the case of cancer spread it is completely unregulated.

Circulation and arrest: during circulation, both mechanical turbulence and the immune surveillance will destroy most cancer cells, probably more than 99.9%. However, some will survive and become trapped in small capillaries of a distant organ or tissue.

Extravasation: the process of intravasation is then carried out in reverse and the cell establishes itself in the new tissue.

Table 3.2

Common sites of metastatic spread	Cancers that commonly spread to these sites
Lung	Breast, colon, bladder, kidney
Liver	Colon, pancreas, lung, breast, stomach
Brain	Lung, breast, melanoma
Bone	Breast, lung, prostate

Growth: further division and establishment of a new blood supply are needed to enable the new tumour to develop and grow.

Note: after many years of remission patients may get a sudden cancer relapse with metastatic cancer. This is thought to be due to dormant micrometastases; metastatic deposits which remain stable due to a lack of angiogenesis for many years, before further genetic changes enable them to grow again.

Treatment implications

The ability to control or prevent metastatic spread would be a major breakthrough in the management of cancer. Cell adhesion molecules, enzymes that cause ECM breakdown and angiogenesis are amongst targets for new cancer treatments (📖 Biological therapy).

Immunology

The links between the immune system and cancer have been long established through a range of different evidence:
- Immune suppression has been shown to directly cause several cancers:
  - HIV and Kaposi's sarcoma or non-Hodgkin's lymphoma.
  - Long-term immunosuppressive therapy and lymphoma.
- Presence of immune system cells in tumour biopsies.
- Spontaneous regression of some primary tumours.
- Effective use of immunotherapy e.g. BCG to destroy tumours.
- Graft vs leukaemia affect in allogeneic transplant (📖 Allogeneic haematopoietic stem cell transplant).

Recent improvements in understanding of cancer biology and immunology have led to increased development and use of biological therapies, e.g. cytokines and gene therapy (📖 Biological therapy).

Understanding the basics of the immune system helps in our understanding of both cancer biology and cancer treatments[1].

Immune system

The immune system exists to defend the body against infectious, e.g. bacteria, viruses, fungi, and parasite invasions as well as malignant transformation. It consists of the following parts:
- Organs: bone marrow, thymus, spleen, lymph, nodes, peyers patches.
- Cells: leukocytes- both myeloid and lymphoid.
- Complement and cytokines. Proteins which have a role in enhancing the immune response.

The immune system consists of two complementary components that closely interact during the immune response.

Innate immunity

This is also known as 'natural', or 'non-specific' immunity. It includes:
- Physical and chemical barriers such as skin, mucosa, mucus secretions, lysozyme, celia.
- Inflammatory response: phagocytes, neutrophils, monocytes, macrophages which directly attack and destroy pathogens and release cytokines which, stimulate further immune response (acquired immunity).
- Other cells, such as natural killer (NK) cells that can directly kill virally infected cells and some tumour cells.
- Complement proteins which enhance the immune response.

Acquired immunity

This is lymphocyte controlled and is a specific response to certain antigens. It has memory, allowing it to respond rapidly in huge numbers on a later exposure to the same antigen. It consists of:
- T lymphocytes: The two main types of T-lymphocytes are:
  - Helper T-cells: recognize foreign antigens, produce cytokines e.g. interleukin/interferon and tumour necrosis factor (TNF). They also have a role in developing antibody response.
  - Cytotoxic T-cells: directly lyse target cells.

1 Sampayrac L M. (2003). *How the Immune System Works*. Oxford: Blackwell Science.

- B-lymphocytes: They produce antibodies in response to certain antigens and present antigens to T-cells, further stimulating the immune response.

The immune response

On encountering a pathogen, e.g. bacterial infection, phagocytes would immediately attack the bacteria, aided by complement. This leads to a release of cytokines, e.g. interleukins, TNF. This stimulates further macrophage and NK cell activation. Through phagocytosis the antigen is degraded and presented to the acquired immunity system. A T-cell and B-cell response occurs, including direct pathogen destruction by cytotoxic T-cells, further cytokine release, and antibody production, leading to enhanced immune response and cell destruction.

On destruction of the antigen the immune system returns to its preactivated state but now has memory T and B cells for that antigen, to enable a more rapid and stronger future immune response[2].

Influences on the immune system

A number of factors impact on the overall functioning of the immune system:
- Age: as we age there is a declining immune response, including reduced T-cell functioning.
- Stress: though it is hard to clearly define, there is increasing evidence that long-term chronic stress has an immunosuppressive effect.
- Exercise: moderate exercise has a generally positive effect, however excessive exercise can reduce immune function.
- Diet: nutrient deficiency, excess alcohol, and smoking all lower immune response.

Immunology and cancer

Several cancers have antigen presentation different from normal tissue, e.g. CA-125 and ovarian cancer, carcinoembryonic antigen (CEA) and colorectal cancer (📖 Diagnosis and classification). These antigen changes can stimulate an immune response, activating NK cells, macrophages and other cytokines. The ability of the immune system to destroy cancer cells is known as tumour surveillance. It is believed that such surveillance can explain spontaneous tumour regression and that the immune system is successfully destroying potential cancer cells throughout our lifetime.

However, tumour antigen presentation may only vary slightly from normal tissue and may not be sufficient to stimulate an effective immune response. Therefore tumours continue to grow. Tumours may also 'down regulate' tumour antigens and other immune system molecules, such as human leukocyte antigens making them more difficult for the immune system to target (📖 Allogeneic haematopoietic stem cell transplant).

2 Moore J S. (2005). The Immunological Basis of Cancer in Kearney N. & Richardson A. (eds) *Nursing Patients with Cancer: Principles and Practice*, pp 303–28. Edinburgh: Elsevier Churchill Livingstone.

Tumour classification

Tumour
A swelling or a mass of tissue that may be benign or malignant.

Benign tumours
Benign tumours cannot spread by invasion or metastasis; therefore, they only grow locally. Because benign tumours do not metastasize or destroy normal tissue they are less likely to be life threatening; an exception is benign brain tumours. Certain benign tumours such as adenomatous polyps in the colon can transform into malignant tumours[1].

Malignant tumours
Malignant tumours are tumours that are able to spread by invasion and metastasis.

Cancer
By definition, the term 'cancer' applies only to malignant tumors.

Main cancer types
There are hundreds of different cancers, due to the many tissue types and points of origin for cancer within the human body. They can be loosely classified into five main types; carcinoma, sarcoma, myeloma, leukaemia, and lymphoma, as well as mixed cell cancers.

Carcinomas are cancers of epithelial tissue and account for 80–90% of all cancer cases. Epithelial tissue lines internal and external surfaces of the body and is found throughout the body. Carcinomas are divided into two major subtypes:
- *Adenocarcinoma*, which develops in an organ or gland and
- *Squamous cell carcinoma*, which develops in the squamous epithelium in many parts of the body.

Most carcinomas affect organs or glands capable of secretion, e.g. the four most common cancers in the UK, breast, lung, colon and prostate.

Sarcomas originate in supportive and connective tissues such as bones, tendons, cartilage, muscle, and fat.

Myeloma is cancer that originates in the plasma cells of bone marrow.

Leukaemias (blood cancers) are cancers of the bone marrow. They are further divided into myeloid and lymphoid types based on the specific blood cell line from which they originate.

Lymphomas are cancers of the glands or nodes of the lymphatic system. They may also occur in specific organs such as the stomach, breast or brain. Divided into Hodgkin's disease and non-Hodgkin's lymphomas.

---

1 Omerod K F. (2005). Diagnostic Evaluation, Classification, and Staging. In Yarbro C.H., Frogge M.H., Goodman M. (eds) *Cancer Nursing, Principles and practice.* 6th edn, pp 153–80. Massachusetts: Jones and Bartlett.

Mixed types: some cancers arise from different aspects of the same tissue e.g. adenosquamous carcinoma. Other cancers arise from the original germ cell layers of tissue and do not have any relationship to their tissue of origin, e.g. teratocarcinomas.

Further reading

Mckinnell R G, Parchment R E, Perantoni A O et al. (2006). *The biological basis of cancer.* 2nd edn. Cambridge: Cambridge University Press.

Pecorino L (2005). *Molecular biology of cancer: mechanisms, targets, and therapeutics.* Oxford: Oxford University Press.

Weinberg R (1998). *One renegade cell: quests for the origins of cancer.* London: Weidenfeld & Nicolson.

Yarbro C H, Frogge M H, Goodman M (eds) (2005). *Cancer Nursing, Principles and practice.* 6th edn. Massachusetts: Jones and Bartlett.

CancerQuest http://cancerquest.org/

Excellent interactive cancer biology website, which assumes no previous knowledge of the subject.

Cancer prevention and screening

Cancer prevention

Though the actual cause of an individual's specifc cancer is often not known, many of the common forms of cancer have causative factors related to lifestyle, such as smoking, sunbathing, and poor diet. They are, therefore, potentially preventable.

Estimates are that over half of all cancers could be preventable; so prevention rather than attempts at cure may have a greater impact on rates of death from cancer[1].

Government targets

In 1999, the UK government set a target of reducing cancer deaths in people under 75 years, by at least a fifth by 2010[2]. The aim is to achieve this mainly through primary prevention (see below). Secondary prevention and improved treatment will also play a part.

Inequalities in cancer health also need tackling. Rates of certain cancers—such as cervical and lung cancer—are higher in deprived areas. For example, smoking rates remain extremely high amongst those living in poverty. Targeted policies aim not only to reduce cancer rates, but also to reduce the gap in cancer incidence and mortality between different groups in society.

> **Key areas of UK government policy on cancer prevention**
>
> - Smoking
> - Diet and nutrition
> - Obesity
> - Physical activity
> - Alcohol
> - Sunlight
> - Radon

This is in line with the European code against cancer (see Table 4.1).

Approaches to cancer prevention

Generally classified as 4 levels:

Primary prevention: strategies that reduce individuals' exposure to carcinogens. These can be **medical** interventions such as immunization against human papilloma virus and hepatitis B, reducing risk of cervical and liver cancer. However, most strategies are **behavioural,** involving health education, lifestyle, and environmental modification.

Secondary prevention: this covers screening (📕 Cancer screening) and early detection measures. Early detection measures include individual and public education about common warning signs of cancer, and recently in the UK referral guidelines for suspected cancer[3].

---

1 Doll R and Peto R (1981). *The causes of cancer: quantitative estimates of avoidable risks of cancer in the United States today.* Oxford: Oxford University Press.

2 Department of Health (2000). *The NHS Cancer plan: a plan for investment, a plan for reform.* London: DoH.

3 National Institute for Health and Clinical excellence (2005). *Referral guidelines for suspected cancer: Quick reference guide.* London: NICE. http://www.nice.org.uk/page.aspx?o=cg027quickrefguide

Tertiary prevention and prevention of suffering: this includes avoiding complications from treatment, rehabilitation, and avoiding recurrence. It is often hard to separate from other aspects of treatment and nursing care. These areas are covered in depth within the supportive and palliative care and symptom management chapters (Sections 4 and 7).

Effective approaches

Evidence on cancer prevention suggests that it is most effective when political interventions are combined with individual interventions, e.g. recent banning of smoking in public places in Scotland and Ireland, combined with well resourced smoking cessation services.

A combination of different approaches is required. These should include:
- Properly resourced health promotion services.
- Skilled professionals who receive training.
- Using the media.
- Targeting services in schools and the community.
- Financial support for those living in poverty.

All health professionals should consider their own role in cancer prevention. For example, nurses may have many opportunities to assess an individual's cancer risk factors, advise smokers on smoking cessation clinics and drug therapy, or give dietary and exercise advice.

Table 4.1 European code against cancer

Adopting a healthier lifestyle
- Do not smoke; if you smoke, stop doing so. If you fail to stop, do not smoke in the presence of non-smokers.
- Avoid obesity.
- Undertake some brisk, physical activity every day.
- Increase your daily intake and variety of vegetables and fruits to at least five servings daily. Limit your intake of foods containing fats from animal sources.
- If you drink alcohol, moderate your consumption to two drinks per day if you are a man and one drink per day if you are a woman.
- Avoid excessive sun exposure, particularly in children and adolescents.
- Apply all regulations and follow all health and safety instructions that restrict exposure to substances that may cause cancer. Follow advice of national radiation protection offices.

Accessing public health programmes
- Women over 25 years, should participate in cervical screening programmes.
- Women over 50 years of age should participate in breast screening.
- Men and women from 50 years of age should participate in colorectal screening.
- Men and women should participate in vaccination programmes against Hepatitis B Virus infection.

Adapted from the European Code against Cancer, Version 3 (2003)
http://www.cancercode.org/code.htm

Cancer screening

Cancer screening involves testing a population of asymptomatic individuals, to find out which members of that group have either cancer or a precancerous condition that might benefit from early treatment. Screening is based on the principle that early disease will respond better to treatment than late disease.

There are three national cancer screening programmes in the UK; for breast, cervical and colorectal cancer (see below). There is no national prostate cancer screening programme; but an 'informed choice' programme of prostate risk management that includes the option for individuals to have a PSA test ([▭] Prostate cancer screening).

Criteria for screening

These criteria (see box opposite) are now widely accepted; and a screening programme should aim to satisfy them all. Many potential screening tests for cancer fail to do this, e.g. prostate cancer screening tests only fulfill the first criterion i.e. it is an important health problem.

Harms and benefits

Screening may seem the right approach to take with many cancers. This is reflected in pressure from the public and the media in many countries to increase screening uptake.

However, screening can be potentially harmful for some individuals. It sometimes produces a false positive or a false negative result (see Table 4.3). At best, screening benefits only a few people. For example, in breast cancer, approximately 500 people are screened to reduce mortality by one. The risks and benefits of population screening are highlighted in table 4.2 opposite.

Evaluating screening programmes

National screening programmes are expensive, and they divert resources away from other health care activities such as primary prevention, or treatment. It can be difficult to measure their cost effectiveness.

A number of inherent biases come into play when evaluating screening tests. Tests tend to pick up the least aggressive cancers, as well as a number of cases that would have regressed naturally, such as cervical dysplasia.

Diagnosis prior to clinical signs, i.e. a screening detected disease, will improve survival statistics, even if those individuals do not live any longer than if they had found the disease through clinical signs at a later date. This is because the individual lives with the 'disease' for a longer period of time (known as lead time bias). Establishing the mortality rates of screened and unscreened groups are the only completely effective way of evaluating screening programmes.

Recall time intervals

Choosing the most effective time interval for some screening programmes is difficult. Reducing the recall interval will generally mean more positive screening results, but will increase costs and the number of false positives. Another approach is more targeted programmes, aimed at those at highest risk (📖 Genetic screening).

Criteria for screening

- The condition being screened for should be an important health problem.
- The natural history of the condition should be well understood.
- There should be a detectable early stage.
- Treatment at an early stage should be of more benefit than at a later stage.
- A suitable test should be devised for the early stage.
- The test should be acceptable to whom?
- Intervals for repeating the test should be determined.
- Adequate health service provision should be made for the extra clinical workload resulting from screening.
- The risks, both physical and psychological, should be less than the benefits.
- The costs should be balanced against the benefits.

Adapted from Wilson JMG and Jungner G (1968). *Principles and practice of screening for disease.* Geneva: WHO.

Table 4.2 Risks and benefits of screening for cancer

Costs involved (cons)	Benefits (pros)
• Morbidity of screening test.	• Life years gained for those with
• Longer morbidity for those with	curable cancers.
unaltered prognosis.	• Avoidance of morbidity from radical
• Over treatment of questionable	treatment.
abnormalities.	• Reassurance with negative results.
• False positives, giving unnecessary	• Reassurance that the disease is at an
treatment.	early stage.
• False negatives, giving false	• Avoid cost of expensive treatment for
reassurance.	advanced cancers.
• Screening expenses.	• Extra years of productivity.
• Cost of additional cases treated.	
• Cost of early treatment and extra	
follow up.	
• Diversion of resources from primary	
prevention and treatment.	

Adapted from Chamberlain J (1988). *Screening for early detection of cancer.* In Tiffany R and Pritchard AP (eds). *Oncology for nurses and health care professionals,* Vol 1, pp. 155–73. New York: Harper Row.

Screening recruitment

A high uptake is required for an effective population screening programme though higher uptake will lead to still greater benefits from these programmes. In the UK, uptake and coverage for breast and cervical cancer screening are above 70%.

Screening uptake

Though overall uptake is high for breast and cervical screening, certain disadvantaged groups are under-represented, such as older women, people from ethnic minorities, and those with high levels of deprivation. In some cases, these groups are at the greatest risk of contracting the targeted disease, e.g. deprivation and cervical cancer are linked.

Reasons for the low uptake of screening in certain groups are complex, and include socio-demographic characteristics, knowledge, attitudes and beliefs, social influences, and health factors.

Many methods have been tried to enhance recruitment. Recommended approaches include:
- Focusing efforts on those who have never been screened.
- Telephone counselling to discuss barriers to screening.
- Reducing economic barriers, such as transportation costs.
- Tagged notes in primary and secondary care.

Some controversy exists where GPs are paid an incentive for increasing cervical screening uptake. This may be seen to go against the principle of informed choice for patients.

Informed uptake

Since screening can harm as well as benefit individuals, information available to those considering screening should clarify both the risks and benefits, including:
- The purpose of screening
- The likelihood of positive and negative findings, including false positive and false negative results (see Table 4.3)
- The risks of the screening process.
- Follow up plans, including counselling and support services.

NHS UK Cancer Screening

Information about the current UK cancer screening programmes, including recent statistics, current studies and patient leaflets can be accessed at NHS Cancer Screening Programmes. http://www.cancerscreening.nhs.uk/

Future directions

The growing emphasis on prevention and early detection, coupled with changes in technology, knowledge of cancer development, and genetics will all create new screening opportunities in the future. Current screening trials that are ongoing include:

- Use of human papilloma virus (HPV) testing in cervical screening.
- Breast cancer screening of women aged 40–49.
- Comparison of faecal occult blood vs. sigmoidoscopy for colorectal cancer.

Table 4.3 Screening sensitivity and specificity

		Disease status	
		+	**−**
Test	+	True positives (TP)	False positives (FP)
Result	−	False negatives (FN)	True negatives (TN)

Sensitivity: an effective test needs to be sensitive enough not to miss actual cases of cancer within the screened group (false negative cases).

Specificity: tests with high specificity will send as few individuals who do not have cancer for further diagnostic procedures, by producing as few false positives as possible.

Sensitivity = TP/(TP + FN) Specificity = TN/(TN + FP)
Positive predictive value = TP/(TP + FP)

Even the best screening tests will produce more false positive results than true positive results. This is due to the low incidence of disease within screened populations. This leads to increased follow-up and anxiety for a large number of individuals.

Further reading

Mackenbach J and Bakker M (eds) (2002). *Reducing inequalities in health: a European perspective.* London: Routledge.

World Health Organization (2004). *Strategies to improve and strengthen cancer control programmes in Europe.* Report of a WHO consultation. Geneva: WHO. http://whqlibdoc.who.int/hq/2004/WHO_CHP_CPM_PCC_04.1.pdf

Breast cancer screening

Breast cancer screening is done by mammogram. This involves taking an X-ray of each breast while it is carefully compressed. Women generally say it is slightly uncomfortable, although about 1 in 14 women find it extremely painful. The radiation dose to the breast is about 5 times that of a chest X-ray.

A mammogram can detect small changes in breast tissue that are too small to be felt by the woman herself, or by a doctor. Two views of the breast are taken at each screening—one from above and one into the armpit diagonally across the breast. Two views increase small cancer detection rates by up to 43%.

Research suggests that out of every 500 women screened, one life will be saved[1].The reduction in breast cancer deaths is attributed to:
- Diagnosis and treatment of asymptomatic pre-invasive disease (ductal carcinoma in situ).
- Diagnosis and treatment of early invasive breast cancer which would otherwise not present until systemic spread had occurred.

None of the trials published so far have shown a mortality benefit for women under the age of 50.

The NHS breast screening programme

This was set up in 1988. Around 1.5 million women are screened in the UK each year. Women aged between 50 and 70 are now routinely invited for screening every 3 years. The age group is based on the average age of the menopause for UK women. Screening is carried out in a specialized screening unit, which can either be mobile or hospital based. It costs about £40 for each woman screened.

Why is there routine screening only for 50–70 years of age?
- Mammograms are not as effective in pre-menopausal women, and show a far higher rate of false positives. The density of breast tissue makes it more difficult to detect problems and these women also have a lower incidence of breast cancer.
- The breast tissue of post-menopausal women is increasingly made up of fat. This is clearer on the mammogram, and makes interpretation of the X-ray more reliable.

Screening for other groups
- Women at moderate–high risk of breast cancer because of their family history, should be offered annual mammography when they are aged between 40–50 years of age. An MRI scan may be of particular benefit in this group.
- Women over 70 are not routinely invited for screening, though they can continue to self refer to the 3-yearly programme. Nurses have an important role in giving these women accurate information about the potential risks and benefits of continuing or stopping screening.

1 International Agency for Research on Cancer (2002). *7th Handbook on Cancer Prevention*. Lyons: IARC.

- Some European countries offer more frequent screening to try to reduce the number of interval cancers (those detected in between screening visits). The cost/benefit of this more frequent approach is currently being evaluated in several trials[2].

Suspicious abnormalities
- If a suspicious abnormality is seen, the woman is recalled to the breast-screening centre.
- A clinical examination is performed with further X-rays, an ultrasound examination, a needle test for cytology, or a core biopsy if appropriate.
- Women thought to have cancer are referred promptly to a breast surgeon who will arrange appropriate treatment.
- 5% of women are recalled for further tests, though only 5 cancers are found per 1000 women screened.

Breast self-examination
- Scientific evidence does not support teaching women to carry out ritualized breast self-examination.
- A more relaxed approach to breast awareness is just as safe and effective.
- Women should be encouraged to check their breasts for what is normal for them, but there is no recommended routine self-examination to a set technique.

2 NHS Breast Cancer Screening website. http://www.cancerscreening.nhs.uk/breastscreen/index.html

Cervical cancer screening

Cervical screening can prevent cancer by detecting and treating early abnormalities, which, if left untreated, could lead to cervical cancer. It is not a direct test for cancer, but picks up early abnormalities on the cervix, which increase the risk of getting cancer. However, it will also detect a cancer that is already present.

Smear and liquid based cytology (LBC) tests

Screening is carried out either through a smear test or LBC. Cells are taken from the cervix using a wooden (Ayers) spatula or brush. Most women consider the procedure to be only mildly uncomfortable.

In a smear test the cells are 'smeared' onto a slide for laboratory examination by a cytologist. In LBC the cells trapped on the brush are placed in preservative fluid, spun and cleaned before being placed on a slide and examined by a cytologist. LBC is starting to replace smear testing in the UK as the standard approach to cervical screening. In pilot sites it reduced inadequate tests from 9% to less then 2%.

National Screening Programme[1]

The NHS cervical screening programme calls all women between the ages of 25 and 64 for a free cervical smear test every 3–5 years (see box below).

Age group	Frequency of screening
25–49	3-yearly
50–64	5-yearly
65+	Only offered to those not tested since age 50 or who have had recent abnormal tests

The programme is carried out through a call and recall system of women who are registered with a GP. It tests almost 4 million women a year and the estimated cost is around £150 million a year in England. Women who have not had a recent smear test may be offered one when they attend their GP or family planning clinic on another matter.

Effective screening interval

There has been a lot of debate about the best interval for cervical screening recall. More frequent screening may slightly reduce the incidence of cervical cancer, but will increase the cost of the programme substantially. It could also lead to many more women facing the anxiety of abnormal smear tests without any actual benefit.

1 NHS Cervical Cancer Screening website. http://www.cancerscreening.nhs.uk/cervical/index. html

Exclusions

Younger women are not tested, as cervical cancer in this age group is very rare. In addition, because the cervix is still developing there is a very high rate of false positives. Women who have never been sexually active with a man are able to withdraw from the call and recall system due to their very low risk of cervical cancer

Abnormal testing follow-up

The test aims to find abnormal cervical cells. Test results are graded borderline (slight dysplastic changes, which normally return to normal), mild, moderate, or severe. Results may also be graded CIN 1, 2, or 3. CIN is Cervical Intraepithelial Neoplasia. CIN 1 is where one third of the cervical epithelium is affected. CIN 3 is where the full thickness is affected. Strictly speaking CIN can only be diagnosed by a biopsy.

Women with a borderline result will be asked to have a repeat smear in 6 months. After 3 borderline results or one mild, moderate, or severe result women will normally be referred for colposcopy (using a low powered microscope). Here the changes can be more closely observed, biopsies can be taken and possible treatment offered.

The usual approach for CIN 2 and 3 disease is colposcopy and loop diathermy, removing the abnormal cells. If CIN 3 disease extends into endocervical canal or there is microinvasion, a cone biopsy is carried out.

Nursing support and prevention advice

If women have an abnormal smear they will naturally feel anxious. It is important to talk through what the result actually means. CIN grades are not cancer, although many women may think they are. The nurse should clarify any increased risk of cancer and the purpose of follow-up. This can also be a good opportunity to talk through other risk factors, such as multiple sexual partners, non-barrier methods of contraception, smoking, and to discuss risk reduction activities.

Human papilloma virus (HPV) testing

Nearly 100% of cervical cancer cases show signs of HPV infection. If women with borderline or mildly abnormal smears do not have high-risk HPV infection (HPV 16 or 18), they have an extremely low risk of developing cervical cancer. HPV testing in combination with standard cervical screening is being trialed in the UK to see if it can reduce the number of repeat tests, and referrals to colposcopy.

Future directions

Increased knowledge about the exact role of HPV in the development of cervical cancer could change current approaches to cervical screening. A clearer idea of high and low-risk individuals may emerge. The use of HPV vaccines may also have a role in preventing the disease.

Bowel and prostate cancer screening

Bowel cancer screening

Trials or pilot studies of different screening methods have been taking place for a number of years in the UK and elsewhere[1]. Overall results have suggested that it was acceptable to the public, could have a high enough uptake, and could reduce bowel cancer mortality by 15% in the targeted group[2].

Faecal occult blood test (FOBT) is not a test for cancer; it tests for a high-risk sign of the disease. About 2% of FOBT tests end up positive. These will be followed up by diagnostic colonoscopy.

National bowel cancer screening programme

The UK's bowel cancer screening programme started in 2006 using FOBT. It will target men and women in their 60s. Tests will be offered via the GP. Flexible sigmoidoscopy trials will also commence, targeting men and women in their late 50s. Exact details of the programme have still to be finalized.

Prostate cancer screening

Currently, prostate cancer only fulfills the first screening criterion; that the condition is an important health problem. The natural history of prostate cancer is poorly understood. There are asymptomatic forms of the disease that would either never prove fatal, or might produce symptoms only very late on in disease development. Autopsy reports also suggest that more men die with prostate cancer, than die from it.

A national screening programme would therefore identify many men who would never benefit from treatment, but who could be harmed both physically and psychologically.

Two methods of screening for prostate cancer exist:
- Digital rectal examination—this is easy to carry out, but has low sensitivity and specificity. It is not recommended in asymptomatic men.
- Prostate specific antigen (PSA) testing.

Prostate specific antigen

PSA is a protein found in a higher concentration in prostate cells than in the blood. It is raised beyond its normal threshold (see box) in about 75% of prostate cancers. It can also be raised in benign prostatic hyperplasia, prostatitis, and urinary tract infections.

If PSA tests are found to be abnormal, then individuals could be referred for transrectal ultrasound and prostatic biopsy (TRUS) as a diagnostic test. About two thirds of men having a TRUS will not have prostate cancer detectable via biopsy.

---

1 UK Colorectal Cancer Screening Pilot Group. (2004). Results of the first round of a demonstration pilot of screening for colorectal cancer in the United Kingdom. *BMJ*, **329**, (7458), 133.
2 Tappenden P, Eggington S, Nixon R, et al. (2004). *Colorectal cancer screening options appraisal. Cost-effectiveness, cost-utility and resource impact of alternative screening options for colorectal cancer.* Report to the English Bowel Cancer Screening Working Group. Sheffield: SCHARR.

Normal PSA levels

There is some controversy about cut off points for normal PSA levels. Some areas use 4ng/mL, where others use age related ranges. The recommended ranges from the Prostate Cancer Risk Management Programme are as follows.

Age (years)	PSA cut-off (ng/mL)
50–59	>3.0
60–69	>4.0
70 +	>5.0

Patient demand

There is considerable demand for PSA testing amongst men concerned about the disease. The current UK strategy is to offer high quality information to men who request this test. This highlights the risks and benefits, and should enable men to make an informed choice.

Information leaflets are available for patients and health professionals via the NHS Cancer screening site at: http://www.cancerscreening.nhs.uk

Persistently elevated PSA

The best management for those men with a persistently elevated PSA, but who have had negative biopsies, is unclear. These men may face prolonged periods of follow up and experience considerable anxiety.

Dietary prevention

Diet has been clearly linked to colorectal, stomach and prostate cancer. Obesity has been linked to post-menopausal breast and endometrial cancer. Inactivity, which can link to obesity, has also been directly linked to increasing risks of colon cancer (📖 Aetiology).

There are clear links between poor diet and social deprivation, highlighting the inequalities that exist in cancer rates within the UK. Barriers to improving diet are:
- Access and availability—whether people have access to good quality, affordable food locally.
- Attitudes and awareness—knowledge, attitudes, motivation and skills concerning the buying, preparation and eating of healthy food.

Advice for improving diet
- Increase intake of fruit and vegetables to at least five portions a day.
- Increase intake of dietary fibre from bread and other cereals (particularly wholegrain varieties), potatoes, fruit, and vegetables.
- Maintain a healthy body weight (within the BMI range 20–25).
- Keep consumption of red meat and animal fat to a minimum (less than 140g per day). This will also have a preventative effect on heart disease.

Strategies for improving diet
Successful strategies include:
- Individual and small group counselling sessions aimed at behavioural change.
- Changes to the local environment, for example in shops and catering outlets.
- National media campaigns, such as the five-a-day fruit and vegetable campaign and the national school fruit scheme.

These strategies can also help with obesity. Combining them with strategies to increase activity is probably more effective in sustaining weight loss than diet or exercise alone in adults.

The National Heart, Lung, and Blood Institute (NHLBI) provides a useful interactive website for both health professionals and patients. It lists a range of useful strategies to help treat obesity. www.nhlbi.nih.gov/health/public/heart/obesity/lose_wt/index.htm

Alcohol
Approaches to reducing alcohol consumption include the following strategies:
- Taxation and pricing.
- Licensing.
- Targeted drink-driving campaigns.
- Controlling the promotion of alcohol: advertising, broadcasting, sponsorship, and packaging.
- Changing attitudes: campaigns to promote responsible drinking.
- Support and treatment, via a range of voluntary and health care organizations.

Brief interventions

'Brief interventions involve opportunistic advice, discussion, negotiation or encouragement. They are commonly used in many areas of health promotion, and are delivered by a range of primary and community care professionals'.

For smoking cessation, brief interventions typically take between 5 and 10 minutes and may include one or more of the following:
- Simple opportunistic advice to stop.
- An assessment of the patient's commitment to quit.
- An offer of pharmacotherapy and/or behavioural support.
- Provision of self-help material and referral to more intensive support such as the NHS Stop Smoking Services'[1].

Brief interventions from health care professionals have been shown to have an important role to play in dietary advice, smoking prevention, and reducing alcohol consumption and improving alcohol related problems.

All health professionals should consider the opportunities they have in their everyday practice to initiate brief health promotion activities.

Reflection points

- How might you introduce cancer prevention strategies into your own practice?
- What potential barriers exist?
- What resources, including training or education might you require?
Find out what resources exist in your own area that promote
  - Smoking cessation.
  - Dietary advice.

1 National Institute for Health and Clinical Excellence (2006). *Brief interventions and referral for smoking cessation in primary care and other settings.* Public Health Intervention Guidance No. 1. London: NICE.

Smoking cessation

- Smoking is the main avoidable cause of premature death in the UK. People who stop smoking live longer than those who don't, and their risk of lung cancer diminishes with time.
- Smoking rates in the UK have steadily declined over the last 30 years. However, this decline has slowed down in recent years. The decline was originally faster in men than women.
- Around 26% of adults now smoke in the UK (27% of men and 25% of women). Smoking among teenagers increased in the 1990s, but has now stabilized at around about 10%, with more girls than boys smoking.
- Socioeconomic trends in smoking behaviour are strong. In manual groups smoking rates are around 32%, while in non-manual groups it is 21%. The gap between socioeconomic groups has increased since the 1970s. Despite a national target of reducing the smoking rate in manual groups from 32% in 1998 to 26% by 2010, there has been little progress[1].

NHS stop smoking services

The NHS Stop Smoking Service provides support to smokers wanting to quit. Most stop smoking advisers are nurses or pharmacists, and all have received training for their role.

This service offers a combination of:
- Group treatment and individual, face-to-face counselling.
- Nicotine replacement therapies (NRT) and bupropion (Zyban).

Evidence from clinical trials suggests that smokers are four times more likely to quit smoking using this combined approach, than by willpower alone. In 2004, around 2 million prescriptions for NRT were dispensed worth a total value of around £44 million.

Long term quit rates for this service show about 15% of people remain non-smokers at 52 weeks. Although this may seem a low rate of effectiveness compared with some treatment successes, smoking cessation treatment is extremely cost effective compared with many other health service interventions. The cost per life year of around £800 is much cheaper than most other medical interventions[2].

Smoking cessation is now permanently funded and organized at PCT level, replacing a previous ad hoc approach. The key aims of the current service are to:
- Increase referral rates via GPs and other members of the primary care team, as these are a major source of recruitment.
- Focus on low-income and pregnant smokers, and ensure the needs of minority ethnic populations are catered for.
- Improve links with acute hospital trusts to ensure patients receive help with smoking cessation while in hospital.

1 Health Development Agency (2002). *Cancer prevention. A resource to support local action in delivering the NHS Cancer Plan.* London: Health Development Agency.
2 Health Development Agency (2003). *Meeting Department of Health smoking cessation targets: Recommendations for service providers.* London: Health Development Agency.

Department of Health position/aims on tobacco use

- Reducing exposure to secondhand smoke—making smoke-free environments the norm at work and at leisure.
- Media/education campaigns—see www.givingupsmoking.co.uk
- Reducing the availability of tobacco products and regulating supply—including action on shops that sell cigarettes to children and further reductions in tobacco smuggling.
- Further improvements to NHS Stop Smoking Services and increased availability of nicotine replacement therapy (NRT) to help smokers quit.
- Reducing tobacco promotion—to include further restrictions on tobacco advertising.
- Regulating tobacco—for example, proposals to put hard hitting picture warnings on cigarette packets.

Useful resources for smokers for easy access advice about giving up smoking

- NHS Giving up Smoking Website: www.givingupsmoking.co.uk
- NHS Smoking Helpline 0800 169 0169.

Skin cancer prevention

Skin cancer is a largely preventable disease. By taking simple measures to protect the skin from the sun, people can substantially reduce their risk of getting skin cancer. Because skin cancers are visible they can also be detected early, and removed, before they pose a threat to life.

Risk factors for skin cancer
- Fair skin which burns easily and tans poorly.
- Personal or family history of skin cancer.
- History of intense or prolonged sun exposure.
- Higher than average number of pigmented skin naevi (moles).

Use of sunscreens
Sunscreens do prevent sunburn, but they may not protect against skin cancer. They may reduce the amount of sunlight reaching the skin's surface, but if they are used to prolong the amount of time a person spends in the sun, they could potentially increase skin cancer risk.

More effective prevention behaviour is to wear a hat, and shirt, stay in the shade and avoid the summer sun in the middle of the day. From a socioeconomic perspective this approach is also much cheaper, as sunscreens can be prohibitively expensive if used as often as recommended.

The sunsmart code [1]

Stay in the shade from 11–3pm
Make sure you never burn
Always cover up
Remember to take extra care of children
Then use factor 15+ sunscreen

Report mole changes or unusual skin growths promptly to your doctor

Skin cancer advice to give about changes in moles

Major risk signs

See your doctor immediately if your mole:
- Is new or growing—moles do change in children, but this becomes less common as we get older and could be a warning sign.
- Has a ragged edge—ordinary moles have a smooth, regular shape.
- Contains different colours—ordinary moles may be dark brown, but are all one shade. A mole containing different shades of black and brown should be checked out.

Minor risk signs

If your mole or dark patch does not return to normal within two weeks, don't ignore it. See your doctor if your mole:
- Is inflamed or has a red edge—ordinary moles are not inflamed.
- Is bleeding, oozing, or crusting—ordinary moles do not do this.
- Feels funny or itches—any change in the feel of a mole should be checked out. Ordinary moles are not itchy or painful.
- Is bigger than all your other moles.

Adapted from Cancer Research UK Sunsmart campaign.http://www.cancerresearchuk.org/
sunsmart/

Further reading

Glaus A, Bialous S A, Rieger P T (2005). Cancer Prevention. In Kearney N and Richardson A (eds) *Nursing Patients with Cancer: Principles and Practice.* Edinburgh: Elsevier Churchill Livingstone.
Greenwald P (2005). The future of cancer prevention. *Seminars in Oncology Nursing,* **21**(4), 296–8.

1 Cancer research UK (2002). Sunsmart. Accessed May 17th 2006
http://www.cancerresearchuk.org /sunsmart/

Cancer genetics

Every cancer arises due to genetic mutations that have occurred within a cell and altered the normal life cycle of that cell. These genetic mutations are usually acquired over a person's lifetime (📖 Cancer biology). However, about 5–10% of cancers are thought to be due to an inherited cancer-predisposing gene.

A number of genes have been identified that confer an increased predisposition to specific cancers. Generally, all people carry two copies of these genes. The predisposition to specific cancers occurs when a person inherits a mutated copy of one of these genes. If a person is known to carry a mutated gene that causes a cancer predisposition, then the risk of their offspring inheriting the predisposing gene mutation is 50%. This is called dominant inheritance (see Fig. 4.1)

Assessment of familial risk

Having one or more relatives affected with cancer raises anxiety for many people suggesting an inherited tendency to cancer in their family. However, for most people it is much more likely that the family history has arisen through chance due to:

- Shared environment.
- Shared lifestyle.
- Cancer being a common disease in the Western population.

A detailed family tree is important for this assessment and should take into account:

- The numbers and relatedness of affected relatives and age at diagnosis.
- The number and relatedness of unaffected relatives.
- The presence of other clues in the family history, e.g. related cancers, bilateral disease.

Key features pointing towards a possible inherited predisposition are:

- Multiple, closely related individuals with cancer.
- Several generations in the family affected with cancer.
- Early age of onset of cancer, e.g. pre-menopausal breast cancer, colorectal cancer age <50 years or childhood tumours.
- Bilateral breast cancer.
- More than one primary in an affected individual.
- Rare cancers, e.g. male breast cancer.

Through this risk assessment, families are usually grouped in one of three categories:

- Low genetic risk.
- Moderate genetic risk.
- High genetic risk.

Genetic testing

Genetic testing is usually only offered to families who fall into the high genetic risk group. Currently genetic testing can only be offered where there is an affected family member who is willing and able to provide a blood sample for testing. The testing process takes a number of months to complete and in many families a causative mutation is not found. All individuals undergoing genetic testing are offered genetic counselling within Clinical Genetic Services to discuss the implications of possible testing outcomes.

In families where a causative gene mutation is found, predictive testing can be offered to at-risk relatives to clarify their personal risk of developing a related cancer. This allows surveillance and surgical interventions to be targeted at those individuals at a high genetic risk. Predictive testing also raises ethical and practical considerations for those individuals considering testing and therefore predictive testing is offered through Clinical Genetics Services.

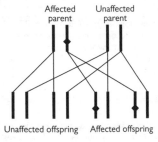

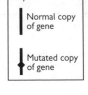

Fig. 4.1 Autosomal dominant inheritance

Common cancers with inherited predisposition

Breast cancer

Around 5–10% of breast cancers are thought to be due to an hereditary factor. Several genes are known to be involved in inherited predisposition—the two most common ones are BRCA1 and BRCA2. A woman who inherits a mutated form of one of these genes will have a lifetime risk of developing breast cancer in the order of 50–80%.

There are other specific cancers that may be associated with inherited mutations in BRCA1/BRCA2:
- Ovarian cancer—lifetime risk 20–60%.
- Male breast cancer.
- Prostate cancer.
- Colorectal cancer.
- Ocular melanoma.
- Pancreatic cancer.

Both men and women can inherit mutations in the BRCA1 and BRCA2 genes, however, men are much less likely to develop an associated cancer than the women in a family. Both men and women can pass on the mutated gene to their offspring (see Fig. 4.1).

Management of familial breast cancer

Individuals and families that fall into the low genetic risk group can be reassured; their risk of developing a cancer is close to that for the general population.

Individuals and families that fall into the moderate and high genetic risk groups should be counselled about their risk. Counselling often takes place in Family History Clinics within Breast Care services for moderate risk women. Counselling for high-risk families takes place within Clinical Genetic Services. Women and families at moderate and high genetic risk are eligible for a number of interventions.

Early detection

Regular surveillance. Current guidelines are:
- Women with a moderate or high genetic risk should be offered a minimum of annual mammography between the ages of 40 and 50 years and then join the NHS Breast Screening Programme (📖 Breast cancer screening).
- Women in the high genetic risk category may be offered earlier mammograms (e.g. from 35 years) and more frequent screening after the age of 50 years (e.g. mammograms every 18 months).

National trials have been underway to assess the efficacy of alternative screening modes, e.g. MRI screening.

Risk-reducing surgery
Women identified to be at high genetic risk for breast and/or ovarian cancer may choose to undergo prophylactic mastectomy, to remove healthy tissue in order to reduce the risk of developing cancer. There is evidence that such surgery does reduce the risk of developing these cancers, but the reduction in risk is not absolute as not all the tissue can be removed. Women considering this intervention are offered genetic counselling within Clinical Genetic Services.

Ovarian cancer
BRCA1 and *BRCA2* gene mutations may also predispose to ovarian cancer. A family in which there are two or more ovarian cancer diagnoses has a high chance of being related to a predisposing gene mutation.

Early detection
Currently there is no surveillance method that has been proved effective in identifying early changes in the ovaries. Women with a significant family history of ovarian cancer or breast/ovarian cancer or colorectal/ovarian cancer may be eligible for a national study looking at annual ultrasound scan and CA125 serum marker, called the UK Familial Ovarian Screening Study (UKFOCSS).

Risk-reducing surgery
See Breast cancer .

Colorectal cancer
Several genes are known to be involved in inherited predisposition to colorectal cancer. The two most important genetic syndromes that predispose to colorectal cancer are:
- Hereditary non-polyposis colorectal cancer (HNPCC).
- Familial adenomatous polyposis (FAP).

HNPCC causes approximately 5–10% of colorectal cancers and confers a 75% risk of developing a colorectal cancer by the age of 65 years. There are other specific cancers that may be associated with HNPCC:
- Endometrial cancer.
- Ovarian cancer.
- Small bowel cancer.
- Stomach cancer.
- Ureteric cancer.
- Renal pelvis cancer.

FAP accounts for less than 1% of colorectal cancers. It confers a 100% risk of developing a colorectal cancer by the age of 50 years. Individuals affected with FAP will develop hundreds of adenomatous polyps in the bowel during their teenage years.

Both men and women can inherit these colorectal cancer predisposing syndromes and can pass on the mutated gene to their offspring (see Fig. 4.1).

Early detection and management

Individuals identified at being at moderate or high genetic risk are offered regular surveillance, usually by sigmoidoscopy or colonoscopy.

HNPCC

- Colonoscopy every 2 years from the age of 25 years.
- Any polyps identified are removed at colonoscopy.
- Endometrial/uterine screening is not routinely offered as there is little evidence of effectiveness.

FAP

- Sigmoidoscopy annually from adolescence.
- Upper gastric endoscopy in known gene carriers.
- Prophylactic colectomy is offered if extensive polyposis is identified.

Further reading

Bleiker E M A, Hahn E E, Aaronson N K (2003). Psychosocial issues in cancer genetics. *Acta Oncologica*, **42**(4), 276–86.

Eeles R A, Easton D F, Ponder B A J, Eng C (eds) (2004). *Genetic Predisposition to Cancer*, Second edition. London: Hodder-Arnold.

Hodgson S V, and Maher E R (1999). *A Practical Guide to Human Cancer Genetics*, Second edition. Cambridge: Cambridge University Press.

Greco K E, and Mahon S (2004). Common hereditary cancer syndromes. *Seminars in Oncology Nursing*, **20**(3), 164–77.

Rare cancer syndromes

A number of rare genetic syndromes can predispose individuals to specific patterns of malignant and non-malignant tumours. Examples include:

Li Fraumeni syndrome
- Early onset breast cancer
- Childhood sarcomas
- Leukaemias
- Brain tumours

Cowden syndrome
- Young-onset breast cancer
- Non-medullary thyroid cancer
- Uterine cancer
- Multiple hamartomatous skin lesions

Von Hippel Lindau syndrome
- Cerebellar haemangioblastomas
- Renal cell carcinoma
- Phaeochromocytoma
- Retinal angiomas

Section 3

The experience of cancer

The personal experience of cancer

Introduction

Government health policy in the UK aims to put the patient, or service user, at the heart of local health services. For this to happen, health care professionals must gain an appreciation of what it is like to be a person with cancer, or a carer of someone with cancer. It is hard to know or understand the experience of another person, but there are various ways that we can gain insights into their experience. This section reviews ways of understanding the experience of cancer, and then goes on to look at different aspects of that experience for individuals, using the words of people with cancer.

Personal accounts of cancer

Personal, autobiographical writing can be a valuable source of personal experience and reactions to cancer. A disadvantage is that it depends on the skill of the writer to convey their experience, so they tend to represent the experience of articulate, middle-class people. Good examples of autobiographical writing include:
- Diamond J (1998). *Because Cowards get Cancer too*. London: Vermillion.
- Picardie R (1998). *Before I Say Goodbye*. London: Penguin Books.

Fictional accounts of cancer, in books and films

Although these can give us insights into the emotions associated with cancer, they will also be selective in what they represent, aiming to tell a good story, or to elicit a specific emotional response from the reader or viewer.

Reflection points
- Have you read a book or seen a film that helped you to understand what it is like to have cancer?
- Was there anything about it in particular that gave you insights?

Research into the experience of cancer

Research can provide us with valuable insights—although these are interpreted by the researcher on behalf of the person with cancer. The advantage of research is that it is rigorous. It is subject to the discipline of scientific method and peer review. Certain research methodologies are particularly suited to the study of human experience. These are Qualitative research methodologies, of which some of the most significant are *phenomenology* and *narrative research*.

One very accessible format for personal stories is available on the internet. The DIPEx (Directory of Personal Experiences of Health and Illness) project includes a range of personal experiences of different cancers collected by interview and shown on the website as written, audio, and video clips. The following pages contain a number of personal accounts taken from DIPEx transcripts. Transcripts are the words of the person, written just as they were spoken at the interview. You are recommended to visit the website and see the original video and audio recordings.

DIPEx website: www.dipex.org

The cancer journey

The term 'cancer journey' has become a popular and useful way of identifying different stages of cancer experience, including diagnosis, treatment, recurrence, dying, and death. By doing this, we can focus on the needs of people at different stages in their cancer journey. These stages have been used in the NICE *Guidance on Supportive and Palliative Care for Adults with Cancer*[1], as points for assessing and re-assessing patients' and carers' needs. Significant stages in the cancer journey are used in the following sections of this book.

Studying personal experiences of cancer helps health professionals to work effectively with patients, and to improve services. Research can involve the use of questionnaires or interviews. Focus group interviews are sometimes used to generate a range of personal experiences and views from people with cancer. An example is the research *Patient-centred Cancer Services? What Patients Say*, published by the National Cancer Alliance[2]. This presents patients' views of their needs and priorities at different stages of their cancer journey.

However, we must bear in mind that these stages may or may not be the most significant experiences for individual patients. Patients themselves may see particular events, both good and bad, as their most important experiences of cancer, and they will view these within the context of their life. As health professionals, we may never know the details of individual lives and families, even if we think we know the patient well.

---

1 Guidance on Supportive and Palliative Care for Adults with Cancer (2004). London: National Institute for Clinical Excellence (NICE).
2 Patient Centred Cancer Services? What Patients Say (1996). Oxford: National Cancer Alliance.

Calendars

Another way of understanding the personal experience of cancer is to see it as a series of overlapping calendars. This places personal experience within a social context. By understanding the overlapping and competing demands on individuals and families, we can gain insights into how they maintain continuity within their lives in the face of illness. They do this by the ways they manage their time, their energy, and their physical resources.

Life calendar

The life calendar represents how we see ourselves over time, in terms of relationships and life events, including births, marriages, and deaths. It also encompasses our personal achievements, at work and at home, our life goals, and future plans.

Personal calendar

The personal calendar represents the schedules of our daily life, the things we do. The personal calendar is the rhythm of our private life, bound by our sense of ourselves and our personal responsibilities.

Illness calendar

The illness calendar begins with the first effects or awareness of the cancer. It then follows the developing understanding of diagnosis and prognosis, and the nature of treatment. It includes the experience of symptoms and side effects, investigations, and results, and continuous changes in life and lifestyle in response to the effects of illness.

Treatment calendar

The treatment calendar follows the phases of treatment regimens, with the demands of surgery, chemotherapy, and radiotherapy. One of the defining elements of the treatment calendar is that it is generally not managed by the patient, but by the professional. In spite of professional management, the treatment calendar is often a series of unpredictable and unforeseen events, including complications, stalls and changes of plan.

Most people strive for their personal aspirations, for stability and personal control. A diagnosis of cancer disrupts both the longer-term aspirations and events of the life calendar, and the day-to-day routines of the personal calendar. The effects of the illness on daily life (the illness calendar) and the demands of particular treatments regimens (the treatment calendar), may come to dominate an individual's life and that of their family. The person becomes a 'patient', and enters a new world of the experience of cancer. Effective health care at this point can make a significant difference to patient's experience of cancer, for example, organized treatment pathways, multidisciplinary team working.

Reflection point

Can you think of a situation where a patient's personal priorities were in conflict with the demands of treatment or the effects of the illness? What was the outcome?

Further reading

Costain Schou K and Hewison J (1999). *Experiencing Cancer*. Buckingham: Open University Press.

Diagnosis

A diagnosis of cancer can be experienced as a single event. However, for many people it will be experienced as a process, or as a series of confusing events, with new information arriving at unpredictable intervals, in an unfamiliar hospital environment, and in unfamiliar medical language. The period prior to diagnosis will have an impact on how it is experienced. For example, if there are pre-existing emotional or social problems, these may be at the forefront of the patient's mind and delay their response to diagnosis. Consider the following scenarios:

Diagnosis of breast cancer by routine mammography: in this case, the patient may be unprepared or only partially prepared for the possibility of cancer. Diagnosis may be dominated by treatment choices and disruption of daily life.

Diagnosis of lung cancer: this may be accompanied by a physical crisis, like breathlessness, making the time of diagnosis a period dominated by symptom distress and functional problems. Adjustment to the diagnosis is accompanied by profound changes to the daily life and outlook of the patient, and their family.

Diagnosis of bowel cancer: this is precipitated by a change in bodily functions, for example, finding blood in the faeces, raising concerns about health. After help is sought, treatment may be radical and disfiguring (e.g. colostomy), leading to profound changes in daily functioning and self-image.

Delay in diagnosis may occur either because the person does not think the problem is serious (e.g. finding a breast lump), or because of a fear of being told the implications of diagnosis. Sometimes, cancers are not identified promptly in primary care. Delays will have an impact on how the diagnosis is experienced. (☐ **Diagnosis, classification, and staging of cancer**). The patient may feel regret at having delayed seeking help, or anger towards health professionals for delays in starting treatment.

The other major challenge for the patient at diagnosis is to begin making sense of the seriousness of the situation, and what the implications will be for the person's hopes and aspirations. This developing awareness can be very difficult. Information is often framed in technical language that the patient may not understand. There is evidence to suggest that some physicians give overly optimistic interpretations of the patient's prospects of cure. We also know that some patients deny the seriousness of their situation. However, in many situations the context of awareness may be ambiguous and contain contradictions. Patients may be told they have a serious illness, but that their prospects for cure are good. Where the information is confusing or ambiguous, patients may 'fill in the blanks' for themselves. It can then be very difficult for the health care professional, the patient, or their carer to know who knows what, or what is the most accurate information.

'...all I've been told is that I've got a lymph node which I don't know what, I don't know what a lymph node is. I'm not very good medically. Some people can ask the questions and they understand the doctor's language, but I don't understand the doctor's language, I don't even know what a lymph node is, even though I've had one before, I've never been explained exactly what it is.

I have, yes I have asked, but whether he's told me in his language and I haven't understood because I'm a bit thick that way inclined I suppose. Perhaps he's told me in his language and I haven't understood what he's told me, if he has told me I haven't understood it.'

DIPEx interview LC27 transcript (lung cancer). Available at www.dipex.org

Reflection point

Think of a patient you have worked with who appeared to have difficulty understanding their diagnosis. Can you think of any factors in the patient or in the situation that made it difficult for them?

Reactions to diagnosis and treatment

People's reactions to the early stages of diagnosis and treatment will be determined by a number of different factors. These include their personal experiences of illness, in themselves and others. People who have not experienced serious illness before may have no personal context within which to understand what is happening to them. On the other hand, experience of cancer in a close relative may predetermine their own reaction. For example, if a woman's mother died of breast cancer under circumstances of pain and distress, the same woman being diagnosed with cancer may fear that this will also happen to her. In fact, developments in palliative care and new treatment options means this need not happen. Other social factors, like newspaper stories of celebrities with cancer, may also have an effect.

Many people do not fully register the reality or the implications of a life-threatening illness at the time of diagnosis. Initial reactions may be of shock, numbness, and disbelief. This can make it hard to take in the volume of new information being presented. For some, possibly as many as 20%, the trauma of diagnosis will lead to an acute stress reaction or disorder (📖 Adjustment, stress reactions, and disorders).

'It was a very strange experience. I felt as though I was sitting in the corner by the window, it was rather like an out of body experience, and when I came back, you know, I came back to reality, I kept trying to put myself back in the seat I was in but I kept going back to the window again. I think everybody thought I was taking it very well, I was very controlled.'

DIPEx interview 02 transcript (breast cancer). Available at www. dipex.org

Others will try to focus on the elements that they can control, or that they feel are the most controllable within their lives. Getting on with the new treatment calendar may be the most effective way for the newly diagnosed patient to manage the new realities of their lives.

'I'm one of these people that's "Right, OK what are we going to do then?" I didn't, I didn't fall apart at all, I thought right OK what have we got to do. Do I, can I go to work, silly things go through your head, can I go to work, I've got to do this and I've got to do that and lets just get on with what, what's got to be done. I just wanted to get over it, I just wanted to sort it out and get rid of it. And because he told me that we caught it fairly early I just wanted to get on with it really.'

DIPEx interview CC13 transcript (cervical cancer). Available at www. dipex.org

Many experience a 'rollercoaster' of new experiences, information, and appointments. For many, the full implications are felt when the rollercoaster ride stops—at the end of the initial period of treatment. Unfortunately, this is often the time when professional support is withdrawn, so the patient can feel isolated or abandoned.

'In fact the other thing I think that, once you've finished your treatment you're just left. Okay, so you've got a breast care nurse you can contact if you want to, but she's busy, she's got other more important things to do. You just feel as though, that you're just dumped basically, you know?

That's it. Treatment's over. Finished, done with. Off you go. See you in four months.

And it's a bit scary. Especially when you've got things like: "Oh God, that pain", you know? "Is that normal?" And things like that.'

DIPEx interview 05 transcript (breast cancer). Available at www. dipex.org

Reflection points

- Can you think of different ways that patients have managed their lives during treatment?
- What options are there in your area of work for supporting patients who have completed treatment?
- Can you think of ways in which these could be improved?

Living with cancer

Living with cancer often involves a personal search for meaning within the cancer experience. The unavoidable question 'why me?' will seldom have a clear answer (though where there is a direct link between behaviour and cancer, e.g. lung cancer, this may be associated with considerable guilt). The answer is more likely to result in a search for new or additional meaning in the person's life. This may involve a spiritual journey, a deepening of personal relationships, or a general re-evaluation of priorities and aspirations.

The unpredictability of disease course, and uncertain prognosis, means that a degree of uncertainty about the future becomes a feature of the lives of those living with cancer. However, accepting a degree of uncertainty into one's life may be a step towards a more positive future.

'Now the future, I'm not really sure what's going to happen. I've got another appointment at the hospital in another month's time just for a check-up to see how things are going. The cancer that I've got in the bones is incurable. ... You can understand that in a way because it's there, it's, they say it's going to be controlled and contained, but nobody will actually tell me, and I think that that's because they don't know, whether I'm going to be back to walking absolutely normally, or whether this is ultimately going to be a further problem and it's going to kill me.'

DIPEx interview 01 transcript (breast cancer). Available at www.dipex.org

'And I do feel very positive. I think, I don't know I don't think cancer will come back, or if it comes back I'll fight it again. So I'm very positive. I do feel very happy. I feel happier than before. And I don't complain about things like bills to pay or because it's cold or because it's raining, I do feel much happier. And I feel much healthier as well. I don't know why but I feel much stronger than before.'

DIPEx interview CC15 transcript (cervical cancer). Available at www.dipex.org

---

Reflection points

- How can we support patients through periods of uncertainty?
- How can we ensure that we do not provide false reassurance?

Fear of recurrence

Fear of recurrence can be a prominent feature of the experience of cancer. Once diagnosed with cancer, one's sense of invulnerability is challenged, the body becomes less reliable, a potential source of threat. It is common for people to check their body for signs of recurrence. This sense of anxiety about any bodily change, and constant self-monitoring involves:

• Interpreting everyday physical sensations as cues that disease may be returning.
• Seeing external cues as significant. This will involve noticing references to cancer in social situations or in the media.

Other factors will contribute to the fear of recurrence:
• The perception of personal risk, based on past experience, knowledge, and beliefs.
• Emotions, such as worry, anxiety, or remorse.

For some the fear of recurrence becomes a problem in itself, characterized by:
• Constant self-checking.
• Seeking further tests.
• Being preoccupied by thoughts of recurrence.

This can become a bigger problem that the cancer itself.

'I became very aware of every ache, pain, itch, lump, bump, you name it, and I probably went backwards and forwards to my GP more during the first couple of years after that than I'd ever been at all in my life, including the time when I went during my pregnancies for ante natal and so on. I'd sort of feel a lump and I'd think well has that always been there or is that new, is it something to worry about or not? And I'd go to the GP and particularly when my new GP was there, I said to her one day "You must think I've turned into a hypochondriac".'

DIPEx interview CC06 transcript (cervical cancer). Available at www.dipex.org

---

Reflection point

How could you help patients find a balance between a healthy concern about their health and a morbid preoccupation with recurrence?

Further reading

Lee-Jones, C, Humphris, G, Dixon, R, Bebbington Hatcher, M (1997). Fear of Cancer Recurrence—a literature review and proposed cognitive formulation to explain exacerbation of recurrence fears. *Psycho-Oncology*, **6(2)**, 95–105.

Recurrence and facing death

Recurrence of disease after treatment brings a new set of challenges. Cure becomes less likely, additional and new effects of the illness may become apparent, and it signifies a new stage in the treatment calendar. If there has been an extended period when the patient has been free of illness, then this may put new strains on family relationships. As initial appraisals of cure can be optimistic, patients may realise more fully at this stage how difficult it can be to treat cancer. Cancer becomes a chronic illness, or a terminal illness. Recurrence can be harder to deal with than the original diagnosis.

The full implications of cancer may be more apparent at recurrence than at diagnosis. Not everyone feels ill at diagnosis, but patients are more likely to be symptomatic at the point of recurrence. Patients can there-fore feel much more vulnerable than they did previously. Recurrence may also trigger a loss of confidence in health professionals. This might lead the patient to express anger, frustration, or disappointment. It may also lead to a loss of faith in conventional medicine. Many people at this point seek alternative approaches to cancer in complementary therapies.

Facing death may be particularly hard if it challenges a person's assumptions about life and death.

'I think probably my attitude at the moment would be anyway, "How could God love me if you know he's made this happen to me?" And, 'Why should, why should this be me? Why me?' That must be the question that everybody that's younger must ask. We expect to live until we are in our 80s or even 90s and the thought I'm going to pre-decease my mother is not a good one. Just comes back to the fact of not being able to accept the fact that I'm dying, just can't accept it. I'm too young. I'm not ready to go. I've got all these lovely babies and it's just not fair but then you know nobody ever said life was going to be fair, I know.'

DIPEx interview LD02 transcript (living with dying). Available at www.dipex.org

For others it is an opportunity for reflection and appreciation.

'Yes. Assess your own lives. Assess your life and what has been. ...What is it your life has been and it's all the positive things. All the times that you've enjoyed. Life is a mixture of all sorts of things. There are sad moments and there are moments when things have gone wrong and there are things when you can be upset and angry about things, but find the positives. And rejoice in those positives and rejoice in the life that you've had. Celebrate the life that you've had and come to terms with the fact that it will ultimately end. The only difference is that you now know and some people ... well it comes to an end and they don't know about it. And I don't know which is worse.'

DIPEx interview LD14 transcript (living with dying). Available at www.dipex.org

Reflection points

- How does your service manage the transition from active treatment to palliation?
- Can you think of any ways of improving the support of patients who have recurrence and are facing the prospect of death for the first time?

Further reading

Dixon, R, Lee-Jones, C, Humphris, G (1996). Psychological reactions to cancer recurrence. *International of Palliative Nursing*, **2**(1), 19–21.

Survivorship

With increasing numbers of people surviving cancer, many are now faced with the long-term consequences of cancer and its treatment. Survival presents an opportunity to return to normal. However, it is also beset with problems. At what point do you become a survivor? Many will see a 5-year survival beyond diagnosis as a significant anniversary. However, anniversaries can also be a grim reminder of the past. Also, life may no longer feel as it did prior to diagnosis. The life calendar, with its hopes and aspirations may have changed. Most people need to adapt to a new 'normal', which may involve:

• New life goals and priorities.
• Changed relationships and new sources of social support.
• Finding new meaning in the cancer experience.

Some survivors will find their employment prospects have become more difficult, because of a lack of understanding from employers, or they may have residual dysfunction or disability that limits their ability to work. Others may encounter frank discrimination or social stigma (Q Threats to personal identity).

Being a survivor can be a very lonely experience. The survivor may have known other patients who died from the same malignancy, and they may experience *survivor guilt*, questioning why they survived when others did not. For others, a sense of being a survivor will be a transformative or liberating experience, allowing them to make positive choices, to retire early or start a new life with new priorities.

'… *your life is really short and it's something like this which is, I'm seeing it now as a wake-up call for my life because to really know where I want to be and what I want to do now. I was at university but I'm going to have to repeat my year next year, but I was also working part time and my part time work was actually taking on sort of more importance over my university job just because you get obsessed with the money side of things and paying for rent at university and that kind of thing and now I'm like no my studies are really important. And in a way, I wouldn't have wished this to happen but in a way it's almost a wake-up call, it's a kind of you can put things in, put priorities and everything straight in your life.*'

DIPEx interview CC11 transcript (cervical cancer). Available at www.dipex.org

Reflection points

- Do you know any patients who are long-term survivors?
- Do you know what sort of problems they have encountered as a result?

Further reading

Dow, K H (2003). Challenges and opportunities in cancer survivorship research. *Oncology Nursing Forum*, **30**(3), 455–69.

Rendle, K (1997). Survivorship and breast cancer: the psychosocial issues. *Journal of Clinical Nursing*, **6**, 403–10.

The social experience of cancer

The family experience of cancer

Most people experience cancer within the context of their family. What constitutes a family varies considerably, but it generally means a household, or those people one is closest to, whether they are related by blood or not. Family members as 'carers' have a significant role in providing physical and emotional care during the cancer journey. The experience of cancer is shared within the family in a number of ways.

The effects of illness and treatment

Partners or other family members are often present when significant news is given, and during treatment. Families experience disruption to their lives because of the effects of symptoms and the side effects of treatment, for example, pain and sleep disturbance. Partners, family members, and friends may have to take on significant amounts of caring work, though in advanced cancer, it is likely that more care will be provided by professionals. Family members, like the person with cancer, will have to make sense of new information and unfamiliar language about the illness and treatment.

Family role changes

Roles within the family have to be re-allocated, either because the person with cancer can no longer continue in their role as parent or carer, or if they need additional care from others. Roles will change sometimes whether family members are prepared, willing, or able to do this. For example, a teenager may have to do additional housework or provide care for younger siblings. This could impact on their ability to maintain friendships with their peers, or to study. Family members share the sense of uncertainty that cancer brings, and communication may become very difficult.

'It was a very strange thing at home. Although I had a lot of support from friends and family, we would say a lot without talking about the issues. …And it's a vicious circle and likewise they wouldn't say anything to me in case it upset or worried me. So there was this, it's a conspiracy of silence, all for the best of reasons, everybody trying to protect everybody else but by the same token there is absolutely nothing that anybody could have said to anybody else that would've made the situation any worse than it already was. But when you go through it you can't see that'.

DIPEx interview CC06 transcript (cervical cancer). Available at www.dipex.org

Children and families

Children experience particular problems when a parent or other adult in the family has cancer.

- The parent may be absent from their lives whilst in hospital, or their presence in hospital brings an unfamiliar and perhaps frightening element to family life.
- There may be breaks in the continuity of parenting, when the parent is too ill to behave in a consistent parental manner.
- The child may be frightened and distressed by seeing their parent weak, distressed, or in pain.
- Problems at home can affect the child's relationships with other children, or disrupt their schooling.

Information and involvement of children

Children vary greatly in their developmental stages and they may have no prior knowledge or context within which to understand what is going on. On the other hand, children can be very perceptive, and sensitive to changes in the emotional life of the family. It is therefore important to involve them in the sharing of information and in the caring process. This must be balanced with an awareness of the needs of the child, bearing in mind their age and their stage of development.

Health professionals who do not work regularly with children may not know how to communicate effectively with them, and should seek supervision from colleagues with more experience of this, e.g. a social worker. It is important to negotiate with the family how they would like the children involved, and what information should be shared with them. This can be as challenging for the family as for the health professional. Many families do not have experience of dealing with serious crises and may need help to do this.

'But I was a bit worried about my son because I did explain everything to him from the first day, I didn't hide anything because I thought, I'm gonna lose my hair so if I don't tell him why, what am I gonna tell him. But luckily I didn't lose my hair with this chemo. But I told him everything; I didn't hide anything from him. I told him everything. And he didn't talk with me, he didn't make any questions so I was a bit worried, but he had a lot of support at school, because I thought it was better if I talk with the teacher and say what's going on and he had a lot of support. ... That was, my main problem was my son because I didn't know what was going inside his head.'

DIPEx interview CC15 transcript (cervical cancer). Available at www. dipex.org

The needs of the child

If children do not get the information or support that they need from family members they may go to friends, or friends' parents to help them understand what is happening. These sources of information and support can be helpful to the child. However, it is important to recognize formal supports, including school teachers, and to liaise with the child's school. If children are being raised in single parent households and the parent is ill or dying, professional support will be essential in giving the child a sense of continuity. If the parent is going to die, legal guardianship arrangements will have to be considered.

Carers

The carer is often the patient's partner, but they may also be a relative, or a friend or neighbour. Carers often share every step of the cancer journey with the patient. They may supply the bulk of the care needed.

Informal care is care that is not paid for, but provided out of love or mutual obligation. It is a significant factor in the overall provision of health care. Increasingly, carers are seen as having distinctive needs of their own, in addition to the needs of the patient.

The demands of caring on the individual are called 'carer burden'. This burden may take a number of forms:

- Physical care, possibly on top of a job (many carers provide more than 20 hours care a week).
- Organizing appointments and travel etc.
- The emotional demands of the illness and treatment.
- Disruption to their own personal needs and social supports.
- Feelings of frustration, or guilt if they are unable to meet all of the patient's needs.

The carer occupies an ambiguous position in the health care system. They can be both users and providers of cancer services; and they have to negotiate their own place in the system. This can be very difficult, as initially, the patient is the focus of attention, and the carer may feel they should be quiet and stand back. If the carer feels they are being involved and invited to participate, they can help the patient to get necessary information and make decisions. It is helpful if they can keep track of progress, and manage the details of treatment regimens and appointments, etc. If the patient's condition deteriorates, they can look after the patient's interests but support their independence as far as possible. Ultimately, carers should be able to recognize their own needs and seek support, whilst balancing these with the needs of the patient.

Further reading

Morris S M, Thomas C (2001). The carer's place in the cancer situation: where does the carer stand in the medical setting? *European Journal of Cancer Care* **10**, 87–95.

http://www.cancerbacup.org.uk/Resourcessupport/Relationshipscommunication/ Talkingtochildren

Employment and finances

Disruption to employment

The work life of both the person with cancer and other family members can be disrupted or have to stop altogether. This will lead to changes in the person's perception of who they are. Our occupation provides us with one of our most significant social roles and social contacts. Future employment prospects can be severely disrupted by cancer.

The cost of cancer

Financial strains are felt by the whole family due to lost income; plus the additional costs associated with treatment. These costs can include travel and parking, diet, and complementary therapies, prescriptions, and increased utility bills. A Macmillan survey found the average cost of breast cancer treatment was £2000 (which does not take into account loss of earnings)[1].

'Uh, they paid my wages, full wages for the few weeks, three weeks I think it was and then they cut my wages down. And then I had pressure put on me to go back to work. And I just told them uh, "I can't come back to work until my doctor says I can go back to work". So they stopped my wages completely and I finished up on Social Benefit like you know. ...I thought it was a bit uh, much of the company doing that to me because we worked, I worked as a manager for 'em thirteen years and never had a day off before I had the operation.'

DIPEx interview 34 transcript (bowel cancer). Available at www.dipex.org (Also see 📖 Social support.)

---

1 http://www.macmillan.org.uk/home.aspx

Culture and the meaning of cancer

Cancer occupies a powerful place in public consciousness. As well as being a dreaded disease, cancer also acts as a metaphor for death. In her analysis of cancer as a stigmatizing condition, Susan Sontag[1] observes that cancer took over the role previously occupied by tuberculosis, as the mysterious bringer of death. Cancer was generally viewed by the public as an incurable illness, a role that has now, arguably, been taken over by AIDS. The use of military metaphors, such as the 'fight' against cancer, suggests that cancer is an enemy to be fought. Within this military vision of cancer, the patient is potentially cast as victim or hero.

More recently, as personal stories or narratives of cancer emerge, the true nature of the cancer experience is presented as more subtle and complex. Examples of recent terminology are 'struggle' and 'survival'. This suggests a challenge to be overcome, rather than a war. Combined with terminology changes, charity fundraising campaigns have emphasized living with cancer, rather than defeating cancer. This acknowledges the reality that, although not all cancers are curable, much can be done to help people live with its effects.

Further reading

Flanagan J, Holmes S (2000). Social perceptions of cancer and their impacts: implications for nursing practice arising from the literature. *Journal of Advanced Nursing*, **32**(3), 740–749.

---

1 Sontag S (1991). *Illness as metaphor; and AIDS and its metaphors*. London: Penguin.

Gender, age, and cancer

Gender

Gender refers to our sexual identity, based on biology, but subject to personal and social factors. Men and women have certain differences when it comes to their experience and use of health services. Women are more likely to seek help if they have a concern about their health. They are also more likely to seek and make use of psychological support. There is no clear biological reason for this; it is likely to be rooted in socially reinforced expectations of gender roles. For this reason, health promotion and screening should take account of men's difficulties seeking or accepting support.

This gender difference is reflected in research; we know more about women's responses to illness because they are more likely to be the subject of cancer care research. This does not suggest men have lesser needs for support, but that it is harder for them acknowledge this or ask for help. However, social changes are taking place which challenge gender roles, for example, more men are now the main carer for a female partner or relative.

Age

Cancer incidence increases with age, and older people are more likely to have multiple, complex health problems. However, there is some evidence that older people are less likely to seek involvement in treatment decisions. Whether this is because of their perception of their entitlement to participate or because of personal preferences, is unclear.

Further reading

Moynihan C (2002). Men, women, gender and cancer, *European Journal of Cancer Care* **11**, 166–72.

Ethnicity and cancer

The UK has an ethnically diverse population, with significant communities of Irish, African-Caribbean, African, South Asian, and Chinese people. In addition, migration for economic reasons continues to bring large numbers of people into the UK, recently from Eastern Europe. There is surprisingly little information on the incidence of cancer in ethnic minority groups. Studies in the USA suggest that African-Americans have poorer survival rates than white Americans, a factor that appears to be related to their lower socio economic status.

Although health beliefs vary across cultures, there is no evidence to suggest substantial cultural differences in understanding about the nature of cancer. However, beliefs about the nature of life, living, and dying, may impact on the behaviour of individuals and families seeking help and accepting treatment and support from health services. Some communities have not made full use of screening for some cancers, and palliative care services are under-used by some ethnic minority groups.

Under-use of services may have a variety of causes. Information about services may not be available in a language understood by a particular ethnic group. Preferences for the place or style of care may be different in different communities. People generally prefer to be cared for by someone who understands their cultural preferences and needs.

We need to understand the diversity of cultural preferences, which go beyond issues of ethnic origin. Where clear cultural differences exist, it is helpful to have advocates or link workers to represent the interests of different communities. This includes having information on services available in different languages, and translation facilities for individuals who are not fluent in English. At difficult times, when significant new information is given, every effort should be taken to provide an independent translator.

Website

🖳 http://www.cancerblackcare.org/

Further reading

Lodge N (2001). The identified needs of ethnic minority groups with cancer within the community: a review of the literature *European Journal of Cancer Care* **10**, 234–44.

Threats to personal identity

There are a number of ways in which people with cancer can feel their identity threatened by the illness and its effects.

The social stigma of cancer

People newly diagnosed with cancer often feel other people respond differently to them. This can include friends becoming distant, or avoiding them. Very often this is because people do not know what to say, cannot deal with their own feelings, or are afraid of cancer.

'And people's reactions to it (cancer) were, sort of: "Ughhh!", you know. They don't like, I mean a lot of people just don't like mentioning the word. Oh, I say, the oncologist didn't. And, sometimes I felt some people avoided me because they didn't know what to say. So that was, that was hard to bear really I think. I mean some people were great but some people, and I mean it wasn't that people didn't want to help, they just didn't know what to say. And so they just avoided it. And avoided me, which was difficult.'

DIPEx interview 17 transcript (breast cancer). Available at www. dipex.org

The social stigma of cancer is made worse by physical manifestations of the disease or treatment. Other people's reactions can be even more difficult if the treatment for cancer leads to visible physical changes, for example hair loss, or the particularly disfiguring changes associated with head and neck surgery. The reactions of others to the patient can be embarrassed, suspicious, or even hostile. Many people find they need to manage the reactions of others, either by using cosmetics, wigs, or by being more selective about where they go and what they do socially. People experiencing stigma may feel the need to re-establish their social identity. This can happen to anyone who has cancer, but is more common in those with changed body image. Support with altered body image is therefore of the greatest importance in managing changes to social role.

'So I came home with the wig before I started to lose my hair. When it did come out it came out fairly quickly and I got [my husband] to shave my hair down to very short and then we sat and shaved it off completely. And I think a lot of people tend to wear the wigs not because they need to, because you do get used to not having your hair and it does grow back very quickly, it actually started growing back before the treatment ended. I think you tend to wear them more for other people because you're not sure how they're going to react.'

DIPEx interview 44 transcript (breast cancer). Available at www. dipex.org

(Also see 📖 Altered body image.)

Other forms of stigma can be seen in the cancer context. Stigma may be attached to certain lifestyles (e.g. gay and lesbian), lower socio-economic groups, travellers, the homeless, or asylum seekers. Health professionals need to be aware of their own potential to stigmatize patients.

Sexuality

Sexuality is part of our identity as a person and it also has implications for the ways in which we interact with other people. This includes our social behaviour, and the way we dress, as well as its effect on our most intimate relationships. These can be severely disrupted during cancer, by the effects of treatment, pain, or just not feeling good.

'I think it's harder for your partner than it is for you. Very hard. I think for [my husband] as well I know he wanted to have sex after the soreness went away. And I said to him, I just didn't feel like sex. I really didn't feel like sex at all, and I still don't. And I think he felt that I was rejecting him and maybe he closed down. And I was in a way, I mean the furthest thing from your mind is having sex. I want a cuddle or just to be held or to talk, you know. I don't feel like sex and I still don't.'

DIPEx interview 25 transcript (breast cancer). Available at www.dipex.org

People who are not in a relationship during treatment for cancer may lose confidence in their ability to find a partner. Those already in a relationship may experience disruption of their sexual activity and physical intimacy. This is usually interwoven with the emotional strains of the illness.

'And I felt and believed that the romance in my life was completely over, and that I was never going to be desired or feel desirable or have any sense of desire myself. That I was going to have something awful done to my breast. I would not be a woman in that sense any more. You feel a sense of invasion and you go through a very bad patch of self doubt. But you come out the other side.'

DIPEx interview 33 transcript (breast cancer). Available at www.dipex.org

It is important to acknowledge the role of sexuality in personal and social identity, and to become comfortable communicating about sexual health and incorporating it into assessment (📖 Sexual health and cancer).

Section 4

Supportive and palliative care

Supportive care

Background

Supportive care is a broad term describing all of the activities that help patients and their families to cope with the cancer and its treatment. Increasingly, this is about engaging in active collaboration with those who use cancer services, i.e. patients and families, to make the best use of both formal and informal resources. Its aim is to maximize the benefits of treatment, but equally to enable the patient and family to live as well as possible with the disease and its effects, achieving optimal quality of life. Supportive care should be provided at every stage of the patient's cancer journey. It includes: user involvement and self-help; coordination of care; communication and information-giving; psychological, social, and spiritual support; rehabilitation; complementary therapies; general and specialist palliative care; and services for families, including bereavement care.

Supportive care is therefore not a specialty in itself, but describes a range of activities and services, some of which are general and some of which are specialist. It falls within the remit of all of the professional groups working with cancer, and requires a range of skills, from, for example, basic communication skills to advanced and specialist psychological skills. It also requires effective communication and continuity of care across different parts of services, and between service users (patients and their families) and service providers (professionals). There is considerable overlap between the concepts of supportive care and palliative care, and they are frequently used together, i.e. 'supportive and palliative care'.

Further reading/websites

Department of Health (2000). *The NHS Cancer Plan: A Plan for Investment. A Plan for Reform.* London: HMSO.

The National Council for Palliative Care. www.ncpc.org.uk/palliative_care.html

National Institute for Clinical Excellence (2004). *Improving Supportive and Palliative Care for Adults with Cancer.* London: Department of Health. Also see www.nice.org.uk/

Communication in cancer care

Communication is a very important aspect of cancer care. Observational studies in the 1980s found that nursing communication was often superficial, routine, and task-related, and that it did not address psychological needs. It suggested that nurses blocked communications by patients that related to emotional aspects of care

This can be a problem in all groups of health professionals—they may avoid difficult topics, or find it difficult to break bad news. Poor communication makes assessment, information giving, and emotional support more difficult.

Communication skills training

Training in communication skills has become a high priority in trying to address these problems. Training programmes often use audio and video recording and feedback, role-play involving actors, and small group work.

It is important to deal with the emotional aspects of communication, and address the attitudes and beliefs underlying practice. Training often focuses on eliciting patient concerns and breaking bad news. Many people gain benefit from these courses, and there are national UK initiatives to promote communication skills training[1]. However, there is limited evidence that these skills are being used in the practice setting after training has taken place. Further research is needed to identify those factors that promote the transfer of communication skills into practice.

> **Reflection points**
> - Have I had adequate communication skills training for my role?
> - What sort of training is available for me in my practice area?

The context of communication

One factor that clearly affects the practice of communication skills is the context within which it takes place. The nursing environment is frequently busy, unpredictable, and nurses are subject to multiple conflicting demands. The type of nursing role is a significant factor in the way a nurse communicates. Ward-based nurses generally care for groups of patients who may have different levels of dependency, whereas clinical nurse specialists often work with a single patient at a time.

Consider the following factors that influence communication in your practice area:
- Staffing levels and workload.
- Distractions and interruptions.
- The need to prioritize different aspects of care.
- Organizational policies and procedures.

wes D, Wilkinson S, Moore P (2004). Communication skills training for health care nals working with cancer patients, their families, and/or carers. Cochrane Review in *The rary*, Issue 2. Chichester, UK: John Wiley & Sons, Ltd.

Reflection point

Are there ways that the environment I work in makes it harder for me to communicate effectively?

A culture of communication

The social environment of care is another significant factor in the style and use of communication skills. If the dominant culture is one of task orientation rather than relationship orientation, then nurses may feel discouraged from communicating with patients on an emotional level.

The attitude of senior colleagues such as ward managers or consultants is a critical factor in determining communication style; and this will also influence the sort of support and supervision that is available. Nurses will not elicit patient concerns if they do not feel able to deal with them, or if they feel they will not be supported with the consequences of emotional disclosure.

Reflection points

- Do I feel supported in my communications with patients and carers?
- What sort of support do I need to communicate effectively?

The patient's view

It is important to be aware of the patient's contribution to communication, a factor that has not been adequately addressed in the research. It is recognized that nurses give 'cues' to their availability, or their willingness to discuss sensitive or emotional issues, and the same is true of patients. Not all patients wish to disclose their personal feelings to nurses, and they may give subtle cues that discourage questioning. Both nurses and patients may want to keep conversations emotionally 'safe'. There is evidence that what patients value most in nurses are competence and knowledge, availability, and approachability.

Reflection points

- Do I know what patients value about the way that I communicate with them?
- How could I find out?

Further reading

Gysels M, Richardson, A Higginson I J (2004). Communication training for health professionals who care for patients with cancer: a systematic review of effectiveness. *Supportive Care Cancer*, **12**, 692–700.

Waterworth S, May C, Luker K (1999). Clinical 'effectiveness' and 'interrupted' work. *Clinical Effectiveness in Nursing*, **3**, 163–169.

Williams A M, Irurita V F (2004). Therapeutic and non-therapeutic interpersonal interactions: the patient's perspective. *Journal of Clinical Nursing*, **13**, 806–15.

Promoting effective communication

Communication is most effective if the nurse demonstrates warmth, empathy, genuine concern about the patient, and a non-judgemental attitude. A warm and confident tone of voice is important. These are also fundamental attributes of skilled counselling (📖 Psychological support).

The following behaviours promote effective communication:
• Space, time, and availability.
• Active listening and attention.
• Assessing and focusing on how the patient is feeling.
• Open questions.
• Focusing, probing, and paraphrasing.
• Clarifying or summarizing.

Inhibiting effective communication

Communication is least effective if the nurse demonstrates a lack of time or attention through their behaviour, is focused inwards on personal feelings such as stress or anxiety, lacks warmth, or is judgemental. The following behaviours inhibit communication:
• Leading or closed questions.
• Premature or false reassurance.
• Advising or blaming.
• Changing the topic or being defensive.
• Judging or placating.
• Focusing on a physical assessment to the exclusion of a psychological assessment.
• Using medical terminology when everyday alternatives could be used.

Non-verbal communication

Communication in nursing is not only verbal. Non-verbal communication is both unavoidable and necessary when interacting with patients. Touch is a fundamental aspect of nursing, and can be used as a therapeutic tool, as well as a means to achieving physical care. It can provide comfort, express warmth and develop rapport with the patient.

Factors to consider in your practice:
• Sensitivity in the use of personal space when providing intimate care.
• Engaging in eye contact, and adopting a warm facial expression.
• Adopting a sensitive orientation in relation to the patient, for example, being face-to-face, or on a similar level, not above.
• Using body movements and gestures that are purposeful, but non-threatening.

Telephone communication

Telephone communication can occur at many points in the patient's care, but it is not always the most effective form of communication. Reactions to information cannot always be judged, as it is not possible to monitor body language or facial expression. Access to specialist advice over the phone can enable patients to feel supported, whilst living independently in their own homes. Significant news about diagnosis or test results should not be given by telephone. Families will frequently make enquiries by phone. This should be encouraged as a means of keeping in contact. It is useful to establish with the patient in advance if there is information that they do or do not wish to be transmitted to the family.

Telephone triage

This system enables patients to gain rapid access to expert advice. Nurses carrying out telephone triage need a range of skills, including clinical knowledge, assessment skills, communication skills, and effective decision making ability. Ideally, staff should be trained for this purpose, and have access to written guidelines or a protocol.

These are guidelines for good practice:
- Clearly state who you are and what your role is.
- Obtain the caller's name and contact number.
- Speak to the person who has the problem.
- Take a detailed history of the presenting problem.
- Give clear advice on the phone, either on what the person can do to deal with the problem at home, or whether they should go to hospital or contact their GP.
- Ensure that the person clearly understand their priorities and options, and what they should do next.
- Document details of the call, including any advice given and any follow up required, and liaise with relevant colleagues.
- Ask if there are any further concerns that need to be dealt with.

E-mail

This is an increasingly popular method for patients to keep in touch with cancer services; particularly if they lead busy work lives.

Imparting significant news (breaking bad news)

Imparting significant information, or breaking bad news, about diagnosis, treatment and prognosis, can be a problematic issue in cancer care, for a number of reasons.

Health professionals may:
- Lack confidence, experience, or training in communication skills.
- Feel personal discomfort dealing with sensitive issues.
- Wish to promote hope, but be unrealistically optimistic.

Most people want to be told the truth. If professionals are not clear, consistent, and open, or do not give sufficient information, there can be a loss of confidence and trust on the part of the patient and their family.

Role of the cancer nurse in giving significant news

At many points, the doctor will give the patient any significant news about cancer and its treatment. However, nurses, particularly specialist cancer nurses, will frequently give information that can have a significant impact on a patient's view of their future, or on their quality of life.

Nurses will often be asked to see a patient after they have been given some news by a doctor. The nurse will also have an important role in ensuring continuity of care between departments or services, and may need to clarify information. The following are guidelines for giving significant information or bad news:
- Ensure there is privacy, time, and space for the consultation.
- Make sure that the patient knows who you are, and what your role is in their care.
- Establish what the patient currently understands their circumstances to be (e.g. diagnosis, prognosis), and who they have discussed it with.
- Allow the patient to express their own narrative of events up to the present, in their own terms, as this will help to establish their context for understanding the new information.
- Inform them that there has been a new development, and give them an initial indication of the nature of the news.
- Note their reaction, and ask them what they now need to know.
- Give information in response to their expressed needs, respecting their preferences to the nature and amount of information they require.
- Allow the patient, and their family, to air their feelings, to express distress, fear, frustration, or anger at the circumstances they find themselves in, without entering into any blame or attribution of fault (unless there is clear evidence of negligence or poor practice).
- Consider what meaning this news has for this patient and their family at this time, and invite them to discuss the implications as they see them.
- Offer additional sources of information if these are available, for example, information leaflets.

- Ensure that the patient knows and understands the next step in their care or treatment, and who they will next have contact with.
- Liaise with all relevant colleagues on the outcome of the interaction, and document this.

It is important to remember that reactions to bad news are hard to predict. You should keep an open mind, and try to understand the impact of the news on the particular circumstances and priorities of this patient and their family.

Further reading

Kaye P (1996). *Breaking Bad News: A 10 Step Approach*. Northampton: EPL Publications.
National Institute for Clinical Excellence (2004). *Improving Supportive and Palliative Care for Adults with Cancer*. London: Department of Health. ▣ www.nice.org.uk/

Information and user involvement

Information

User involvement in cancer services operates at two levels:
- Providing information and involving patients and carers in decision-making about their own care.
- Involving patients and carers in decisions about the development and management of cancer services.

The amount and type of information that an individual patient wants will depend on a number of factors, including their age, gender, education, and personality. Their needs may also change at different stages of their illness. The priorities for most people are:
- Extent of the disease.
- Outcome of treatment and prognosis.
- Types of treatment available.
- Side effects of treatment.
- Effects of treatment on social life and activities.
- Personal autonomy and return to normal life.

Ways of providing information
Verbally
In cancer care, information is usually given verbally and face-to-face with the patient. This allows interaction between the patient, family, and the nurse. The patient can ask questions, gain clarification and support. It also allows the health professional to adapt information to the needs of the patient, to monitor their response, give explanations, and respond to questions.

In writing
There is a wide range of information now available in written form. Some of it is provided by charitable organizations, and is written in everyday language. Many cancer services have information centres where patients can access written information, or information on audiotape, video, CD or the Internet. Some cancer services provide written information on their own services.

The advantage of written information is that it can be taken away, studied at leisure, and shared with family and friends. It is important to match the nature or level of written information with the needs of the audience, although this can be more difficult than in verbal information.

Patient-held records
In some areas, patients are offered their own record of their illness and treatment. This offers the opportunity for written information to be accumulated, for professionals to make entries in the record, and for patients to record their own experiences in diary form.

Reflection points
- What sources of information do you offer your patients?
- How can you match the information to their needs?

Information technology

The Internet enables patients to access information on cancer from sources all over the world. This can include personal accounts of cancer, support groups, technical information on research and treatments and alternatives to conventional treatments.

Use of the Internet is limited to those who have access to the necessary technology, and this can exclude those with limited financial resources. However, many information centres in hospitals enable patients to have access. It is often hard to establish the status of information on the Internet, that is, how accurate or reliable it is, or whether it is a commercial site.

Chat rooms are another way that the Internet can be used. Both patients and carers can correspond with people in a similar position, and use them as a source of support.

Further reading

Mills M E, Sullivan K (1999). The importance of information giving for patients newly diagnosed with cancer: a review of the literature. *Journal of Clinical Nursing*, **8**, 631–42.

National Institute for Clinical Excellence (2004). Supportive and Palliative Care: Research Evidence. User Involvement in Planning, Delivering and Evaluating Services. In: *Improving Supportive and Palliative Care for Adults with Cancer*, pp 29–45, London: Department of Health.

Patient and family involvement in decision-making

The evidence suggests that most people want to take an active role in making decisions about their care and treatment. However, this varies from person to person. More people want to be fully informed than to be fully involved in the decision-making process itself.

It is the responsibility of all nurses working in cancer care to involve the patient and their family as fully as possible in the process of clinical decision-making.

Consent and competence

Consent is the most basic level of involvement in decision-making. To give informed consent, the patient needs sufficient information, to be free from coercion, and to be competent. Competence means that the patient must be able to understand the nature and purpose of the treatment, its risks and benefits, and be able to retain the information for long enough to make the decision (📖 Ethics in cancer care).

Choice and shared decision-making

Choices should always be offered where these are possible. It is also important to be clear when choices are limited. Decision-making should be viewed as a shared responsibility. For example, the patient and their family need to be involved in decisions about whether to proceed with adjuvant therapy. However, care needs to be taken to ensure that they do not feel decisions are being pushed onto them, creating an additional burden for the family. The extent to which a patient wants to be involved will be influenced by a number of personal factors. They may have other concerns that distract them, or they may have difficulty taking in the information offered.

Problems with information and decision-making

The following conditions impair decision-making:
- Anxiety.
- Pain.
- Nausea.
- Fatigue, malaise.
- Depression.
- Drowsiness—may be due to sedation.
- Family conflict.

Key issues

- Be clear what the treatment or care options are.
- Outline the implications of the options in terms of likely outcomes.
- Offer additional sources of information, e.g. support groups, websites.
- Advise on what to do when the patient is feeling tired or unwell, e.g. focus on current priorities.

Key questions
- What information do you need in order to make this decision?
- How would you like to be involved in the decision-making process?
- What sort of support do you need to help you make this decision?
- Who is the key person to contact for information/support?

Decisions can be particularly difficult when active or curative treatment is no longer an option. This can represent a difficult period of transition for the patient and family. At times of transition, it can be particularly important to 'have someone on the end of the phone', to talk things through and offer support. Specialist nurses are often well placed to provide this sort of support.

Further reading
Coulter A, Entwistle V, Gibert D (1999). Sharing decisions with patients: is the information good enough? *BMJ*, **318**, 318–22.

Ford S, Schofield T, Hope T (2003). Are patients decision-making preferences being met? *Health Expectations*, **6**, 72–80.

NHS centre for reviews and dissemination, University of York (2000). Informing, communicating and sharing decisions with people who have cancer. *Effective Health Care Bulletin* **6**(6).

Patient involvement in evaluating and managing health care

The Department of Health document, *Patient and Public Involvement in the New NHS*[1], identifies the benefits of user involvement as, '*promoting the individual's perspective, improving services, improving public understanding,* and *improving health*'.

What level of involvement?

Basic levels of involvement include providing information, seeking feedback on services, and consulting on developments to services. This can be done through questionnaires, surveys, meetings, or focus groups.

Participation or partnership involves service users as participants in the process of planning, managing, or evaluating services. This can be achieved through having service users as members of committees, or employing them as consultants to services.

User involvement: issues to consider

Meaningful involvement

In order for involvement to be meaningful, the role of the service user must be clear, with an agreed sharing of responsibilities between the service and the service user. Otherwise there is a danger of only token involvement.

Representativeness

Individuals best represent their own personal experience. Service user groups will be better able to represent a range of views. When involving a service user, consider how representative their voice will be.

Education and payment

User representatives may require preparation and payment for the role.

Minority or disadvantaged groups

Special efforts may be needed to involve groups such as ethnic minorities, who may not feel fully integrated into the systems that manage health care. Efforts should also be made to involve the physically ill, and socially and financially disadvantaged groups such as the homeless, who often feel disempowered.

Language

This should be inclusive, avoiding medical jargon and technical terms wherever possible.

Reflection points

- What level of involvement do service users have in your service?
- How could you improve user involvement?

Further reading

Tritter J, Daykin N, Evans S, Sanidas M (2004). *Improving Cancer Services through Patient Involvement*. Abingdon: Radcliffe Medical Press.

1 Department of Health (1999). *Patient and Public Involvement in the New NHS*. London: Department of Health.

Psychological, social, and spiritual support

Therapeutic relationships with people with cancer

There has been increasing research evidence suggesting that nurses use subtle and complex skills, both verbal and non-verbal, in their interactions with patients. Skilled nurse-patient interaction involves using opportunities to shift between focusing on a task and focusing on the relationship, integrating physical and psychological care. This has the capacity to help the patient feel secure and cared for, and part of a warm and inclusive therapeutic environment. Many nurses feel that an emphasis on therapeutic relationships with patients also brings them satisfaction with their role and underlines the intrinsic value of nursing work.

Closeness and intimacy

- Skilled nursing care can create a unique therapeutic relationship between nurses and patients, characterized by physical and emotional closeness and intimacy.
- This involves the skilled use of touch, humour, and metaphor, using physical proximity and a relaxed posture to enable a sense of closeness. The skilled nurse can make a potentially embarrassing situation comfortable. This should give the patient an enhanced sense of well-being.
- Closeness and intimacy can make the ward environment feel more familiar and *'domestic'*. The ward can feel like a 'home from home' for patients who return regularly for treatment[1].

Advocacy

Advocacy can be viewed as a moral or ethical dimension of nursing care. It involves the nurse representing the patient's interests, or providing care that respects their wishes or interests. It acts in different ways depending on the level of dependency and the participation of the patient. It can involve protecting, supporting, or educating the patient, or empowering the patient and promoting self-determination.

Reflection point

How do I know when to be protective towards a patient and represent their interests, and when to change the emphasis to empowering them to make their own decisions?

1 Savage J (1995). *Nursing Intimacy*. London: Scutari Press.

Emotional labour and stress

Nurses are expected to be warm and spontaneous with patients, whatever their own personal feelings. The act of caring in nursing is associated with the suppression of the nurse's personal feelings, to produce an outward appearance to the patient of being cared for.

The management of feelings within a professional caring role can be described as 'emotional labour'. This involves a form of professional 'acting'. 'Surface' acting requires the presentation of a suitable expression to fit the situation, e.g. warmth and concern. 'Deep' acting requires a modification of inner feelings and portraying these on the outside as facial expression, e.g. smiling whilst suppressing feelings of discomfort in the presence of pain or distress.

Although emotional labour is often recognized as a feature of nursing, it is not formally taught, and it is not always valued by health care employers. It may be seen as an extension of the traditional role of women in society, both undervalued and emotionally demanding. For some nurses, this emotional aspect of the role can seem limitless—where does the role end?

Managing stress

There is limited evidence of the effects of this suppression or modification of feelings on the nurse. However it is clear that working with patients who are distressed, in pain, or dying can be very stressful for nurses. In terms of occupational demand, three factors are significant in predicting the ability to cope: work demands, the degree of control over demand, and personal and professional support.

In addition to the emotional demands of the work, sources of stress can include:
- High turnover of staff, vacancies.
- Conflicts with colleagues.
- Poor management or leadership.
- Role ambiguity or role conflict.
- Lack of support.

Working environments that are supportive and where relational care is valued, are likely to be less stressful for nurses, and emotional labour more effective.

Burnout

In its most extreme form, the effect of work stress is called 'burnout'. Burnout is characterized by the following:
- Emotional exhaustion.
- Demoralization and personal isolation.
- Loss of job satisfaction.

Other signs of stress and burnout include:
- Poor sleep, poor concentration, chronic tiredness.
- Increased reliance on drugs, such as alcohol, cannabis, tobacco, coffee.
- Tension and irritability.
- Work problems spilling over into the home and social life.

How to cope with stress and prevent burnout
Develop support systems
- Work stresses should be dealt with at work—teams should develop systems for mutual support and dealing with stress. Examples include regular individual or group supervision (Psychological support), or discussion during handover periods. This helps to reduce any sense of personal isolation.
- Debriefing, a meeting of those involved in a difficult or distressing incident, preferably with a facilitator, provides an opportunity to air feelings, share support, and learn lessons for future practice.
- It is also important to take breaks during the working day.

Personal autonomy and control of workload
When work demands are high, having a sense of personal control over one's own workload aids coping. Individuals should be able to monitor their own workload, and regularly appraise this in consultation with their manager.

Role clarity
Role ambiguity, for example, having a role with no limits, is associated with burnout. Roles should be defined, with any overlap between roles clarified.

Manage the work/home boundary
Take care not to use friends as the primary means of coping with work. Develop interests and social contacts that are separate from work. Live a healthy lifestyle, with adequate exercise, and monitor the use of drugs, including alcohol and coffee.

Education and personal development
Having regular access to education that fits with an overall plan of personal development, keeps practice fresh and motivates the individual.

Reflection points

- Have I ever had problems coping with work?
- How did I deal with this at the time, and what helped most?

Further reading
Aldridge, M (1994). Unlimited liability? Emotional labour in nursing and social work. *Journal of Advanced Nursing*, **20**, 722–8.

Bottorff J and Varcoe C (1995). Transitions in nurse-patient interactions: a qualitative ethology, *Qualitative Health Research*, **5**, (3), 315–31.

Psychological support

The NICE *Guidance on the Supportive and Palliative Care of Adults with Cancer* identifies four levels of professional assessment and support[1]. This is a useful model for understanding the contribution of different professionals. There is the potential for overlap between levels, and individuals may function on different levels at different times (see Table 9.1).

Psychological support: level 1

All health professionals should be able to provide basic psychological support: listening and communicating effectively, developing supportive relationships with patients and carers, and responding to distress.

Psychological support: level 2

Professionals with additional training, experience, or supervision may provide more specific or skilled support. This can include dealing with adjustment difficulties and loss, offering supportive counselling, problem solving and supporting the patient's ability to cope.

Psychological support and psycho-oncology services: levels 3 and 4

Level 3 involves a working knowledge of specific counselling or psychotherapy models. This may be done by a CNS with additional training, or by psycho-oncology services.

Psycho-oncology is the term used to describe psychological services specializing in the care of people with cancer. It may be provided by individuals or teams. These teams will typically be comprised of some of the following: a psychiatrist, a clinical psychologist, a mental health nurse, or a social worker. Some of these may only work part-time within psycho-oncology.

Psycho-oncology services operate on levels 3 and 4 of the NICE model of psychological assessment and intervention, and typically provide:
- Psychological assessment and psychiatric diagnosis.
- Psychological treatments, typically counselling and cognitive behaviour therapy.
- Consultation and liaison—advising on the management of psychological problems in cancer services.
- Clinical supervision of cancer care staff.
- Education in psychological aspects of care.

1 National Institute for Clinical Excellence (2004). *Improving Supportive and Palliative Care for Adults with Cancer*. London: Department of Health.

Table 9.1 Levels of psychological support (adapted from NICE 2004)

Level	Group	Intervention
1	All health care professionals	Effective information giving, compassionate communication, and general psychological support
2	Professionals with additional expertise	Psychological techniques such as problem solving
3	Trained and accredited professionals	Counselling and specific interventions, e.g. anxiety management and solution-focused therapy, delivered according to an explicit theoretical framework
4	Mental health specialists	Specialist psychological and psychiatric interventions such as psychotherapy, including cognitive behavioural therapy

Counselling and psychotherapy in the cancer care setting

Counselling is frequently available within cancer services. Many services are provided by professional counsellors with training and supervision, practicing at NICE level 3. However, there can be considerable variation in the level of training or experience of individual counsellors. Nationally, within the UK, counselling is a largely unregulated activity.

Many nurses have undertaken some form of counselling training, but it can be very difficult to practice as a counsellor within a nursing role. There are a number of reasons for this:
- Counselling is characterized by clear boundaries—contact takes place at set times and places, without interruption. A nurse's contact with patients is usually more fluid than this; it is harder to keep to set times or to guarantee privacy.
- Nurses usually see their patients either in hospital wards, busy outpatient departments, or in the patient's home.

For these reasons, it is more common for nurses to use counselling skills such as active listening and attending, or to see counselling as an aspect of their role (for example, breast care nurses), than to work specfically as a counsellor.

Websites
The British Association for Counselling and Psychotherapy. www.bacp.co.uk/
Westminster Pastoral Foundation. www.wpf.org.uk/

Specific psychological interventions

Cognitive behaviour therapy
Cognitive behaviour therapy (CBT) or cognitive therapy, is useful in mood disorders like depression. It is based on the idea that people develop characteristic patterns of thinking and feeling about life (schemas). The therapist works collaboratively to help the patient develop more positive ways of dealing with the problems they encounter in life.

Problem solving
Problem solving is a specific cognitive behavioural technique that aims to help people clarify what their problems are and what potential solutions there may be.

Solution-focused therapy
Solution-focused therapy is a brief interactive therapy. It is similar to problem solving in its collaborative nature, but it focuses on solutions rather than problems.

Group therapy
This involves groups of patients, or carers, meeting regularly with a therapist. It is good for sharing feelings and reactions to cancer, generating support, and maintaining morale.

Psycho-educational interventions
These usually combine education about cancer and its effects, group support and help with coping strategies such as relaxation training and stress management.

Further reading
National Institute for Clinical Excellence (2004). Supportive and Palliative Care: Research Evidence, Psychological Support Services. In: *Improving Supportive & Palliative Care for Adults with Cancer*, pp.115–48. Department of Health: London

Roberts, D (2002). Mental Health Liaison in Cancer Care, In: Regel S, Roberts D (eds). *Mental Health Liaison. A Handbook for Nurses and Health Professionals*, pp.127–154. London: Bailliere Tindall.

Sanders, D, Wills, F (2005) *Cognitive Therapy. An Introduction*. London: SAGE Publications.

Social support

Social support is composed of the following elements:

Emotional support

This involves the expression of positive feelings, like concern and affection, resulting in feeling that one is cared for, loved, or esteemed. Mostly, patients will get this from their family and friends, but nurses can help by acknowledging the patient's feelings, and encouraging the open expression of feelings. Consideration should be given to people with no clear supportive network, bearing in mind their personal preferences. Questions about the patient's social support should be included as a part of assessment (📖 Assessment).

Informational support

Informational support is usually sought and valued from professionals, and may take the form of advice or guidance, in addition to information about illness and treatment, side effects etc. (📖 Information).

Instrumental support

This includes material or financial aid and services. Professionals frequently overlook these areas; they may simply attend to and prioritize the medical aspects of the patient's life when this type of support may be the highest priority for the patient and their family. It is therefore important to be sensitive to the full range of patients' concerns (📖 Employment and finances).

Social work support

Social workers are trained to provide support to the family as a system, and to see the patient's needs within the social and family context. They will often work as part of the specialist oncology or palliative care team; and to some extent their role will overlap with others, in that they provide general psychosocial support.

Specific aspects of the social work role include:
- Supporting families with particular social problems or with young children.
- Helping to prepare families for bereavement.
- Arranging packages of care or access to specialist social facilities.
- Advice on finances and benefit entitlements.

Priorities for referral to a social worker:
- Families or family members believed to be at risk.
- Individuals or families who lack social support, or have clear financial difficulties.

Financial entitlements

Patients' needs for financial assistance have become more significant, and many centres are now employing staff to advise and support patients with their financial entitlements. These include:

- *Attendance Allowance*—a non means-tested benefit for people over 65 with disabilities.
- *Disability Living Allowance*—a non means-tested benefit for people under 65 with disabilities.
- *Carer's Allowance*—a benefit for carers who spend over 35 hours a week caring for someone.
- *The Hospital Travel Costs Scheme*—a means-tested benefit for people attending hospital for NHS treatment.

See the Macmillan benefits webpage: www.macmillan.org.uk/abetterdeal/benefitsavailable.htm

Further reading

Krishnasamy M (1996). Social support and the patient with cancer: a consideration of the literature. *Journal of Advanced Nursing* **23**, 757–62.

National Institute for Clinical Excellence (2004). Supportive and Palliative Care: Research Evidence, Social Support Services. In: *Improving Supportive and Palliative Care for Adults with Cancer* pp.149–70. London: Department of Health.

Spiritual support and chaplaincy

Spirituality

The experience of spirituality includes personal faith and religious affiliation, a sense of inner strength, of hope or purpose in life, and a search for meaning at times of illness, loss, or when facing death.

Support for spirituality can be seen as an essential part of cancer nursing. It is also a specialist activity that is undertaken by trained professionals such as chaplains.

Spiritual aspects of care should be based on good communication, an ability to listen to the patient, and be with them at times of pain, distress and fear. This can be similar to other aspects of psychological and social support, but deals with a more intangible area of human experience. Suffering and spiritual pain are two terms often used to describe personal experiences of existential distress, of fear, despair, or hopelessness in the face of illness. These can include the person's whole being, and transcend the physical or material aspects of life.

A person who is suffering may need to re-examine their inner sources of strength, and their most fundamental beliefs about life. Supporting someone through this requires the nurse to be available, but not to impose any preconceptions, to affirm the patient's beliefs, but not to impose their own. To do this ideally requires an understanding of one's own beliefs and spirituality, a degree of self-awareness, and an ability to learn and grow in response to the experience of suffering in others.

Assessment should include questions that open up the subject of spirituality for the patient, allowing them space to discuss their concerns. Rather than being structured, spiritual assessment is best seen as part of an ongoing relationship, in response to the patient's perception of their needs (Assessment).

Religious faith and chaplaincy

Religious faith is an important part of how many people cope with illness, so access to specialist spiritual support is an important aspect of care. In doing this, it is important not to make assumptions about faith or religious practices. People with no regular religious affiliation may wish to have support from a chaplain, whilst members of a religion may not always want to practice it. Helping people to practice their faith can include helping them to make a place for religious symbols within a ward setting, e.g icons, books, or pictures. Some patients will have religious dietary requirements, or need uninterrupted time for prayer or meditation. Many hospitals and hospices have a chapel, or a multifaith room, which serves as a place of peace and contemplation for all.

Hospital and hospice chaplains usually represent the main Christian denominations, so it is important that contact details are maintained for members of other faiths as well. Many hospital chaplains will see their role as going beyond direct religious ministry, to providing support to both patients and staff, and they may also provide counselling.

Further reading

Marie Curie Cancer Care (2003). *Spiritual and Religious Care Competencies for Specialist Palliative Care*. London: Marie Curie Cancer Care.

National Institute for Clinical Excellence (2004). Supportive and Palliative Care: Research Evidence: Spiritual Support Services. In: *Improving Supportive & Palliative Care for Adults with Cancer* pp.171–92. London: Department of Health.

Wright MC (2001). Chaplaincy in hospice and hospital: findings from a survey in England and Wales, *Palliative Medicine*, **15**, 229–42.

Rehabilitation of the cancer patient

Rehabilitation of the cancer patient

Disability is a major but often under recognized problem for people with cancer. The illness itself and the treatments given can cause short-term problems such as restricted shoulder movements following mastectomy. It can also result in more prolonged disabilities such as paraplegia, from spinal cord compression.

Most cancer patients are likely to need rehabilitation at some point in their illness. For patients with advanced disease, the focus of rehabilitation will shift from improving function—usually in the early stages of the illness—to finding alternative ways to achieve satisfaction and fulfillment in daily activities. At the end of life, rehabilitation interventions must take account of rapidly changing needs, and be led by the priorities of patients and their families. At all times, rehabilitation aims to maximize the potential for health, and support adaptation to changes and limitations imposed by the illness and its treatment.

The importance of rehabilitation

Many cancer patients find the thought of progressive disability and future dependence on their carers worrying and distressing. Rehabilitation can engage patients and their families in an active process of achieving goals that are meaningful to them, so that decline does not have to be associated with helplessness and hopelessness.

The process and aims of rehabilitation

The process of rehabilitation includes:
- Assessment to identify the nature and extent of functional difficulties and factors that will contribute to their resolution.
- Working with the patient to set goals.
- Identifying and implementing strategies to achieve these goals.
- Constantly monitoring progress and adapting plans to incorporate changes.

Rehabilitation aims to:
- Maximize social participation—role, function and social status.
- Maximize well-being—physical and emotional.
- Achieve satisfaction—adaptation to disability.
- Minimize carer stress and distress.

Effective rehabilitation of the cancer patient is a team effort. It cannot be accomplished by any one professional working in isolation. Each discipline will have its own contribution; those of the occupational therapist and physiotherapist are outlined below.

Allied health professionals (AHPs)

Rehabilitation is a multiprofessional activity carried out by a range of AHPs, and other health and social care professionals. These will include, for example, occupational therapists, physiotherapists, speech and language therapists, therapy radiographers, and stoma therapists.

Occupational therapy

Occupational therapists address the impact of disability on the patient's everyday life[1].

This involves:
- Assessment and analysis of the person's activities—those which are necessary for basic daily living, and those which are creative and pleasurable.
- Making suggestions about alternative ways of managing, or providing resources—such as equipment or a wheelchair—that might make life easier.
- Anxiety and fatigue management—for example, teaching relaxation techniques (📖 Anxiety, 📖 Fatigue).

Physiotherapy

Physiotherapists use a range of treatment approaches to reduce the effect of symptoms such as pain, fatigue, dyspnoea, and neurological impairment on the patient's quality of life. These include:
- Non-pharmacological approaches to pain management such as TENS, electrotherapy, heat, and ice (📖 Pain management).
- Manual therapies such as massage, acupressure, manual lymphatic drainage (📖 Lymphoedema), and joint mobilizations (📖 Complementary therapies).
- Exercise and movement.
- Positioning and relaxation.

Referrals for rehabilitation

Any patient whose ability to carry out daily activities is compromised by their illness, should be referred to a suitable therapist for rehabilitation. Rehabilitation takes place in a variety of settings including hospitals, hospices, the community, and specialist rehabilitation units.

In any in-patient setting (with the exception of patients requiring terminal care) discharge planning is likely to supersede rehabilitation as the focus of care. Once the patient is at home, it is essential to consider their longer-term rehabilitation needs and to make the appropriate referrals.

Ongoing rehabilitation is usually provided by community-based primary care rehabilitation teams. Care for patients with specialist palliative care needs is given by the local palliative care provider.

Referral to a specialist rehabilitation unit may be considered for patients with a prognosis of three to six months or longer, who need to adapt to living with a long-term disability, and are motivated to engage in a structured rehabilitation programme. For example, a patient who is hemiplegic, and who has cognitive and perceptual problems as a result of a brain tumour, may benefit from the input of a physiotherapist to work on mobility, and an occupational therapist to develop strategies for managing daily tasks such as dressing and shopping.

1 College of Occupational Therapists (2004). *Occupational Therapy Intervention in Cancer: Guidance for Professionals, Managers and Decision-makers,* London: College of Occupational Therapists.

Nurses play an active part of the rehabilitation process, and can contribute by making the appropriate rehabilitation referrals when the need for specialist intervention is identified, and by working with AHPs to encourage and enable patients to maintain their independence and control in their daily activities. This can involve goal setting, and working collaboratively in the management of specific problems such as breathlessness. The 4-level model opposite (Table 10.1) shows how different members of the MDT can work together to enable the greatest patient benefit from rehabilitation (adapted from NICE[2]).

2 National Institute for Clinical Excellence (2004). *Improving Supportive and Palliative Care for Adults with Cancer*. The Manual. London: Department of Health.

Table 10.1 Recommended model of rehabilitation (adapted from NICE)

Level	Patient need (examples)	Professional group	Assessment/intervention
1	• Energy conservation techniques • Dietary advice • Advice on skin care	• Patients and carers • General nursing staff • Therapy radiographers • Support workers	• Recognition of needs for help based on assessment of function. • Basic interventions, including self-management and care strategies
2	Post-operative physiotherapy following breast surgery	General AHPs	• Routine assessment of rehabilitation needs. • Routine interventions including postoperative input + management of common side effects
3	Dietary advice for patients having enteral feeding regime	Experienced senior AHPs with basic level training in cancer rehabilitation.	• Specialist assessment. • Interventions requiring specialist knowledge of cancer treatment and aetiology, and impact of disease

4	• Management of patient with spinal cord compression
	 • Swallowing assessment for patient after radical head and neck surgery
	 • Management of severe or complicated lymphoedema
		Advanced practitioner AHPs working mainly with cancer + higher level training	• Highly specialized assessment from expert AHP.
			 • Highly specialist interventions for patients:
			   • Having radical surgery
			   • With advanced disease
			   • With severe functional impairment
			   • Undergoing combination therapies
			   • With complex end of life issues

Further reading

Doyle L, McClure J and Fisher S (2004). The contribution of physiotherapy to palliative medicine, In D Doyle, G Hanks, N Cherney and K Calman (eds) *The Oxford Textbook of Palliative Medicine* (3rd ed), pp.1050–56 Oxford: Oxford University Press.

National Council for Hospice and Specialist Palliative Care Services. (2000). *Fulfilling Lives. Rehabilitation in Palliative Care.* London: NCHSPCS.

Complementary therapies

Complementary therapies

Complementary therapies are gaining popularity with both the public and health professionals and as a result are finding a more substantial place in a number of areas of mainstream health care provision. One of these areas is that of cancer care. Patients are accessing a wide range of therapies including acupuncture, homeopathy, aromatherapy, reflexology, and massage. Complementary therapies are used in addition to, and complementing, conventional therapies for cancer or other illnesses. Increasingly, the term *integrated* or *integrative health* is used to describe an approach that combines elements of both.

In the UK a variety of models are in operation to provide complementary therapies. For example, in hospices volunteer therapists give treatments, in some hospital settings, nurses with specialized training integrate therapies within their nursing role. However, the most common way that people living with cancer access complementary therapies is via independent practitioners.

Commonly used therapies

The literature suggests that people living with cancer find the following therapies helpful (the list is not exhaustive):

Acupuncture

Acupuncture has been used quite extensively for control of chronic and treatment-related cancer pain. Use of the traditional point PC6 on the inside of the wrist, seems to be an effective anti-emetic technique in the early stages during chemotherapy. There is also some evidence to show that acupuncture can relieve dyspnoea. Patients taking tamoxifen have found acupuncture helpful in reducing hot flushes.

Aromatherapy

Aromatherapy is a therapy that systematically uses essential oils derived from plants in treatments to improve physical and emotional well-being. Most of the evidence suggests that essential oils applied via massage can be helpful in a number of ways including the reduction of anxiety, improved relaxation, and emotional symptoms. Quality of life enhancement has also been reported. Despite the lack of a clear evidence base for the effects of aromatherapy, it remains one of the most widely used therapies in cancer care.

Massage

Massage is a term for a number of techniques that include touching, kneading, and manipulation of the soft tissues for therapeutic purposes. The use of massage within cancer care is often integrated within nursing as skillful touch and a technique to enhance communication. It has been shown to be effective, although only short-term, in reducing anxiety and pain perception. Foot massage has been shown to have a positive effect on reducing pain and nausea and encouraging relaxation.

An important aspect of this therapy is the element of focussed touch. Patients have described relief from suffering, feeling good in spite of the cancer and its treatment, and feeling 'special' and empowered. The process of massage also contributed to the development of a positive relationship with the nurse. One study also suggests that massage combined with listening—being there for the patient—could help with aspects of adjustment to having a mastectomy.

Reflexology

This therapy is based on the principle that there are areas in the feet that correspond to all of the glands, organs, and parts of the body. The language of reflexology is not easily understood within orthodox health care and may be more readily accepted if it is viewed as a specific system of touch. Patients have reported benefits that include relief of pain and anxiety, and improved quality of life. As with massage the benefit of focussed touch by the practitioner is probably a significant part of the therapeutic process.

Homeopathy

This is the treatment of illness by using remedies prescribed according to the principle that 'like cures like'. The remedies are derived from plant, animal, and mineral sources, which, through a process of serial dilution and agitation, become extremely dilute. There is limited rigorous evidence of effectiveness, but patients show high satisfaction when homeopathy is included in their package of care. Some of the symptoms that have been helped are the dermatological adverse effects of radiotherapy, anxiety, and depression, positive effect on mood disturbance, and improvement in quality of life.

Herbal medicines

Herbal medicines are readily available over the counter but there are potential risks concerning the safety of remedies and the possibility of interactions with conventional drug regimens. Patients are encouraged to inform their health care practitioner about the herbal preparations they are taking.

Reiki

Central to this system of healing that originated in Japan, is the concept that an energy flow exists within living beings which supports life by helping to maintain homeostasis. This energy is known as Ki and when diminished ill health can arise. Alongside this is the concept that Ki can be channelled from its originating source by a reiki practitioner and passed on to a recipient. A treatment consists of the practitioner placing their hands either on or just above certain points on the patient's body. Despite the lack of scientific evidence on the effects of reiki there is anecdotal evidence to show that this therapy can assist in the care of patients with cancer and this is usually around improvement in quality of life.

Spiritual healing

This is the channeling of healing energies through the healer to the patient. Healers do not generally relate to the disease specific symptoms but aim to help the patient in more general terms such as increasing well-being. Despite a lack of evidence for its effectiveness, spiritual healing remains a popular therapy with people living with cancer.

Regulation and training

The House of Lords Select Committee on Science & Technology produced a report in 2000 that has provided a framework for the potential integration of complementary therapies into orthodox care. A range of areas was covered including research, regulation, training, and delivery models.

Lack of an evidence base is one of the biggest hurdles to integration, but successive surveys show that in spite of this, patients are increasingly vociferous about having access to complementary therapies.

Safety was seen as an important focus of the Select Committee report and this is a key factor in the development of appropriate regulatory systems that will protect the patient. Many therapies are working towards voluntary self-regulation and are supported by the Prince of Wales's Foundation for Integrated Health. This process includes a review of the quality of education and training.

The Prince of Wales's Foundation for Integrated Health has produced a booklet that is a valuable resource. *Complementary Health Care: a Guide for Patients* is designed to help people choose a suitable therapy and find a properly trained, qualified and registered practitioner and can be downloaded from www.fihealth.org.uk.

Nurses' role

The key role that nurses have in relation to complementary therapies is to provide support to people who are exploring ways of coping with the symptoms of cancer. Nurses need to be comfortable in discussing therapies and be able to direct patients to the best sources of information. There may also be a need to modify unrealistic expectations, that is, to be clear about the benefits and limitations of therapies.

The most popular websites on complementary therapies for cancer offer information of variable quality. Many websites endorse unproven therapies and some have the potential to be dangerous. Nurses have a valuable role in helping patients to make sense of the information.

When patients are admitted to hospital, find out if they are having any complementary therapies, in particular any supplements and/or herbal medicine they are taking. This is important from a safety perspective, and is helpful in understanding how the patient is coping.

Patients' reasons for using complementary therapies include seeking an alternative to conventional medicine, or they may wish to improve the quality of their lives. An advantage of complementary therapies is that they are generally perceived as treating the whole person. Making a positive decision to access a complementary therapy can facilitate empowerment and a sense of control and choice.

Accountability issues and complementary therapies

Where nurses provide a therapy within clinical practice they must be confident that the training they have undertaken is appropriate—that they are fit to practice. Until regulation issues are resolved it is difficult to determine the quality and standard of currently available training courses in areas such as aromatherapy and reflexology. Nurses need to be clear about what they want to achieve in delivering a therapy or part of a therapy and then make diligent inquiries. The RCN provides guidelines on choosing a course. (See 'Useful websites' below).

Nurses also have a duty to ensure that the patient gives informed consent before a therapy is given.

Significantly, studies suggest that the patient–practitioner relationship is an important component of the therapeutic process and that the use of complementary therapies serves a variety of functions beyond the explicit relief of symptoms. Many patients report that the process of receiving a complementary therapy from an independent practitioner makes them feel cared for. This implies that their contact with orthodox practitioners is less satisfactory.

Example of integrated care provision

The Breast Care Unit, Queen's Hospital, Burton-on-Trent, is an integrative breast care service with a team consisting of surgeons, radiologists, nurses, pathologists, a plastic surgeon, oncologists, a genetics specialist, a psychotherapist, an aromatherapist, a reflexologist, an acupuncturist, and a homeopath. The two consultant surgeons set up the unit in late 2003. The consultants, junior doctors, and nurses make referrals to the therapists. The complementary therapy policy in place for the hospital ensures practitioners are working to the standards set by the relevant complementary therapy regulatory bodies. Response to the service has been very positive from patients and staff. For further information contact Sally Hughes, homeopath at the clinic via sally@sallyhughes.org.uk.

Further reading

Tavares, M. (2003). *National Guidelines for the Integration of Complementary Therapies into Supportive and Palliative Care*. London: Prince of Wales's Foundation for Integrated Health. www.fihealth.org.uk

RCN (2004). *Complementary Therapies in Nursing, Midwifery and Health Visiting Practice: RCN Guidance on Integrating Complementary Therapies into Clinical Practice*. London: Royal College of Nursing. Pub code 002 204.

House of Lords Select Committee on Science & Technology. (2000). *Complementary and Alternative Medicine*. HL Paper 123. November. London: The Stationary Office.

NMC (2005). *Position Statement on Use of Complementary and Alternative Therapies*. London: Nursing and Midwifery Council.

Websites

The following organizations offer information on a variety of therapies

Bristol Cancer Centre: www.bristolcancerhelp.org/
Cancerbackup: www.cancerbackup.org.uk
Macmillan Cancer Support: www.macmillan.org.uk
Royal College of Nursing: http://www.rcn.org.uk/

Palliative care

Background

The practice of palliative care aims to enhance the quality of life of people experiencing life-threatening illnesses and their families. The principles on which palliative care is based suggest that it[1]:

- Affirms life and regards death as a natural process.
- Provides relief from pain and other distressing symptoms.
- Integrates the psychological and spiritual aspects of care.
- Offers support to enable people to live as actively as possible until their death.
- Offers a support system to enable families to cope during the illness and after the person's death.
- Applies early in the course of illness, in conjunction with other therapies that are intended to prolong life, such as chemotherapy or radiation therapy, and includes those investigations needed to manage distressing clinical complications.

Palliative care services utilize the skills and knowledge of a multiprofessional team to support people who are experiencing a life-threatening illnesses, and their family members. This care may start at the diagnosis of an illness and continue during treatment until death, and for the family, into the bereavement period. One of the key themes of palliative care is working in partnership with people and their family members, to enable their remaining life to be as fulfilling as possible. The philosophy of palliative care can be applied across a variety of illnesses, settings and contexts. Within practice settings, palliative care will be provided by

- Staff who provide palliative care as part of a more general role.
- Specialists who have particular expertise in the provision of palliative care.

General palliative care

General palliative care refers to a core set of skills and knowledge, based on a philosophy of care, which can be used by any health or social care professional. Given that people with life-threatening illnesses can be cared for in any health care setting, these skills and knowledge should be part of any health or social care professional's repertoire. Practitioners utilizing this approach might include staff working on oncology or surgical wards in the acute hospital setting, or community nurses for whom palliative care is a part of their work. General palliative care will include: holistic assessment and effective communication, basic symptom control, and psychological, social, spiritual, and practical support.

---

1 World Health Organization (2002). *Definition of Palliative Care*. www.who.int/cancer

Specialist palliative care

Specialist palliative care refers to services for patients and their families with moderate to complex needs provided by practitioners with specialist qualifications and experience, e.g. clinical nurse specialists in palliative care. Specialist palliative care services might include hospice inpatient care, community palliative care teams, acute hospitals teams, or teams with a particular focus, for example paediatric palliative care. This care may take place within the acute hospital, the community, nursing homes, or in a hospice setting. In the UK some specialist palliative care services will be NHS funded; others will be voluntary or charity funded and have independent status. However, most contribute to NHS work.

Specialist palliative care services may be provided on a consultation or advisory basis, or can involve the direct care of the patient and family. Most services also include in their remit people with any life-threatening illness with palliative care needs, for example, people with HIV, heart disease, or other chronic conditions, in addition to people with cancer. Not everyone with cancer will need specialist palliative care. Only those with complex palliative care needs will require the specialist services. Individuals with difficult to manage pain and symptom problems, complex family dynamics and spiritual or psychosocial distress may require referral to the specialist services.

Palliative care: terminology

The terms used to describe palliative care vary depending on the context within which they are used. For example, in some parts of the world, services describe themselves as a palliative care service but do not regard symptom management as part of their role. There is a lack of agreement about the use of terms internationally. In the UK services are recognized by the Strategic Health Authorities and Cancer Networks as providing specialist palliative care particularly in terms of practitioner's skills and knowledge.

There is also considerable overlap between the terms *supportive* and *palliative* care. However, the role of specialist palliative care is well established in the management of patients with advanced disease and end of life care, where there are complex psychosocial and symptom management issues, and in the care of the bereaved.

Interface between cancer and palliative care services

Current policy in the UK suggests the introduction of specialist palliative care services at any stage of the illness, from diagnosis to the end of life, where patients would benefit[1,2]. In the UK it is not uncommon for patients to have palliative care and cancer care in tandem, however in other parts of the world, notably in the USA, patients may have to make a choice about not seeking further treatments like chemotherapy.

Referral to palliative care services

A key part of the specialist palliative care role is to support the delivery of general palliative care to patients and families in their own settings (e.g. hospital or community). Requests for help with difficult clinical situations are common. Referrals can usually be made to specialist palliative care services by GPs, nurses, other professionals or sometimes by the patient themselves. Most services will have clear referral criteria. These will often ask colleagues to identify the reason for the referral and the area they need support in. This might, for example, be pain or symptom management, family support, or spiritual support.

The specialist palliative care team often includes a number of different professionals. Teams vary, but may include some or all of the following: nurses, doctors, social workers, psychologists, occupational therapists, physiotherapists, chaplains, art therapists, and music therapists.

Referrals to a specialist palliative care team will commonly result in a full assessment and advice will be given to the referring team. If ongoing contact is needed teams will often work in partnership to meet the needs of the patient and family.

1 Department of Health (2000). *The NHS Cancer Plan: A Plan for Investment, A Plan for Reform.* London: HMSO.
2 National Institute for Clinical Excellence (2004). *Improving Supportive and Palliative Care for Adults with Cancer.* London: Department of Health.

Caring for dying people

The end of life is a unique moment for each individual, which will stay in the memory of family members and carers who witness it. It is an opportunity to enhance the experience of dying and to promote dignity and comfort. It is an important time for those soon to be bereaved to prepare for death of a loved one, as the moment of death can contribute adversely to the bereavement experience.

The key aims of care at the end of life are:
• To enable the person to die as comfortably as possible.
• To manage pain and distressing symptoms.
• To enable the family to make the most of the time left, to minimize regrets.
• To meet the needs of both the dying person and their family, including emotional and spiritual needs, and make the memory of the death as positive as possible.

Recognizing the terminal phase

Recognizing the end of life helps practitioners to meet the patient's needs and prepares their family for the reality of death. However, there is commonly a reluctance to 'diagnose dying' or to state verbally that someone is dying.

The signs of approaching death are:
• Deterioration in condition.
• Gaunt appearance.
• Pallor.
• Cool or clammy skin.
• Diminished intake of fluid and food.
• Reduced fluid output.
• Profound weakness.
• Difficulty swallowing.
• Person becomes bed-bound.
• Changes in breathing pattern.
• Reduced consciousness.

If these signs appear suddenly in a person not expected to die, it is important to rule out other potentially reversible causes of deterioration, for example infection, hypercalcaemia, or haemorrhage.

Communication at the end of life

The focus of communication at the end of life, or during the dying phase, is on providing opportunities for, and demonstrating a willingness to talk about, issues related to death and dying. It is also an opportunity to clarify what the patient's key concerns are. For example, this may be concern about their family and what will happen after their death, it may be concerns about physical symptoms and the actual process of dying or it may be concerns around unfinished business related to relationships.

It is important to ask for the person's views on any care or treatments during the dying phase that would take place after they are no longer able to take decisions themselves (📖 Ethical issues in cancer care). Anxiety and fear associated with the process of dying is common. Voicing these anxieties and fears and breaking them down into specific issues may be helpful. Specific issues to consider are:

- Identifying where the person wishes to be cared for.
- Involving the person in decision-making for as long as possible.
- Assisting the dying person to put their affairs in order, involving other members of the team who have specific expertise.
- Considering spiritual needs (📖 Spiritual support).
- Letting the dying person know that their family will be supported in bereavement, and what support is available.
- Answering any questions honestly. Be prepared to repeat any explanations.
- Providing privacy and opportunity for families to be together and make the most of the final days or hours.

Caring for families at the time of death

A common concern of families when a family member is dying is meeting their needs for comfort. In particular, in ensuring that everything possible has been done to manage pain and distressing symptoms. If there have been problems and unmet needs around the time of the death this may make the subsequent bereavement more difficult. It is therefore important to try to meet the needs of both the person who is dying and their family.

Inevitably there comes a time at the end of life when the focus of care shifts from the patient to the family's needs. As the dying person deteriorates, the family's and practitioner's, role in advocating on behalf of the person becomes greater. Families will have their own needs for information and support and may need to be informed that death is close. Some family members may wish to be actively involved in the physical care of the dying persons, whilst others may find this very difficult. Support should be given to the decisions made by family members, in an inclusive and non-judgemental way.

Care pathways

Many services use care pathways as a way of addressing the variation in the standard of care at the end of life. These are multiprofessional tools that provide a focus for integrated care. The Liverpool Integrated Care Pathway for the Dying Patient has become well established as a template for the delivery of care. There is some controversy over whether this allows for tailored, individualized care, or is overly prescriptive. It can enable teams to audit their practice, identify measurable outcomes, and it can also be a focus for education.

Further reading

Ellershaw J E, Wilkinson S (eds) (2003). *Care of the Dying: a Pathway to Excellence*. Oxford: Oxford University Press.

Bereavement

Bereavement is the experience of loss, particularly of someone close. Grief is the associated emotional reaction. Bereavement and the grief response are a feature of the cancer experience at many different stages of the journey. There are numerous losses, associated with treatment (e.g. mastectomy), the effects of the illness (e.g. altered body image), and the overall effects on the patient's life (e.g. loss of function, social activity, occupation). Within the context of palliative care, bereavement is frequently encountered in the families of patients in the period prior to and after death. Although the nurse's immediate responsibility may end with the patient's death, it is important to anticipate the family's needs, be aware of potential problems, and identify services that can help, where these are available.

Features of grief

Grief can be associated with the following features:
- Feelings of shock, disbelief, numbness, and derealization (feelings of unreality).
- Being preoccupied with the deceased, or feeling they are seeing them or hearing their voice.
- Being sad and tearful.
- Disturbed sleep and appetite.
- Feelings of anger or guilt.
- Physical feelings of anxiety, emptiness, tiredness, breathlessness, sighing.
- Social withdrawal, restlessness.

The nature and scale of these features varies from person to person, and duration varies considerably.

Websites

🖳 Cruse Bereavement Care: www.crusebereavementcare.org.uk/
🖳 The Child Bereavement Trust: www.childbereavement.org.uk/
🖳 Winston's Wish: www.winstonswish.org.uk/

Models of bereavement

Bereavement is a very complex phenomenon with physical, psychological, social, cultural, and spiritual elements. There are a number of models of bereavement that help us to understand the grief experience and how it can be helped. No one model has pre-eminence, these should be judged for their usefulness in practice:

Stress and coping

One way of understanding bereavement is that is a form of stress or trauma and the grief reaction is an attempt to cope with it (📖 Adjustment, stress reactions, and disorders)

Psychosocial transition

Parkes[1] suggests that bereavement is a period of adjustment to a new reality that has long-term consequences for the assumptions the person has about their world (📖 Stress and coping).

Continuity

This emphasizes the nature of the continuing bonds that link the bereaved with the person who has died. The period of bereavement involves a reinterpretation of the relationship, and its implications for the life of the bereaved[2].

Dual process

Stroebe and Schut[3] conceptualise the bereavement processes oscilating between loss-oriented activity (acknowledging the nature and meaning of the loss) and restoration-oriented activity (rebuilding life and moving on).

Anticipatory grief

If death is anticipated, this gives the family some time to prepare emotionally for the death. There is evidence that some family members go through features of bereavement prior to the death, and that this may help with the later bereavement process. Nurses can work with the family to prepare for the process of dying, and support emotional adjustment. This involves communicating effectively about dying, helping the family to make decisions.

Complicated grief reactions

Complicated or abnormal grief reactions are characterized by greater intensity or duration of the features of grief. This can also include reactions that do not appear to acknowledge the bereavement, or are delayed. Some people will become clinically depressed. They may be associated with long-term difficulties of adjustment, and may require intervention from specialist psychological or bereavement services.

1 Parkes, CM (1996). *Bereavement*, 3rd edn. London: Routledge.
2 Klass D, Silverman P, Nickman S (eds) (1996). *Continuing Bonds*. London: Taylor & Francis.
3 Stroebe M, Schut, H (1999). The dual process model of coping with bereavement. *Death Studies*, **23**, 197–224.

Support for the bereaved

Support for a bereaved person requires a sensitive, facilitative approach, indicating availability to listen, talk about the deceased, encouraging the expression of feelings, and supporting a healthy lifestyle:

• Maintaining outside interests.
• Avoiding reliance on drugs, e.g. alcohol.
• Acknowledging the loss and its implications for every aspect of life.
• Providing information on the nature of bereavement, what to expect and where to get specialist help.

It is important to let the bereaved person know that everyone grieves in their own way and in their own time. There are a number of local and national support groups for the bereaved, e.g. Cruse (see website below), which can be accessed directly by individuals.

Specialist bereavement services are frequently available in hospices. There should be clear criteria for referral to these services, some of which may be accessible to families who have not had direct contact with the hospice. Many hospices also offer commemorative services and events that provide support and put bereaved people in touch with others in a similar position. Some bereaved people find ongoing links with services (including volunteer work) very comforting. However, caution should be taken engaging with the bereaved on an ongoing basis, as they must balance their need for support with their need to move on.

Children

Children will have particular needs after the death of a loved one. This will depend on their age, any previous experience of losses, and the ongoing relationships within the family. As with adults, children will benefit from being given time and space to adjust to changes, and may also need answers to questions that the bereavement raise for their understanding of the world. (See websites The Child Bereavement Trust and Winston's Wish below).

Further reading

Komaromy, C (2004). Nursing care at the time of death. In Payne S, Seymour J, Ingleton C (eds) *Palliative Care Nursing: Principles and Evidence for Practice*, pp.462–71. Buckingham: Open University Press.

Stroebe, MS, Stroebe, W, Hansson, RO (1993). *Handbook of Bereavement. Theory, Research and Intervention*. Cambridge: Cambridge University Press.

Websites

▣ Cruse: www.crusebereavementcare.org.uk
▣ The Child Bereavement Trust: www.childbereavement.org.uk
▣ Winston's Wish: www.winstonswish.org.uk

Ethics in cancer care

Introduction and overview of ethical guidance

Ethical and moral values affect all aspects of cancer care, including treatment, management of symptoms, end of life care and participation in research. With advancing medical technology and developing evidence-based practice, ethical issues in cancer care are increasingly complex.

Much of what has been written underpinning ethics is guided by a principle-based approach incorporating the 'Four Principles'[1].

Four principles of biomedical ethics

- **Autonomy**—*self-determination, the capacity to think, decide and act on the basis of such thought, freely and independently.* A person has the right to have control over his/her life, including decisions about how it should end. It is therefore acknowledged that persons should be able to refuse life saving or prolonging treatment.
- **Beneficence**—*to do good; the principle refers to the moral obligation to act for the benefit of others.* In treatment decisions at the end of life this principle revolves around what will be in a person's best interests and being able to balance the benefit and harm of continuing treatment. A person's perception of their quality of life is important here in determining best interest.
- **Non-maleficence**—*not to harm; the principle asserts an obligation not to intentionally inflict harm.* The harmful effects of a treatment may outweigh the benefits and debate may arise as to the benefit or futility of treatment.
- **Justice**—*to be fair, equitable and provide appropriate treatment in light of what is due or owed to persons.* The distribution of resources is central to this debate.

It can be difficult to apply this approach within the complexity of everyday practice. For example, conflict can arise between two or more of these principles. Does the benefit of a treatment (beneficence) outweigh the risks (non-maleficence) or threats to the patient's autonomy? It is not enough, therefore, to rely solely on a principled-based approach. It is equally important to take into account the personal and social context of caring for patients and families, which will enhance our understanding of a person's experience of illness. This involves:

- Open communication enabling the development of a therapeutic relationship and expression of individual wishes and values.
- Teamwork that incorporates the patient, family and professional relationship.
- Attention to the patient and family experience of illness and their feelings about this.

---

1 Beauchamp T and Childress J (1994). *Principles of Biomedical Ethics*, 4th Edition. Oxford: Oxford University Press.

Guidance for decision-making: questions to consider (adapted from Edwards and Mauthner[2])

- Who is involved and affected by the ethical dilemma?
- What is the context—the situation and available knowledge?
- What are the social and personal elements?
- What are the needs of those involved?
- What is your role within the decision-making process?
- What is the balance of personal and social power of those involved?
- How will those involved understand our actions? Are these in balance with our own judgements?
- How can we best communicate the ethical dilemma to those involved?

These contextual elements stress the importance of individual values and skills (virtue ethics), with an emphasis on care and relationships (feminist ethics), and provide additional considerations when dealing with ethical dilemmas. This emphasizes active participation in decision-making for patients and their families, and involvement with their own care (📖 Patient and family involvement in decision-making).

What to do in situations of conflict or uncertainty?

Initially, any ethical dilemmas should be discussed within the multidisciplinary team, ensuring that senior members of the clinical and managerial staff, who carry responsibility, are actively involved. It is important to keep communications within the team open. Further advice may be sought from colleagues with particular expertise (for example, in some areas medical ethicists are available for consultation). If the situation is ongoing, or represents a recurring ethical dilemma, it may be possible to consult the local clinical governance department or ethics committee.

Further reading

Gillon R (2003). Ethics needs principles—four can encompass the rest—and respect for autonomy should be 'first among equals'. *Journal of Medical Ethics*. Oct. 29, 307–12.

Harris J (2003). In Praise of unprincipled ethics. *Journal of Medical Ethics*. Oct. 29, 303–6.

2 Edwards R and Mauthner M (2002). Ethics and Feminist Research: Theory and Practice. In Mauthner M, Birch M, Jessop J, and Miller T (eds). *Ethics in Qualitative Research*. London: SAGE Publications.

End of life issues

Ethical issues are prominent in end of life care. Patients and families face significant challenges about the meaning of life and death. There are difficult decisions to be made about how best to provide care at the end of life. This requires a sensitive, holistic, and comprehensive approach that involves the patient, family, and health professional.

Advance directives (living wills)

An advance directive (advance decision, statement, or living will) is a written or verbal statement made by a competent individual, which states their intention to accept or refuse care. It enables the expression of choice in the management of their illness, if in the future they lack the ability to decide for themselves.

An advance directive is a way of prolonging autonomy and enables patients to request care that they feel is in their best interests. This enables open discussion and forward planning. Advance directives can be very general, providing an overview of a person's values and preferences, or they can be more specific, expressing preferences for particular treatments or care.

The legal status of advance directives varies in different countries. In England and Wales, advance directives are currently recognized by common law as legally binding and should be respected by health professionals. From April 2007 The Mental Capacity Act (2005) will be implemented and become their legal basis.

In order for advance directives to be valid the patient must be:
• Mentally competent and free from mental distress at the time
  the advance directive was made.
• Acting free from pressure.
• Have been offered sufficient, appropriate information about treatment
  options and their implications.

The patient must also have some idea of the type of situation for which the advance directive is being written. At the time of reading, the advance directive should be clearly applicable to the patient's present circumstances and there should be no reason to believe the patient has changed his/her mind. An advance directive cannot authorize a doctor to do anything that is illegal or provide treatment that in their professional view is clinically inappropriate.

Problems with advance directives can include:
• Treatment decisions are complex and it is not always possible to
  foresee all the options.
• The possibility that patients may change their minds because of a
  change in circumstances.

Therefore an advance directive may help in decision-making but must not be a substitute for effective communication.

Reflection point

Consider for yourself what you might write in an advance directive for your own end of life care.

Euthanasia

The term euthanasia has a Greek root, meaning a *good* or *easy death*. Contemporary understanding describes euthanasia as the *deliberate ending of life*. Several different types of euthanasia are recognized.

Definitions
- **Euthanasia:** a deliberate act or omission that shortens the life, or hastens the death, of a person.
- **Active euthanasia:** the purposeful shortening of life through active or direct assistance e.g. administering a lethal injection.
- **Passive euthanasia:** the purposeful omission (withdrawing or withholding) of life-sustaining measures e.g. withdrawing or withholding artificial nutrition and hydration.
- **Voluntary euthanasia:** freely given consent of the individual to his/her death.
- **Involuntary euthanasia:** purposeful shortening of life without the individual's consent.
- **Nonvoluntary euthanasia:** when a life is taken when it is impossible to ask for an individual's consent e.g. incompetent or unconscious persons.

Currently within the UK, active euthanasia is illegal, even if it is voluntary. However there is ongoing debate, which may lead to a change in the law (◻ Physician assisted suicide below).

Factors supporting the use of euthanasia
- Symptom burden.
- Pain and suffering.
- Worries and anxieties about the future.
- Lack of hope.
- Fear of poor quality of life and loss of control (a life 'not worth living').
- Fear of being a burden on others.
- Fear of death.
- The right to dignity.
- The right to choose (the right to die).

Arguments against euthanasia
- Everyone has the right to access and receive expert palliative care.
- Faith/religious objections to shortening life.

Although it may be difficult to deal with all of these issues in practice, it is important to offer patients and their families the opportunity to talk through their fears and concerns about care at the end of life within a supportive and caring relationship.

Other concepts that influence the euthanasia debate
The slippery slope

The main emphasis of the slippery slope argument is that if we agree to requests of death from patients, we find ourselves sliding down a slope that leads to unnecessary and unwanted killing. Euthanasia might be extended beyond those who are capable of requesting it.

Sanctity of life

This is the belief that there is an intrinsic value of being alive. Some people believe that life should be sustained at all costs no matter what the quality and therefore, prolonging life always provides a benefit despite any other factors. Sanctity of life may also be understood not in terms that life is an absolute good, but that life may never be intentionally taken.

Doctrine of double effect

This principle determines an action to have both good and bad consequences, but that you act with the intention to provide a good result even if you foresee a harmful effect. Providing pain relief that in large doses may shorten a person's life is an example of the doctrine of double effect in practice. However it is important to recognize the evidence that suggests the therapeutic levels of morphine for achieving pain relief, are not the same as those that would result in respiratory failure for a patient.

Reflection points

- Should patients be kept alive as long as technology allows?
- Is it ethical to keep someone alive just because we can, and is it morally acceptable to let someone die?

Physician assisted suicide

Physician assisted suicide is the result of a deliberate medical act or omission taken by a doctor that shortens the life (hastens death) of a patient. Current debate in the UK is driven by the Assisted Dying Bill (Lord Joffe 2005), which advocates the rights of the individual who is suffering unbearably as a result of a life-threatening illness, to seek medical assistance to die at their own considered and persistent request.

The arguments and questions arising against legalising physician assisted suicide are;

- Where would we draw the line?
- The fear of the elderly, disabled, mentally ill—that they are a burden to society and their lives less worthy.
- The fear of being a burden to carers.
- Difficulty in trusting doctors and nurses.
- Effects on bereaved families and friends.

Reflection point

Can you consider situations you have encountered in your practice that raised ethical questions for you about assisted suicide?

Further reading

Finlay IG, Wheatley VJ and Izdebski C (2005). The House of Lords Select Committee on Assisted Dying for the Terminally Ill Bill: implications for specialist palliative care. *Palliative Medicine*, **19**, 444–53.

Hendrick J (2004). Death, dying and the incurably ill patient. In *Law and Ethics* pp.239–263. Nelson Thornes Ltd: Cheltenham.

Johansen S, Chr. Holen J, Kassa S, Havard Loge J and Materstvedt LJ (2005). Attitudes towards, and wishes for, euthanasia in advanced cancer patients at a palliative medicine unit. *Palliative Medicine*, **19**, 454–60.

National Council Hospice and Specialist Palliative Care and The ethics Committee of the Association of Palliative Medicine (1997). *A Joint Working Party: Ethical Decision Making in Palliative Care: Cardiopulmonary Resuscitation for people who are terminally ill.* London: NCHSPC.

⌨ www.ageconcern.org.uk Advanced statements, Advance directives and Living Wills (October 2005).

Withdrawing and withholding treatment

At the end of life, decisions have to be made about whether to start, continue, stop, or withhold treatment. Such decisions are complex and can be the most difficult for patients, their families, and health professionals to make. The reasons for withdrawing or withholding treatment may be either to respect the wishes of the patient and family, or that further treatment has no potential benefit.

To propose the withdrawal and withholding of treatment can however be very emotive and challenging for all involved. Should treatment be prolonged indefinitely when it has ceased to provide any benefit for the patient? Should treatment commence if it is deemed to be futile?

There is the potential for conflict and misunderstanding where terminology is unclear. The following are commonly accepted definitions:
- In English law there is no distinction between withdrawing and withholding treatment. Both can be viewed in law as an omission of care.
- Life-prolonging treatment refers to all treatment which has the potential to postpone the patient's death, including cardiopulmonary resuscitation, artificial ventilation, artificial nutrition, and hydration.
- Treatment should not be withheld or withdrawn if there is a possibility that it will provide some benefit, unless this is requested by the patient.
- Basic care means the procedures essential to keep a patient comfortable, and can include warmth, shelter, pain relief, management of distressing symptoms, hygiene care, and the offer of oral nutrition and hydration.
- Whilst treatment may be withheld or withdrawn, basic care should always be provided unless the patient makes a competent decision to refuse it.

Artificial nutrition and hydration

Artificial nutrition and hydration refers to techniques such as nasogastric tubes, gastrostomy, subcutaneous hydration, and intravenous cannula to provide a patient with nutrition and hydration when they have difficulty taking food and fluids orally. Artificial nutrition and hydration is regarded and classified by the British Medical Association as medical treatment and not basic care, and the withdrawal or withholding of either is therefore legally acceptable if seen to be in the patient's best interests.

Discussion surrounding artificial nutrition and hydration may be difficult and contentious, with differing opinions as to the appropriate management of terminally ill patients who are unable to eat and drink. For some families, not taking nutrition and hydration may be seen as part of the natural dying process. For others, providing nutrition and hydration may be seen as a basic human need and right, and should be provided even at the end of life. Another potential problem is if attempts to provide artificial nutrition and hydration appear to cause distress and suffering rather than relief.

For this reason, decisions about providing appropriate artificial nutrition and hydration must involve the patient, family, and health care team and include an appropriate and balanced assessment to determine the patient's condition, their requirements, needs and views.

Reflection point

Can you think of ways of enabling patients and families to discuss their wishes for withdrawal or withholding of artificial nutrition and hydration?

Cardiopulmonary resuscitation

Cardiopulmonary resuscitation (CPR) can be attempted on any person whose cardiac or respiratory functions cease. A few patients will make a full recovery, some recover but have a number of health problems and in many cases it is unsuccessful. For patients in poor health and those with serious conditions it is known to have a low success rate.

Discussions regarding CPR raise sensitive and difficult issues for the patient and those close to them. Ideally resuscitation should be discussed with patients in advance. The nature of cardiopulmonary resuscitation and its consequences for the patient should be fully explored, within the context of end of life care. In making advance decisions about whether or not to attempt CPR, the values, wishes, and illness experience of the patient must be taken into account.

The views of the medical and nursing team immediately involved in the patient's care and those of the patient's family are valuable in forming a decision. It is also important to assess the clinical situation and be guided by local policy:

- Is CPR likely to restart the patient's heart and breathing?
- Would restarting the patients heart and breathing provide any benefit (taking into account the patients views)?
- Do the expected benefits outweigh the potential burdens and risks of the resuscitation process?

Decisions should be based on the best evidence available and agreed within the team. The decision-making process should be shared and all details of the discussion documented.

Reflection points

- Consider what you think patients understand by cardiopulmonary resuscitation.
- What level of involvement do patients have in order to express their views on cardiopulmonary resuscitation in your practice area?

Further reading

British Medical Association (1999) *Withholding and Withdrawing Life-prolonging Medical Treatment. Guidance for Decision Making*. London: British Medical Journal Books.

British Medical Association (2001). *Decisions Relating to Cardiopulmonary Resuscitation*. Model Information Leaflet. London: BMA.

British Medical Association, The Resuscitation Council and Royal College of Nursing (2001). *A Joint Statement: Decisions Relating to Cardiopulmonary Resuscitation*. London: BMA/RCN.

Section 5

Clinical management of cancer

Diagnosis and staging

Diagnosis, classification, and staging of cancer

Early diagnosis still offers the best opportunity for cure or extended survival for many types of cancer. Therefore, fast and accurate diagnosis is essential to ensure the most effective and appropriate approach to managing cancer.

Cancer classification

Classifying cancers into specific histology (grade) and extent of spread (stage), allows for prognostic information and planning of appropriate treatment, as well as comparison of treatment results, e.g. survival, cure, and quality of life, within countries and worldwide (☐ Cancer Biology for classification of main tissue types).

Cancer diagnosis

The chosen approach depends on the presenting signs and symptoms, clinical performance status (see box opposite), the anticipated goal of treatment, availability of equipment and the patient's and their family's own expectations and wishes. It is essential to consider how an individual will cope with going through a whole host of invasive tests and also whether or not it would be worthwhile.

There are no single tests specific and sensitive enough to determine the exact diagnosis of an individual cancer. Therefore a range of tests, both invasive and non-invasive, need to be carried out before an individual patient can have an accurate diagnosis.

Advances in diagnosis

Improved CT and MRI scanning, the introduction of PET scans, and use of ultrasound guided biopsies have all led to more accurate diagnosis and staging of many cancers. This has led to more effective targeting of treatments, for example reducing futile surgery in both lung and rectal cancer. In the future, more accurate diagnosis of cancer at a cellular and genetic level will improve staging and treatment planning further. For example, the expression of specific gene products will be used to predict responses to treatment, and biological markers will elucidate whether a drug is working on the target.

Areas that need explored during the diagnosis process are covered on the following pages under the headings.
- Patient history.
- Presenting signs and symptoms.
- Laboratory studies.
- Surgical/specialist viewing.
- Radiological imaging.
- Staging and grading.

Performance status (PS) is an attempt to quantify cancer patients' general well-being. This measure is often used to determine whether they can receive chemotherapy, whether dose adjustment is necessary, and as a measure for the required intensity of palliative care. Clinical trials often include performance status as one of the criteria patients must meet for joining.

The main scales are WHO/ECOG scales, summarized below. Performance status is referred to in this book mainly in Management of major cancers (Section 6) and occasionally in Supportive and palliative care (Section 4) and Symptom management (Section 7). Other scores such as the Karnofsky score, after Dr David Karnofsky, are also in use. This runs from 100% 'perfect' health to 0% death, in intervals of 10%.

Grade	ECOG/WHO performance status scores
0	Fully active, able to carry on all pre-disease performance without restriction
1	Restricted in physically strenuous activity but ambulatory and able to carry out work of a light or sedentary nature, e.g., light house work, office work
2	Ambulatory and capable of all self-care but unable to carry out any work activities. Up and about more than 50% of waking hours
3	Capable of only limited self-care, confined to bed or chair more than 50% of waking hours
4	Completely disabled. Cannot carry on any self-care. Totally confined to bed or chair
5	Dead

Diagnosis: multidisciplinary evaluation

Many members of the health care team will be involved. Diagnosis can be a point for potential delays, which can impact on overall survival and cause high levels of anxiety. Effective coordination of the MDT is essential to ensure an efficient and well-supported patient journey through this difficult time. Patient pathways have been designed for many cancers to reduce diagnostic and treatment delay.

Nurses are heavily involved in this process. Nurses will support the patient with information and symptom management. Clinical Nurse Specialists may coordinate the MDT and evaluate the patient pathway. Some specialist nurses may also be involved in actual diagnostic tests such as digital rectal examination, and cystoscopy or in telling patients their actual diagnosis (□ Patient experience).

Further reading

Gupte C, Padhani A R (2004). New imaging techniques in cancer management. *British Journal of Cancer Management,* **1**, 4–7.

Omerod K F (2005). Diagnostic evaluation, Classification and Staging. In Yarbro C H, Frogge M H, Goodman M (eds). *Cancer Nursing, Principles and practice,* 6th edn, pp. 153–80. Massachusetts: Jones and Bartlett.

Souhami R L and Tobias J S (eds) (2005). Staging of tumours. In *Cancer and Its Management.* 5th edn, pp.42–56. Oxford: Blackwell.

National Cancer Institute. Cancer Imaging Programme imaging.cancer.gov/imaginginformation/cancerimaging/page

Patient assessment

Patient history

Past medical history, family history, risk factors, and physical examination are all an essential part of diagnosis. A thorough history needs to be taken, including the duration and speed of progression, and general and specific symptoms. Cancer can take years to progress so signs/symptoms may have been there for many years.

The patient's own expectations, beliefs, physical, social, spiritual, and emotional needs all need to be assessed and discussed. This may take time and should be a part of an ongoing assessment process (Assessment).

Presenting signs and symptoms

Screening has increased the number of non-palpable lumps seen at diagnosis. However, more typically, other signs and symptoms of disease take the individual into the health care system. Common presenting symptoms are shown in Table 14.1.

Knowledge of the common presenting signs/symptoms of each cancer, gives health care professionals a benchmark to screen patients against. In the UK, the Department of Health has produced referral guidelines for all cancers. These highlight patient signs and symptoms that should be referred urgently to cancer specialists.[1]

Laboratory studies

These include tests such as full blood count, liver and renal function tests, blood chemistries, urinalysis, faecal occult bloods, and specific tumour markers (see below).

Tumour markers

These are hormones, enzymes, or antigens produced by tumours or by tissue stimulated by tumours. They vary in sensitivity and specificity. Many tumour markers are highly sensitive, i.e. they are generally identifiable if tumour is there. However, they are often not very specific, i.e. they are often present when the disease is absent, but other non-malignant causes account for the marker's presence. This reduces their use as a diagnostic test. However, some can be useful in assessing response to treatment (see Table 14.2).

Surgical evaluation

This is where the cancer is looked at macroscopically and a biopsy may also be taken. Obtaining an accurate tissue sample is essential in establishing cancer diagnosis. Different cancers in the same organ may require very different treatment approaches, e.g. small cell and non-small cell lung cancer.

Other tests that are also carried out include paracentesis, or lumbar puncture (see Table 14.3).

NICE (2005). *Referral guidelines for suspected cancer*. London: NICE www.nice.org.uk/page. ?0=cg027niceguideline

Table 14.1 Common presenting symptoms

- Weight loss
- Persistent pain
- Unexplained fever
- Unusual bleeding or discharge
- A sore which does not heal
- Change in bladder and bowel habits

- Fatigue
- Painless lump
- Obvious change in wart or mole persistent cough/hoarseness
- Indigestion/difficulty in swallowing

Table 14.2 Some commonly used tumour markers

Marker	Indications	Uses
CEA (carcinoe mbryonic antigen)	Breast, colorectal, lung	Monitoring patients with known disease
PSA (prostate specific antigen)	Prostate cancer, benign prostate enlargement	Initial screening, response to treatment, recurrence
HCG (human chorionic gonadotrophin	Germ cell tumours (testicular, some ovarian), pregnancy	Diagnosis, prognostic indicators
AFP (alpha-fetoprotein)	Germ cell tumours, liver, cancer, pregnancy	Diagnosis, monitoring, response to treatment
CA-125	Ovarian, colorectal, gastric cancers	Monitoring response to treatment

Table 14.3 Common diagnostic tests and indications

Diagnostic test	Common indications
Core or fine needle aspirate	Breast or thyroid cancer
Excision biopsies	May be used for malignant melanoma, other skin cancers and some breast cancers
Endoscopy (± biopsy)	Lung, gastrointestinal, genitourinary cancer
Laparoscopy	Lymphoma, gastrointestinal, urological, gynaecological cancer
Bone marrow aspirate	Haematological cancers, or suspected spread to bone marrow
Colposcopy	Cervical and vaginal cancer

Radiological imaging

Imaging aims to demonstrate the anatomy of a particular area of the body and detect any abnormalities. It is used within oncology to provide a detailed understanding of primary tumours, their likely routes of spread and their response to treatment.

Main imaging modalities (see Table 14.4)
- Plain X-rays.
- Fluoroscopy.
- Computed tomography (CT).
- Magnetic resonance imaging (MRI).
- Nuclear medicine (NM) and ultrasound (US).
- More recently, positron emission tomography (PET) is being introduced into UK practice.

These modalities can be used either alone or in combination to produce an image that can be interpreted.

The dose of radiation received from radiological imaging should be kept to a minimum (📖 Radiation protection). US and MRI are the preferred imaging modalities where possible, as neither uses ionizing radiation.

It is important to select the correct imaging tool for the examination required, based on efficiency of detecting lesions and least risk and discomfort to the patient. Cost will also be a factor.
- MRI and CT are particularly effective at imaging soft tissue abnormalities, and for imaging bony structures.
- A combination of imaging tools can sometimes give the health care professional a clearer understanding of any abnormalities present. In some cases it is now possible to fuse different types of images together (📖 Radiotherapy: 'advances in technology').

Diagnosing different cancer sites

Several different modalities may be used to assist in accurately diagnosing and staging a specific cancer. The actual diagnostic and imaging modalities used for individual cancers are listed within each cancer site section.

Contrast media

Contrast media are substances that are used in conjunction with some imaging modalities, to help visualize anatomical structures. For example, when imaging the urinary system, the introduction of a contrast agent enables the radiographer to visualize the kidneys more easily, and can track the flow of urine through the system. An allergic reaction can occur when a contrast medium is used. Emergency drug therapy must therefore be readily available to treat reactions (📖 Anaphylaxis).

In an ideal situation, a patient would be transferred to the imaging department for their investigation, however it is possible for some imaging to be carried out on the ward. Mobile X-ray units and portable ultrasound equipment can be used at the bedside.

Note: it is important that appropriate radiation protection procedures are followed when mobile X-ray units are used (📖 Radiation protection).

Table 14.4 Types of imaging and specific indications

Imaging modality	Clinical indication
Plain X-ray Use of X-rays to produce an image on film or digitally	Chest: e.g. lung lesions/pleural effusions/infection Abdomen: e.g. blockages Skeletal system: e.g. bony abnormalities such metastatic disease.
Flouroscopy Continuous use of low dose X-rays to produce a dynamic image	GI tract abnormalities. Often contrast media such as barium is used to outline the GI tract. Arteriography Has been superseded by CT guided biopsy/ultrasound guided biopsy.
CT scan The use of X-rays to produce transverse sections of the head and body. The X-ray tube rotates around the patient	Any region of the body can be scanned. Can be used for diagnosis, staging, radiotherapy planning.
MRI scan Images produced by applying a pulse of strong magnetic energy to tissue. The energy released is processed into high quality images	CNS, musculoskeletal, cardiac, breast, abdomen, and pelvis. Not useful for lung imaging. Some patients unable to have MRI as the magnetic field may displace any metallic implants or foreign bodies
Nuclear medicine The use of radio-isotopes injected or inhaled into the body, imaged using a gamma camera. Typically shows abnormal physiology of the body rather than anatomical detail, e.g. bone scan	Skeletal: bone metastases Thyroid: focal nodules Respiratory: pulmonary embolus
PET scans PET and its fusions with other imaging modalities helps health care professionals to see not only the blood flow and metabolism of the tumour, but also the anatomical location in the fused image	It offers improved accuracy in staging several cancers, including non-small cell lung, upper GI, lymphomas, and recurrent bowel cancer. It has reduced the futile thoracotomy rate in non-small cell lung from about 40% to about 20%
Ultrasound High frequency sound waves are used. Different tissues transmit different sound waves that are converted into an electrical current and subsequent image. Bone and air are poor conductors of sound. Fluid is a good conductor	Abdomen: liver, gall bladder pancreas and kidneys, testes Breast and ovary: distinguish between solid and cystic mass Thorax: confirms pleural effusions and plural masses

Staging and grading cancer

Grading

This is a method of classifying tumour cells based on cellular differentiation or resemblance to their normal cell of origin, in terms of behaviour, structure, and maturity (see Table 14.5).

Grading can be very important, indicating the potential for spread or likely rate of growth of a particular tumour.
- High-grade tumours tend to be fast growing and more 'aggressive' and are more likely to spread quickly.
- Low-grade tumours tend to be slower growing and less likely to spread quickly.

Examples of grading systems include the Gleason System used to grade prostate cancer and the Fuhrman system used for kidney cancer.

Staging

Staging is a classification system based on the anatomical spread of a cancer. The most commonly used system is tumour node metastasis (TNM). This was set up by the International Union Against Cancer (UICC) nearly 50 years ago and has been regularly updated. Stage classifications have been determined for most cancer sites by the American Joint Committee of Cancer[1]. TNM assesses,
- **T**: size of primary tumour.
- **N**: absence or presence of regional lymph nodes.
- **M**: absence or presence of distant metastases.

Information from each part is combined together to determine the stage of the cancer. Most cancers are then staged from stage 1–4, though there may be further subdivisions e.g. into stage IIIa and IIIb. The stage should be given at diagnosis, if possible, but often changes after surgery as a more accurate picture of extent of disease emerges (see Table 14.6).

Limitations

There are limitations with the TNM system. It is not always sensitive enough to accurately determine prognosis or treatment. It is also not useful in several cancers. For example it cannot be used for haematological cancers. Leukaemias are classified according to cell type and differentiation. Acute leukaemias are further subdivided by the French American British (FAB) classification. Hodgkin's and non-Hodgkin's lymphoma are classified by cell type and then through a system, based on the areas or region of lymph node involvement plus presence or absence of 'b' symptoms[2].

---

1 American Joint Committee on Cancer (2002). *Cancer Staging Handbook.* 6th edn New York: Springer-Verlag.
2 Hoffbrand A V, Pettit J E, Moss P A H (2001). *Essential haematology* 4th ed. Oxford: Blackwell Science.

Table 14.5 Cancer grading

Grade	Differentiation	Appearance
Grade 1 (low grade)	Well differentiated	Mature cells—resembling normal tissue
Grade 2	Moderately differentiated	Cells with some level of immaturity
Grade 3	Poorly differentiated	Little resemblance to normal tissue
Grade 4 (high grade)	Undifferentiated	No resemblance to normal tissue

Table 14.6 General TNM definitions

	Stage designation	Definition
T	**Primary tumour**	**Size or depth of primary tumour**
	Tx	Cannot be assessed
	T0	No evidence of primary tumour
	Tis	Carcinoma in situ
	T1–T4	Increasing size or depth of primary tumour
N	**Regional lymph node spread**	**Extent and location of lymph node involvement**
	Nx	Cannot be assessed
	N0	No regional lymph node involvement
	N1–N3	Increasing number and size of involved regional lymph nodes
M	**Metastasis**	**Absence or presence of distant metastases**
	Mx	Cannot be assessed
	M0	No distant spread
	M1	Distant metastatic disease present

Other staging systems sometime run alongside TNM, for example Duke's (colorectal cancer) and Clark's (malignant melanoma). In central nervous system (CNS) tumours the system is based on the biological behaviour of the tumour (grade), size, and location. A higher grade is more malignant. N is not used, as the brain is not supplied with lymphatic drainage.

Other prognostic factors

As cancer biology and genetics becomes more fully understood the range of prognostic factors becomes more complex. Oestrogen and progester-one receptors, Her-2/Neu and vascular endothelial growth factor (VEGF) are examples of cell surface receptors that are important prognostic factors, and which also now offer specific targeted therapy options.

In the future, specific cell and molecular biology may become more important in helping treatment to be tailored to the individual, replacing the current less specific staging and grading systems.

Further reading

National Institute for Health and Clinical excellence (2005). *Referral guidelines for suspected cancer*. London: NICE www.nice.org.uk/page.aspx?0=cg027niceguideline

Surgery and cancer

Cancer surgery

Although there has been development in radiotherapy, chemotherapy, and other drug therapies in the last two decades, surgery remains a major treatment modality. Surgery offers the best hope of a cure for many patients with many different types of tumour.

Traditionally surgery was the mainstay of cancer treatment. It can still be used as a single treatment, e.g. removing a very small breast cancer lump or colonic polyps. However, it is now more usually combined with other treatments such as radiotherapy or chemotherapy (see box below).

Surgery is used in a number of different ways in managing cancer.
- Diagnosis, e.g. tissue biopsy of primary tumour.
- Staging, e.g. lymph node sampling.
- Tumour excision: primary cancer or metastatic disease with intention to cure, e.g. colorectal cancer with single liver metastases.
- Palliative surgery (see below).
- Supportive procedure, e.g. central venous catheters, PEG tubes.
- Reconstructive surgery (see below).
- Stoma formation (📖 Care of the patient with a stoma).

Multiple treatment modalities

Breast cancer is a good example of the multimodality treatment of cancer. A woman with breast cancer may typically have the following treatment pathway.
1. Surgical removal of the primary disease and sampling of lymph nodes.
2. Radiotherapy to the affected breast, to reduce the risk of local relapse.
3. Adjuvant combined chemotherapy treatment to reduce distant metastatic recurrence. (Some women with a large tumour or small breast may have chemotherapy prior to surgery—neo-adjuvant).
4. Endocrine therapy (if oestrogen or progesterone receptor positive) to reduce recurrence.

Principles

Effective surgical removal of a tumour relies on a key number of principles.

Accurate staging

If the tumour has metastasized from the original site, has become too large to be removed or involves, or is adjacent to vital structures, then surgery alone may not be successful. Accurate staging prior to surgical intervention can also prevent futile surgery on widespread disease.

Good excision margins

If a tumour can be removed completely with a buffer of unaffected tissue around the excised tumour then surgery is likely to be more successful. A larger margin will generally be more successful in reducing relapse, however this increases the surgical morbidity for the patient, i.e. more mutilating surgery.

Co-morbidities

If the patient is fit and well and able to tolerate surgery then a surgical plan is more likely to be successful.

Quality of life (cost/benefit)

If surgical treatment is liable to seriously effect the ability of an individual to function in society and drastically reduce their quality of life, then the wisdom of surgery needs to be considered within the multidisciplinary team setting and through discussion with the patient.

Adjuvant and neo-adjuvant treatments

Chemotherapy and radiotherapy can be employed prior to surgery. This is termed neo-adjuvant treatment and is normally employed to reduce the size of a tumour to make excision easier or the margins more accessible (📖 Chemotherapy). More commonly, adjuvant treatments are utilized following surgery and are used to prevent the tumour metastasizing. The primary tumour site and lymph nodes can be irradiated to reduce the risk of local metastases and chemotherapy can be given to treat systemically to eradicate any existing micrometastases.

Developments in surgery

In recent years there have been some major developments in surgery. Increased knowledge of cancer biology, improved surgical techniques, and technological advances in imaging equipment have all combined to improve patient outcomes in a number of settings. Breast cancer surgery has become less mutilating, with more use of breast conserving surgery. In rectal surgery total mesorectal excision (TME) has improved survival rates and quality of life for a number of patients. There has also been an increased use of less invasive surgery, using endoscopic/laparoscopic approaches, both for staging and disease excision.

In the UK, guidelines suggest a minimum number of specific surgical cases that each surgical team should see. The aim is for surgeons to have sufficient expertise in their particular cancer surgery. In theory this should lead to better patient outcome, though evidence for this is not strong in most cancer sites. This can have other impacts on patients and their families, with many having further to travel for treatment, which is now based in larger regional centres.

Further reading

Cassidy J, Bissett D, Spence R A J (2002). *Oxford Handbook of Oncology.* Oxford: Oxford University Press.

Gillespie T W (2005). Surgical Therapy. In Yarbro C H, Frogge M H, Goodman M (eds) (2005). *Cancer Nursing, Principles and practice.* 6th edn, pp.212–28. Massachusetts: Jones and Bartlett.

Kearney N. & Richardson A (eds) (2005). *Nursing Patients with Cancer: Principles and Practice.* Edinburgh: Elsevier Churchill Livingstone.

Preparing patients for cancer surgery

Prior to patients undergoing surgery there are a number of important issues that need to be addressed.

Staging

Prior to a full surgical assessment it is vital that the multidisciplinary team are aware of the size, position, and pathology of the tumour and the presence of any local or distant metastatic spread. This is normally evaluated by radiological methods. It is increasingly possible to assess tumours with a high degree of accuracy due to the greater availability of very sensitive diagnostic imaging techniques such as MRI scanning and, increasingly, PET scanning (Diagnosis and classification).

Lymph node assessment

An important aspect of any staging investigation is to determine whether cancer may have spread to the lymph nodes. This is important as lymph nodes may be able to be removed during surgery and adjuvant treatment (e.g. radiotherapy) can be employed to treat any affected nodes. A relatively new technique used to assess spread of cancer to lymph nodes is sentinel lymph node biopsy.

Sentinel node biopsy

This technique is increasingly employed in order to accurately assess the spread of a cancer to surrounding lymph nodes. It has proven particularly useful in treating melanoma, and, more commonly, breast cancer. The tumour site is infused (normally by injection) with a radiological marker and/or a blue dye. Time is allowed for the marker to diffuse to the first, or 'sentinel', lymph node. This equates to the first node that cancer cells would diffuse to. Once identified this node is then removed and examined for the presence of cancer cells. If it is clear then it is almost certain that other nodes will not have been affected and need not be removed. If the sentinel node is positive then this node, and other nodes further up the chain are removed.

The technique allows surgeons to preserve lymph nodes wherever possible and spares patients the possible side effects of lymph node removal, such as lymphoedema (Diagnosis and classification—for more information on staging systems).

Pre-operative assessment

A good pre-operative assessment is vital. It determines whether an individual is able to tolerate surgery both physically and psychosocially. It will also help determine if a patient will tolerate any long-term side effects from the surgery itself and therefore the overall viability of a surgical approach. It is useful to have a wide-ranging spectrum of assessments if surgery is likely to be complex and have long-term side effects. For example an anaesthetist, a specialist nurse, and a dietician may assess a patient. The individual's social situation may also have to be taken into account and may be highly relevant, for example an elderly frail person who lives alone being assessed for formation of a permanent ileostomy.

Multidisciplinary team (MDT) discussion

In situations where complex surgery may be required it is important that any decisions made at an MDT meeting are based on the assessments of the whole MDT. It is also important that the decisions made are fully discussed with the patient. Details of the proposed treatment plan should be disseminated to all the clinicians caring for the patient. This ensures a consistent approach.

Information giving

Once a proposed treatment plan has been formulated then it is vital that information is passed onto the patient and family prior to consent being sought for the operation. A valuable role in supporting the patient and their family through this process will be that of the clinical nurse specialist, or key worker. The information that an individual and their family requires in order to make decisions about surgery needs to be tailored according to their own specific needs (☐ Patient decision making).

Consent for surgery

Although the issue of consent is important when considering any cancer treatment, it has particular relevance in surgery, since surgery often results in major, and sometimes permanent, changes to an individual's body image, functional ability, and quality of life.

The consent procedure should ideally address issues around treatment intent (whether curative or palliative) the need for further adjuvant treatments and the benefits of any surgery weighed up against any possible long-term side effects and other risks.

Perioperative care of patients

There are a number of perioperative risks associated with surgery, which require careful management to minimize risks. Cancer surgery sometimes requires large excisions around other complex physiological structures to remove tumours that may also be highly vascular. Tumours can also alter blood chemistry and disrupt the clotting cascade. A patient's nutrition may also be poor and many cancer patients have major comorbidity, such as cardiorespiratory limitation. This can increase the number of perioperative complications and reduce effective recovery and wound healing.

These risks and their management are summarized in the Table 15.1.

Palliative surgery

As well as being a curative treatment, surgery can be used to palliate symptoms or reduce discomfort. A full discussion with the patient about the realistic risks and benefits is essential. The clinicians need to be mindful that the patient may decline palliative surgery and should openly discuss other possible palliative support. Some of the areas where surgery can be used palliatively are:

- Removal of a tumour which is causing pain or psychological distress, i.e. a fungating lesion (□ Skin and mucosal alterations).
- Relieving an obstructive process in the intestinal tract e.g. stenting an oesophageal lesion or removing a tumour causing a bowel obstruction.
- Decompressing the spinal cord. (□ Spinal cord compression).
- Providing haemostasis in a tumour that is causing high levels of blood loss.
- Managing airway obstruction by forming a tracheostomy.
- Debulking a large tumour, even when not all the tumour can be removed, e.g. in ovarian cancer this can both prolong survival and improve symptoms such as pain.

Reconstructive surgery

Surgery can also be used to restore form and function following excision of a tumour. Good examples of this are

- Breast reconstruction following mastectomy (□ Breast reconstruction).
- Facial and oral reconstruction following surgery for head and neck cancers.
- Skin grafting following removal of lesions.
- Surgery which allows or facilitates the use of prostheses.

This form of surgery has developed rapidly over the last two decades with vascular microsurgery being employed to utilize 'free flaps' (moving tissue, complete with its own vascular network, from another site in the body) to repair deficits left by tumour excision. This has led to improvements in breast reconstruction, reducing the long-term impact on body image. Developments in flap repair of the tongue or mandible has improved long-term function for many patients.

Table 15.1 Perioperative risks and their management

Risk	Management
Nutrition	• Refer to dietician pre-operatively for full nutritional assessment • Maximize calorie intake preoperatively • Assess for tube-feeding or parenteral nutrition throughout perioperative period • Monitor weight and protein levels regularly
Wound healing	• Monitor and maintain adequate oxygen perfusion • Assess cardiac and pulmonary function preoperatively—administer O_2 as required • Ensure adequate nutrition (see above) • Reduce risks of infection (see below)
Bleeding/DVT	• Correct blood chemistry preoperatively where possible • Utilize anti-embolus aids • Help the patient to get back to normal levels of mobility as quickly as possible postoperatively • Regular postoperative observations • Observe wound site regularly postoperatively • Monitor any blood loss carefully
Infection	• Good hygiene and technique throughout the perioperative period • Administer preoperative and postoperative antibiotic regimens • Thorough and regular postoperative observations • Observe wound site regularly for signs of infection
Pain	• Detailed preoperative pain assessment and education • Manage postoperative pain with infusional analgesics, which should preferably be 'patient-controlled'. • Regular assessments of pain • Ensure that the period of transition between the acute postoperative pain and longer-term postoperative pain is well managed • Manage patients anxiety effectively (see below)
Anxiety	• Give good and clear information throughout the operative period • Information should be given regularly and be in response to the patients needs • Involve specialist teams where pain is not adequately controlled

Psychological effects of surgery

Despite reconstructive surgery being more widely available and accessible, not all surgical side effects can be resolved and many patients suffer from short- and long-term effects of cancer surgery. These can range from shorter-term side effects such as wound infections and seroma formation (collections of fluid post breast surgery) to long-term body image alteration such as the loss of a breast or facial disfigurement. Even short-term problems or slight changes in appearance and function can have a profound effect on an individual's body image causing a loss of confidence and a range of psychosocial difficulties from sexual problems to social withdrawal. The greater the postoperative changes the greater the difficulties are likely to be (📖 Body image).

Radiotherapy

Principles and uses

Radiotherapy works by destroying cells within the body. It is delivered in as uniform a dose as possible to an accurately defined target to minimize physiological and psychological consequences for the patient. The aim is to kill the tumour cells whilst avoiding as much normal tissue as possible

When radiation is directed at tumour cells, it damages vital structures such as the cells' DNA or enzymes. Cells are generally more vulnerable to the lethal effects of radiation when they are dividing, therefore the rate of cell division within a tumour will have an impact on its response to that treatment. Cells may also repair themselves. Cancer cells are generally less effective at repairing themselves than cells in normal tissue. This, in part, accounts for the ability of radiotherapy treatment to destroy a cancer whilst enabling normal tissues repair. (See 4 R's opposite).

Radiosensitivity

Different types of tissues and organs have different tolerances to radiation. Lymphoid tissue, haematopoietic tissue, ovaries, testes, and lenses of the eye are the most sensitive, requiring a smaller dose to cause lethal damage. Lung, liver, gut, and skin are moderately sensitive. Muscle, bone, and connective tissue are the least sensitive. The tolerance of normal tissues to radiation is one of the main dose-limiting factors of radiotherapy.

Use of radiotherapy

Approximately 60% of patients with cancer will have radiotherapy as a treatment.

- *Primary treatment:* for some disease e.g. skin, prostate, head and neck cancer and Hodgkin's disease radiotherapy can be the primary treatment. Radiotherapy has increasingly become used to treat primary tumours instead of surgery.
- *Adjuvant:* more commonly it is given as an adjuvant with surgery and/ or chemotherapy, e.g. breast, head and neck cancer, to cure or control a cancer.
- *Palliative:* palliative radiotherapy is used frequently to manage a range of symptoms in many cancers including metastatic bone disease, spinal cord compression, haemorrhage, and fungating tumours.

Fractionation

The amount of times a dose of radiation is delivered is known as the number of fractions. The number of fractions will vary depending on whether the patient is having radical or palliative treatment.

- *Radical:* a high dose of radiation divided into small fractions, delivered daily over several weeks, to eliminate a tumour and minimize side effects, but remaining within the tolerance of normal tissues.
- *Palliative:* a smaller amount of radiation is given in a short number of fractions over a shorter time span with few acute side effects.

Chemo-irradiation

Concurrent chemotherapy and radiation treatment (particularly with radiation sensitizing drugs) is increasingly used as a major radical treatment modality in a number of cancers, including oesophageal, head and neck, and cervical. (📖 Chemotherapy: concurrent chemo-irradiation).

The 4 'Rs' of radiotherapy

There are four main principles that influence the biological response of a tumour and normal tissue, and these help guide the planning of radiotherapy treatment.

Repair

Radiation has two main damaging effects—direct breaks to DNA and indirect effects, where it interacts with water molecules and oxygen to create free radicals. Free radicals are highly reactive molecules, which can oxidize and damage DNA synthesis. Most cells do not die immediately but instead die after several divisions, due to damaged DNA and cell mechanism such as apoptosis (Cell biology). The ability of cells to repair this damage will impact on the effectiveness of radiotherapy as a treatment. Fractionating the dose aims to take advantage of the ability of normal tissue to repair itself more effectively than the cancer[1].

Repopulation

During radiotherapy, tumour cells not destroyed by the treatment begin to grow to replace the damaged cells. Some fast growing cancers show accelerated growth. Reducing the overall treatment time of radical treatments and ensuring that there are no delays in treatment schedules are important. In tumours with fast growth some patients may have more than one treatment a day. This is known as hyper-fractionation, which has been used in both head and neck cancers and lung cancer.

Reoxygenation

Oxygen has an important role to play in the effectiveness of radiotherapy. The more oxygenated the tumour cells are when irradiated, the more effective the radiation is at destroying the DNA. Many tumours have areas of reduced oxygen (hypoxia) due to poor vascularity. This makes them more resistant to radiation damage. Ways of improving oxygenation include ensuring patients are not anaemic (having a Hb of above 12g/dl), and the development of drugs that can sensitize hypoxic cells.

Fractionating radiotherapy increases the chance of killing cells that have already survived one treatment, as with each fraction, the tumour becomes less hypoxic and more oxygenated.

Redistribution

Cells that are initially destroyed by radiotherapy will have been dividing (in the cell cycle). Over time cells moving from G_0, into the cell cycle, replace these cells (Cancer biology). Therefore fractionating radiotherapy allows a greater chance of damaging cells at a sensitive stage of the cell cycle (particularly mitosis-M phase).

1 Kearney N and Richardson A (eds). *Nursing Patients with Cancer: Principles and Practice*, pp.265–82. Edinburgh: Elsevier Churchill Livingstone.

Treatment modalities

External beam radiotherapy

The main treatment machines used today are called external beam megavoltage linear accelerators. These produce extremely accurate, high energy beams under computer control, that are able to destroy cells. The unit of radiation dose is known as a Gray (Gy). This is the amount of energy that is absorbed per unit mass so $1Gy = 1Joule/Kg$.

Unsealed sources

These can be administered directly via either oral or intravenous routes. They are used to treat specific cancers, such as thyroid cancer, where radioactive iodine is given orally and is taken up by the thyroid gland.

Brachytherapy (sealed source)

Radiotherapy can also be delivered via a radioactive source placed inside a body cavity or directly into a tumour (see table below).

The main treatment modalities available are shown in Table 16.1.

Radiation protection

Radiation is potentially dangerous. It can cause cancer, although the chance of this being caused by diagnostic X-rays is small, due to the low dose used.

In order for radiotherapy treatment to be safe, a maximum 'tolerance' dose should not be exceeded, as above this dose there is an increased chance of permanent damage to tissues. Radiotherapy must only be used when there is a benefit for the patient.

The Ionising Radiation (Medical Exposures) Regulations 2000 [IRMER], specifies responsibilities for staff and employers using radiation on patients. It sets training requirements, and it requires justification of exposures for individuals. The employer has to provide a safe framework for staff to work with, including lists of trained staff and written procedures.

Table 16.1 Radiotherapy: main treatment modalities

Superficial and Orthovoltage	Uses low energy X-rays to treat superficial skin legions such as basal cell carcinomas and squamous cell carcinomas. These modes of treatment are being replaced by electron treatment.
Megavoltage (external beam)	For deeper structures in body. Uses a range of X-ray energies produced from an external electrical source. Patients may require complex planning of treatment using a range of imaging modalities to help localize the tumour. Patients require simulation (□ Treatment planning).
Electrons	For skin lesions and scars. Particularly useful for treating skin lesions and areas overlying bony structures as the energy of the beam is lost rapidly upon interaction with tissue, producing a high dose close to the skin surface.
Unsealed source	Radioactive isotopes administered intravenously or orally, e.g. iodine I^{131}, which is used orally to treat thyroid cancer. I^{131} is taken up selectively by the thyroid gland.
Brachytherapy	Treatment using a radioactive source element such as iridium 192 or caesium 137, that is placed inside a body cavity e.g. the cervix or use of radioactive wires, needles, or seeds that can be inserted directly into a tumour e.g. tongue, breast, penis, prostate (□ Treatment planning).

Radiation protection issues

- All personnel who may come into contact with a patient who could be radioactive (e.g. radioactive iodine patients, brachytherapy patients, patients having a radio-isotope scan) must wear a radiation dose monitor, usually at waist level.
- It is advisable for staff who are pregnant or breast feeding to avoid prolonged contact with a patient who is radioactive.
- Radiation protection equipment (e.g. mobile thick lead screens) should be used when nursing patients who are radioactive. The intensity of radiation decreases with distance, and so the further you are away from the source of radiation, the safer you are.
- All radioactive waste should be disposed of in accordance with the local rules governing each oncology ward/department.
- Once a patient who has been radioactive leaves the ward, the area should be monitored using a Geiger counter to ensure no residual radioactivity is present.

Treatment planning and delivery

Treatment planning

Radical radiotherapy

Planning generally happens in two stages: localization and verification.

1a. Localization: planning imaging

- CT/MRI/US/plain film is used to locate the tumour for planning purposes.
- Wire markers or 'permanent body marks' are placed onto the patient's skin as reference points to aid the planning of treatment. These will be clearly visible on the scan(s).

1b. Localization: computer planning

- The planning image is loaded into a planning computer. This enables the treatment area to be accurately defined, and is known as the planning target volume (PTV). From this, the size of the area to be treated can be determined. The aim is to treat the tumour to the maximum dose, whilst minimizing the dose to surrounding tissues and organs.
- Planning determines the number, location, shape, and size of the treatment fields, as well as the need to shield any sensitive structures such as the spinal cord or the lens of the eye.
- The prescribed dose is calculated and checked several times to ensure accuracy.
- The amount of treatment is determined by the size and tolerance dose of the area being treated, and the sensitivity of any surrounding structures (📖 Radiation protection).

2. Verification

Once the planning process has been completed, the patient will be given a dummy run of the treatment in a simulator (see below), to ensure that all of the treatment parameters that have been planned are correct. This is known as verification, and any fine-tuning to the treatment plan can be done at this stage, before the patient starts treatment.

The simulator is a diagnostic X-ray machine that enables the radiographer and oncologist to screen an area of the body. It simulates the movements and parameters of a treatment machine. Recording this information allows radiographers to deliver the treatment exactly as it was simulated.

Treatment delivery

Megavoltage treatment delivery (external beam)

- Information from the treatment planning stage is put into the treatment machine's computer.
- The patient is positioned underneath the treatment machine, reproducing the radiotherapy planning. Lazer lights and the field light in the machine are used to line up with the marks and permanent body marks drawn on the patient.
- The treatment is accurately delivered using a computer controlled system. All staff leave the treatment room during delivery of the treatment, due to the high level of radiation.

Note: in many solid tumours patients may have a second phase of treatment that focuses more specifically on the tumour, known as a boost. This requires a further planning session during treatment.

Brachytherapy/radioisotope/interstitial treatment delivery

Treatments can last several hours or even days.

- The patient will be required to remain in a specially designed room for the duration of their treatment, usually on an oncology ward.
- Nursing staff are responsible for checking that the treatment is being delivered. This may involve checking to make sure the source of radiation has not moved out of place, or checking for machine failure. Any changes must be reported to the radiotherapy team.
- Any nursing procedures that need to be carried out must be done as quickly and efficiently as possible and utilize any radiation protection equipment as appropriate (🕮 Radiation protection).

Advances and new technology in radiation therapy

Radiotherapy planning

Virtual Simulation: a patient's radiotherapy planning procedures can all be done by a computer programme. This eliminates the need for the patient to attend the planning department for several visits (as is the case with most conventional planning and simulation). Virtual simulation is only available in a minority of departments and is unlikely to be in widespread use for several years.

Radiotherapy treatment

Conformal treatment: this involves shaping the beam to 'fit' the shape of the tumour, using individual leaves of lead in the head of the machine. This aims to:

- Minimize the amount of normal tissue in the treatment field.
- Enable a higher overall dose to be delivered to the tumour, as the size of the beam is reduced, and less normal tissue is within the treatment field.

Intensity modulated radiotherapy (IMRT): this allows the beam to fit the 3-dimensional shape of the tumour and to take account of any inconsistency within the tumour volume to improve the beam shape and profile.

Management of radiotherapy treatment and its side effects

Undertaking a course of radiotherapy can be an emotionally and physically demanding time for patients and their families. It may last several weeks plus the initial planning time, requiring daily travel, often over a long distance. Radiotherapy treatment may occur after or alongside other treatments, adding to the potential for debilitating side effects.

Many patients have fears of radiotherapy and its side effects. They may also have misunderstandings about the nature of the treatment. Media coverage of nuclear accidents and weapons raise concerns about radioactive fallout, dangers of getting other cancers or being a danger to others e.g. 'will I be radioactive?'

Initial assessment needs to
- Clarify the individual's beliefs and concerns about radiotherapy treatment.
- Explain the actual treatment process, potential side effects and management of these.

After treatment is completed patients may still face acute and long-term side effects (📖 Community support).

Side effects

Radiotherapy side effects occur because of radiation damage to the cells (📖 Principles and uses). As the radiation cannot distinguish between normal and cancerous cells, it is inevitable that some normal cells will be damaged. This may lead to the patient experiencing radiation side effects. These side effects are generally localized to the area being treated. The main systemic side effect is fatigue (📖 Fatigue).

Table 16.2 highlights the main side effects from radiotherapy to different body areas.

Acute and long-term side effects

Side effects occur at different stages of the treatment, depending on the amount of treatment being delivered, and the duration of the course of treatment. Side effects can be acute or long-term. Acute side effects can continue to worsen after treatment has been completed for up to 2–3 weeks. Most acute side effects will disappear a few weeks after treatment has been completed, though some may take longer and continue, becoming long-term[1]. Symptom management is therefore a key element of continuing care and follow-up.

Knowledge and understanding of the tolerance dose of radiation treatment that a normal tissue or organ can withstand, and the advances in treatment planning and delivery, greatly reduces the risk of long-term side effects occurring.

---

1 Faithfull S (2005). Radiotherapy. In Kearney N and Richardson A (eds). *Nursing Patients with Cancer: Principles and Practice*, pp.265–82. Edinburgh: Elsevier Churchill Livingstone.

Multidisciplinary team

The management of radiotherapy side effects often involves many health care professionals including: an oncologist and their medical team, oncology nurses including CNS, therapeutic radiographers, dieticians, speech and language therapist (SALT), occupational therapist, physiotherapist, phychologists, counsellors, G.P., and other community health care professionals.

Table 16.2 Side effects of radiotherapy

Area being treated	Acute side effects	Long-term side effects
Brain/CNS (including spinal cord)	Raised ICP, headache, nausea, blurred vision, unsteady gait, tiredness, dysphasia	Neurological defects including CNS necrosis, cognitive dysfunction, neuro-edocrine abnormalities CNS: spinal cord myelopathy
Head and neck	Pain, dysphagia, mucositis, skin reaction, xerostomia, fungal infection, weight loss	Pain, bone necrosis, dysphagia, xerostomia
Breast (including axilla)	Pain, skin reaction, tiredness	Brachial plexopathy, skin telangiectasia and pigment changes (rare with modern linear accelerators), lymphoedema, bone necrosis (ribs), lung fibrosis, psychosocial problems
Thorax	Breathlessness, pain, haemoptysis, dysphagia, weight loss, tiredness	Pericardial complications, lung fibrosis, pneumonitis
GI tract (including oesophagus, small and large bowel)	Nausea, vomiting, pain, diarrhoea, weight loss, tiredness	Oesophagus: dysphagia, oesophageal ulceration/perforation. Small bowel: malabsorption syndromes, hypermotility, diarrhoea, pain, ulceration, fistulas, perforation, ischaemia, bleeding. Large bowel: colitis, stricture, bowel obstruction, ulceration, fistulas, perforation, ischaemia, tenesmus, bleeding
Pelvis (including bladder/prostate, gynaecological)	Pain, difficulty in micturition, frequency, nocturia and urgency, cystitis, haematuria, proctitis, diarrhoea, tiredness	Bleeding, scarring, vaginal stenosis and vaginal dryness, fibrosis, cystitis, urinary incontinence, erectile dysfunction, urethral dysfunction, large bowel complications (see above)

Note: please refer to the appropriate topic of Section 7, Symptom management, for detailed management of the main side effects listed in the table above.

Skin toxicity

The basal layer of the epidermis is sensitive to radiation because of its high proliferation rate. Radiotherapy treatment prevents cell division within the basal layer, therefore preventing re-population.

- The dose of radiation needed to induce a skin reaction depends on the amount of dose delivered each time, the duration of the course of treatment, and the energy of dose used.
- The degree of skin reaction will vary depending on the area of the body being treated. Common areas that experience acute skin reactions include the breast, head and neck, groin, or areas where there are skin folds.
- For radical treatments, skin reactions tend to occur 2–3 weeks into a course of treatment (Table 16.3). Most skin reactions will heal within a few weeks of radiotherapy being completed.

The evidence base for managing skin reactions is limited and practice varies. However, the following skin care advice is recommended for all radiotherapy patients by the Royal College of Radiographers[1]. Patients should be given this advice in written and verbal form, clearly stating:

- How, why, when, and where skin reactions are likely to occur.
- What they look and feel like.
- Risk factors for them occurring.
- How they will be treated and self-care strategies.

Community support

When patients finish their radiotherapy treatment many are still experiencing the physical side effects of the treatment. However, many can also experience emotional, social, financial, and spiritual difficulties. This is not only due to the effects of treatment but also the process of returning to 'normal'.

Assessing the need for follow up and community support is an important part of supporting patients post-treatment. Patients should receive advice and information on the support services that are available to them. There should be a coordinated care package for each patient that should include the contact details of their cancer nurse specialist.

The department/ward must work in partnership with primary care staff to ensure the patient's needs are met following completion of radiotherapy treatment. Communication between the radiotherapy centre/ward and primary care should be initiated early on and protocols should be in place that ensures any post radiotherapy problems are dealt with promptly. Understanding and awareness of the roles and contribution hospital and community health care professionals have will help ensure a collaborative approach to care post radiotherapy is achieved.

---

1 College of Radiographers (2001). *Summary of Intervention for acute radiotherapy induced skin reactions in cancer patients, A Clinical guideline for use by The College of Radiographers.* London: College of Radiographers. www.sor.org/public/pdf/skinreact.pdf

Table 16.3 Skin reactions to radiotherapy treatment

Skin reaction	Management and patient advice
No visible skin reaction	For the duration of treatment: • Avoid friction. • Wear loose, natural fibre clothing (cotton). • Gentle washing of the treatment area with warm water using a mild non-perfumed soap, pat skin gently dry. • Avoid shaving the treated area if possible. • Do not expose the treated area to the sun, or harsh weather conditions. • Avoid use of deodorants/perfumes/aftershaves in treated area. • Apply a simple emollient (aqueous cream) sparingly to the treated area twice a day. This may help delay reactions. • Increase fluid intake to ensure adequate hydration.
Erythema (reddening of the skin in the treated area)	• Continue to use aqueous cream, increasing the frequency of application to soothe and moisturise. • If the skin begins to itch then 1% hydrocortisone cream can be applied sparingly.
Dry desquamation (red, dry, flaky skin in treated area)	As for erythema. If the skin breaks down, then discontinue cream (s) and follow advice for moist desquamation.
Moist desquamation (skin peeling, pain, weeping with exudate in treated area)	• Dress the area with a hydrogel, hydrocolloid or alginate dressing. • Avoid the use of adhesive tape in the treated area. • Take a swab if there are any signs of infection. • Aqueous cream can still be used on areas that have not broken down. • Pain medications as required.

Further reading

Department of Health (2000). *Ionising Radiation (Medical Exposure) Regulations 2000, Statutory Instrument No. 1059*. London: HMSO.

Devereux S, Hatton M, and Macbeth F (1997). Immediate side effects of large fraction radiotherapy. *Clinical Oncology*, **9**, 96–9.

Faithfull S. and Wells M (2003). *Supportive care in radiotherapy*. Edinburgh: Churchill Livingstone.

Maher K E (2005). Radiation Therapy: Toxicities and Management. In Yarbro C H, Frogge M H, Goodman M (eds) (2005). *Cancer Nursing, Principles and practice*. 6th edn, pp.283–314. Massachusetts: Jones and Bartlett.

Stone H, Coleman C, Ansher M et al. (2003). Effects of radiation on normal tissue: consequences and mechanism. *Lancet Oncology*, **4**, 529–36.

Symonds R P (2001). Recent advances: Radiotherapy *BMJ*, **323**, 1107–10.

Chemotherapy

ples and uses

otherapy can be used with curative or palliative intent, either alone
n conjunction with other treatment modalities. Cytotoxic drugs disrupt
ell division and replication with rapidly proliferating cells being most
susceptible to their action. As cytotoxic drugs are unable to distinguish
between cancer cells and normal cells, rapidly proliferating cells of the
bone marrow, gastrointestinal tract, reproductive system and hair follicles
are particularly vulnerable to their effects, resulting in many of the common
side effects of chemotherapy. Normal cells have a greater capacity for
repair and renewal than cancer cells. Some of the newer anti-cancer
drugs (📖 Biological therapies) have a more sophisticated selective
approach with the capability to target specific tissues.

Cancer cell growth

Chemotherapy aims to reduce the number of actively dividing cells in a
tumour thereby reducing the growth potential. Smaller tumours tend to
have a faster growth rate, are likely to have more actively dividing cells
and are therefore more susceptible to chemotherapy.

Effects of cytotoxic drugs on the cell cycle

Cytotoxic drugs have the greatest effect on actively dividing cells. Many
cytotoxic drugs act on specific phases of the cell cycle e.g. S phase (cell cycle
specific drugs) while others act on cells in any phase of the cell cycle (cell
cycle non-specific drugs). Drugs acting on a specific phase of the cycle will
only affect cells that are in that phase at the time of administration. Cell cycle
non-specific drugs affect both cells that are actively cycling and quiescent
cells. Multiple courses of chemotherapy are required to affect cells entering
different phases of the cell cycle at different times. Examples of cell cycle
specific and cell cycle non-specific drugs are shown in Table 17.1.

Classification of drugs

Cytotoxic drugs have differing modes of action, which are not yet fully
understood. Most disrupt cell reproduction either by damaging DNA or
affecting mitosis and are categorized according to their mode of action
(see Table 17.2).

Table 17.1 Examples of cell cycle specific and cell cycle non-speci.
drugs

Cell cycle specific drugs	Cell cycle non-specific drugs
Cytosine arabinoside, 5-fluorouracil, gemcitabine, methotrexate, thioguanine (S phase)	Chlorambucil, doxorubicin, daunorubicin, procarbazine, cisplatin, cyclophosphamide, ifosfamide, melphalan.
Bleomycin, etoposide, irinotecan, topotecan (G_2 phase)	
Vincristine, vinblastine, docetaxel, paclitaxel (M phase)	
L-asparaginase (G_1 phase)	

Table 17.2 Classification of cytotoxic drugs

Classification	Mode of action	Examples
Antimetabolites	Replace or compete with naturally occurring purines, pyridamines, or folates necessary for synthesis of nucleic acids	Methotrexate, cytosine arabinoside, 6-mercaptopurine, 5-fluorouracil, gemcitabine, 6-thioguanine, capecitabine, cladribine, fludarabine
Anthracyclines (cytotoxic antibiotics)	Inhibit synthesis of RNA and DNA by different mechanisms, e.g. breaks and cross-links in strands of DNA, intercalation of base pairs	Doxorubicin, daunorubicin, epirubicin, idarubicin, dactinomycin, mitoxanthrone
Alkylating agents (plus platinum agents)	Cause breaks and cross-links in the strands of DNA	Chlorambucil, cyclophosphamide, ifosfamide, melphalan, dacarbazine, busulphan, cisplatin, carboplatin, carmustine, lomustine, procarbazine, amsacrine
Mitotic inhibitors: Vinca alkaloids	Inhibit mitosis by binding to tubulin an essential component of the mitotic spindle	Vincristine, vinblastine, vindesine, vinoralbine
Taxanes	Cause mitotic arrest by binding to microtubules	Paclitaxel, docetaxel
Topoisomerase inhibitors	Inhibit topoisomerase enymes necessary for DNA replication. Causes single strand breaks in DNA strands	Etoposide, topotecan, irinotecan(drugs from other categories e.g. doxorubicin, mitoxanthrone, amsacrine are also topoisomerase inhibitors)

motherapy regimens

erent cytotoxic drugs with proven efficacy against a particular cancer e combined in different chemotherapy regimens. Other agents with anti-cancer activity e.g. hormones and biological therapies, may also be included in these regimens. The dose and combination of drugs aims to achieve the maximum therapeutic effect with acceptable toxicity levels. A fine balance exists between the therapeutic dose of a cytotoxic drug and a lethal dose.

Combination chemotherapy

Combinations of drugs are used to overcome problems associated with single agent drug resistance. Most chemotherapy regimens include a combination of cell cycle specific and non-specific drugs to increase malignant cell destruction. Drugs with different but complementary actions and efficacy are combined. Drug toxicities should differ or occur at different times so that maximum tolerated doses of drugs can be administered without severe toxicity.

Scheduling and sequencing of drugs

The order in which drugs are given can either affect their efficacy or cause increased toxicity e.g. clearance of paclitaxel is significantly decreased if it is administered after cisplatin leading to increased myelosuppression[1]. Other drugs are synergistic, enhancing each others effect, e.g. cisplatin and etoposide.

Intervals between pulses of chemotherapy

The time interval between pulses of chemotherapy is important; too short and normal cells will not have recovered resulting in increased toxicity; too long and cancer cells may regrow between treatments. The interval between pulses is the period of time required for the most sensitive normal cells (usually the bone marrow) to recover. Most chemotherapy regimens are therefore repeated every 3–4 weeks. However, this is dependent on the toxicity of the drugs used.

Modes of use

Chemotherapy can be used in different ways and with different intent.
- *Curative:* chemotherapy is used as first line treatment to cure a number of cancers particularly haematological and lymphatic cancers.
- *Adjuvant:* following surgery to remove the primary tumour adjuvant chemotherapy is used as a means of destroying micrometastases.

Neo-adjuvant

Neo-adjuvant chemotherapy is used before surgery to:
- Reduce the size of the primary tumour.
- Reduce metastatic potential.
- Measure tumour response to chemotherapy.

1 Fischer D S, Knobf M T, Durivage H J, et al. (2003). The Cancer Chemotherapy Handbook. (6th edn). Philadelphia: Mosby.

It is used to treat various cancers including head and neck, bladder, non-small cell lung (NSCLC), and early breast cancers. Clinics continue to investigate the effectiveness of neo-adjuvant chemoth for different cancers.

Concurrent chemo-irradiation

Chemotherapy is administered concurrently with radiotherapy to increase the effectiveness of radiotherapy while reducing the potential for metastatic disease. Certain cytotoxic drugs, e.g. cisplatin, 5-fluorouracil and gemcitabine, are known to have radiosensitizing properties, increasing the sensitivity of cancer cells to radiotherapy and increasing therapeutic potential. The use of concurrent radiotherapy has been investigated for various cancers including: colorectal, cervical, oesophageal, laryngeal, pancreatic, cervical, NSCLC, and stomach (☐ see specific disease sections).

Optimal dose, schedule, and combination of drugs to use concurrently with radiotherapy have yet to be established. Ongoing clinical trials are investigating effects on both survival and toxicity profiles. Concurrent therapy may increase treatment toxicities e.g. haematological and gastro-intestinal in cervical cancer, neutropenia and acute oesphagitis in NSCLC and severe mucositis in head and neck cancer.

High dose therapy

High dose therapy involves increasing the dose of cytotoxic drugs to a point where they are lethal to the normal bone marrow. Bone marrow then has to be replaced by haematopoietic stem cell transplant (HSCT). High dose therapy and HSCT are used mainly for haematological and lymphoid cancers (☐ High dose therapy).

Palliative

Palliative chemotherapy is used to control symptoms, improve quality of life and treat oncological emergencies e.g. superior vena cava syndrome. Traditionally, no survival benefit has been associated with palliative chemotherapy and its use has been controversial because treatment toxicities may impact on quality of life. The costs of chemotherapy need to be balanced against the survival benefit and compared to the cost of best supportive care[2].

2 Archer V R, Billingham L J, and Cullen M H (1999). Palliative Chemotherapy: No Longer a Contradiction in Terms. The Oncologist, 4, 470–7.

andling

oxic drugs are known to be teratogenic, mutagenic, and carcino-
ic and therefore are potentially hazardous to patients, staff, and the
nvironment. Exposure can occur through ingestion, inhalation, and
absorption through the skin. Exposure can occur at all stages of preparation,
administration, and disposal of drugs, most notably when reconstituting
or mixing drugs, connecting and disconnecting intravenous tubing and
disposing of used equipment and patient excreta[1].

It is vital that health care professionals involved in the preparation,
administration, and disposal of cytotoxic drugs and waste adopt safe
handling procedures to protect themselves and others from the potential
health risks associated with exposure.

Legal requirements

The preparation, administration and disposal of cytotoxic drugs and
waste must comply with the relevant legislation:
- Medicines Act (1968).
- Environmental Protection Act (1990).
- Management of Health and Safety at Work Regulations (1999).
- Control of Substances Hazardous to Health Regulations
  (COSHH) (2002).

Pregnant workers

EEC Council Directive 92/85/EEC (EEC, 1992) identifies cytotoxic
drugs as potentially hazardous to pregnant workers. Employers have a
duty to assess the risk to health and decide what measures should be
taken. Pregnant workers can choose not to be involved in activities
involving exposure to cytotoxic drugs.

Measures to reduce exposure to cytotoxic drugs

The evidence supporting safe handling practices is incomplete. However,
various guidelines exist based on the available evidence and expert opinion.

Preparation

Cytotoxic drugs should be reconstituted by appropriately trained personnel, wearing personal protective equipment, under aseptic conditions
in a biological safety cabinet or isolator within a pharmacy department.
Cytotoxic drugs should only be reconstituted outside pharmacy departments in exceptional circumstances.

Transport and storage

Cytotoxic drugs should be transported and received in patient areas by
staff trained in safe handling and safe storage procedures. Cytotoxic
drugs should be securely stored in appropriate conditions in a clearly
marked location separate to other medicines.

Personal protective equipment

Gloves should be worn at all times when handling cytotoxic drugs and
excreta. No gloves are completely impermeable to cytotoxic drugs.

Permeability of gloves increases with time and gloves should be on a regular basis to reduce the potential for exposure.

Eye and respiratory protection are advised when there is a risk of splas or if the risk of generating an aerosol exists[1,2]. Aprons and gowns c protect clothing and subsequent skin exposure. A COSHH risk assessment should be undertaken for each handling activity to assess whether a gown or plastic apron offers the most protection.

Administration

Drugs should be supplied ready for administration and not require any further mixing or reconstitution. Oral preparations should not be handled. Tablets should not be crushed and capsules should not be opened.

Disposal of waste

Gloves and aprons should be worn when disposing of used intravenous equipment, excreta, blood, and body fluids. Contaminated needles, syringes, and intravenous giving sets should be disposed of intact. All waste should be placed in clinical waste bags and clearly marked cytotoxic. Patient excreta may contain traces of cytotoxic drugs for up to 72 hours following administration.

Spillage

Procedures should be in place for preventing and dealing with spillage. Spillage kits should be available in all areas where cytotoxic drugs are administered. Any spillage should be dealt with promptly. A warning sign should be in place to indicate the spill and prevent exposure and contamination, measures taken to contain the spill and protective clothing worn. Contaminated materials should be clearly labeled and packaged for disposal. Porters and laundry staff should be aware of procedures for handling and disposing of contaminated materials.

Copious amounts of soap and water should be used for skin contact. Eyes should be flooded with water or an isotonic eye wash solution for at least five minutes and medical advice obtained[2]. Spillage of a large amount of cytotoxic drug incurring exposure to people should be reported to RIDDOR (Reporting Injuries, Diseases and Dangerous Occurrences Regulations 1995).

Cleaning

Drug residue may be left on work surfaces in drug administration areas. All staff involved in cleaning areas where cytotoxic chemotherapy is administered should have training in minimizing exposure. Procedures for minimizing exposure should also be in place[3].

1 Health and Safety Executive (2003). *Safe Handling of Cytotoxic Drugs*. HSE Information Sheet MISC615 www.hse.gov.uk (Accessed Feb 2006).
2 Royal College of Nursing (1998). *Clinical Practice Guidelines: The Administration of Cytotoxic Chemotherapy. Recommendations*. London: RCN.
3 Scottish Executive Health Department. HDL (2005). 29. *Guidance for the Safe Use of Cytotoxic Chemotherapy*. Edinburgh: SEHD.

administration

...toxic drugs can have severe and potentially fatal consequences if ...ninistered incorrectly. Prevention of errors and patient safety are of ...aramount importance and policies and procedures relating to cytotoxic drug administration should be adhered to at all times. All practitioners involved in chemotherapy administration must have undertaken specific education and training, be knowledgeable about the drugs they are administering and their side effects and have demonstrated competence in their role.

- Patient consent should always be obtained and documented before the administration of chemotherapy.
- Cytotoxic chemotherapy should be administered during normal working hours, in a specifically designated area.
- Administration should not be rushed and care should be taken to avoid distraction during administration.
- Practitioners should be aware of emergency situations which may occur during and following administration of cytotoxic drugs e.g. allergic reactions, anaphylaxis, and extravasation, and be competent in managing them.
- Resuscitation equipment, emergency drugs, and extravasation kits should be available in all areas where cytotoxic drugs are administered.

Before administering drugs, practitioners should be familiar with the individual patient's:

- Blood count and general physical condition. Neutropenia or thrombocytopenia may mean that chemotherapy is delayed. Abnormal liver or renal function may require dose modification.
- Allergy history.
- Any contraindications to chemotherapy administration.
- Any drugs they are taking (including non-prescription drugs) and any possible interactions.
- Recommended dose range and maximum dose of drugs.
- Route of administration.
- Potential adverse reactions.
- Short and long term side effects.
- Route of excretion.
- Compatibility of any drugs or IV fluids to be administered in conjunction with cytotoxic drugs.

Note: the *British National Formulary* and specific drug information sheet should always be consulted before drugs are administered.

Chemotherapy guidelines for safe practice

The Manual of Cancer Standards (England and Wales)[1] and Gui
for the Safe Use of Cytotoxic Chemotherapy (Scotland)[2] set o
guidelines for the administration and handling of chemotherapy. Loc
trusts are able to adapt these to their own local circumstances where
appropriate.

All staff must follow their local trust guidelines on administration and
handling of cytotoxic chemotherapy at all times. These guidelines must
be available in any area where cytotoxic drugs are administered.

1 Department of Health (2004). *Manual of Cancer Standards*. London: DH.
2 Scottish Executive Health Department. HDL (2005). 29. *Guidance for the Safe Use of Cytotoxic Chemotherapy*. Edinburgh: SEHD.

s of administration

xic drugs can be administered by a number of different routes.
oute of administration is chosen to achieve maximum cancer cell
ath by optimizing the bioavailability and exposure of cancer cells to
drugs thereby improving efficacy.

Main routes of chemotherapy administration

- Intravenous (IV)
- Intrathecal (IT)
- Intracavity e.g. intravesical, intraperitoneal
- Subcutaneous (SC)
- Intramuscular (IM)
- Intra-arterial
- Topical
- Oral

Intravenous

The intravenous route is the most commonly used route for the administration of cytotoxic drugs[1]. It is the most reliable route as the drug is delivered systemically. Drugs can be delivered through a variety of venous access devices (VAD).

Venous access devices

The choice of device depends upon the condition of the patient's veins, the drugs to be administered, and the length of treatment. For those having lengthy courses of treatment a central VAD (CVAD) should be considered. Choosing the right VAD for the treatment to be administered is important in reducing potential complications. Prevention of infection is vital and strict asepsis is required irrespective of the choice of VAD. Extravasation and subsequent tissue damage are major potential problems with the IV route (see below).

Peripheral cannulation

Careful placement of any peripheral VAD is required and nurses administering chemotherapy need to be skilled in cannulation. Individuals with cancer may have veins difficult to cannulate.

- Patients may have experienced previous problems with venous access and should always be asked if they have a preferred choice of arm for cannulation.
- Limbs affected by lymphoedema, dermatitis, cellulitis, skin grafts, previous fractures, stroke, arteriovenous fistulae, or wounds should be avoided. The forearm is the cannulation site of first choice. Joints such as the ante-cubital fossa and wrist should be avoided as there is greater chance of dislodging the cannula.
- If the first cannulation attempt is unsuccessful a subsequent one should be proximal to the first.
- The smallest gauge of cannulae should be used and be firmly secured.
- Pre-existing intravenous lines should be avoided for chemotherapy administration wherever possible.

1 Dougherty L (2005). Intravenous Management In: Brighton, D. Wood, M. (eds), *The Royal Handbook of Cancer Chemotherapy*, pp.93–111 Edinburgh: Elsevier.

Table 17.3 Venous access devices

Type of cannula	Use
Winged infusion device 'butterfly'	Bolus injections only. Steel needles should never be used for vesicant administration
Peripheral cannula	Short term use
Mid-line cannula	Medium term use 2–4 weeks
Peripheral IV central catheter	Can be used for several months
Central venous access device (e.g. Groshong and Hickman catheters)	Long term use
Implantable port (e.g. Port-a-cath)	Long term use

Administration

Drugs may be administered by direct bolus injection, bolus injection into the side arm of a fast-running infusion of 0.9% normal saline or by infusion. The choice of method depends upon the pharmacological properties of the drug (e.g. whether it is a vesicant, requires dilution, stability, osmolarity, and pH of the drug) and the type of VAD used. Any prescribed pre-hydration fluids or anti-emetics should be given before chemotherapy is commenced.

Before any drug is administered, the patency of the VAD should be assessed by withdrawing blood and then flushing with 0.9% sodium chloride. If a peripheral cannula is being used the site should be closely observed throughout the infusion for signs of tissue infiltration or extravasation e.g. resistance, swelling, pain or discomfort, redness, or signs of leakage. Cannula dressings should allow clear visibility of the insertion site and surrounding area. Cannulae should be flushed between drugs and after completion of drug administration with a compatible fluid.

Note: sodium chloride is not compatible with all drugs.

...al

...totoxic drugs are unable to cross the blood–brain barrier and ...rathecal route is used in the treatment of acute lymphocytic leu-...nia and some lymphomas. Cytotoxic drugs are injected into the ...rebral spinal fluid usually into the subarachnoid space via a lumbar puncture but drugs can also be injected into a ventricular space. Only certain drugs can be safely administered intrathecally: methotrexate, cytosine arabinoside, and thiotepa.

The box below highlights the key recommendations for prescribing, issuing, dispensing, transport, storage, and administration of intrathecal chemotherapy.

Fatal vinca alkaloid administration

Since 1985 at least 13 patients in the UK have died or been paralysed due to the erroneous intrathecal injection of vinca alkaloids (usually vincristine) causing severe or fatal neurotoxicity. Strict guidelines for everyone involved in intrathecal administration of cytotoxic drugs have now been implemented.

Full details of guidance for intrathecal administration can be found on www.dh.gov.uk. The implications of these guidelines for Scotland[1] are outlined at www.show.scot.nhs.uk/publicationsindex.htm

---

Intrathecal chemotherapy guidelines[2]

- A written local protocol must be in place.
- A register of named people trained and authorized to prescribe, dispense, issue, check, or administer IT chemotherapy must be kept and only those on the register can undertake these procedures.
- Those on the register must have specific education and an annual review of competence.
- Drugs should be transported by the administering doctor or designated pharmacist.
- IT drugs should be stored in a dedicated lockable container or refrigerator.
- IT drugs should be administered after intravenous drugs.
- IT drugs should only be issued following written confirmation that IV chemotherapy drugs have been administered.
- A specific area should be designated for IT administration.
- All IV vinca alkaloids should be clearly labelled. Avoid negative labelling.

---

1 Scottish Executive Health Department. HDL (2004). 30. *Safe Administration of Intrathecal Cytotoxic Chemotherapy.* Edinburgh: SEHD.
2 Department of Health. HSC 2003/010. (2003). *Updated National Guidance on the Safe Administration of intrathecal chemotherapy.* London: DH.

Intra-cavity

Cytotoxic drugs are instilled into body cavities such as the bladder (intravesical) and peritoneum. Malignant cells are therefore exposed directly to the drug maximizing effectiveness.

Intravesical

Intravesical chemotherapy is used following surgery to treat bladder cancer (📖 Bladder cancer). Patients are catheterized, residual urine in the bladder drained and the cytotoxic drug instilled slowly. The drug is retained for 2 hours either by clamping the catheter or removing it and asking the patient not to pass urine for 2 hours. Patients should be encouraged to change position every 15 minutes from back to front and from side to side so that all of the bladder mucosa is exposed to the cytotoxic drug. Drugs most commonly used are mitomycin C and doxorubicin.

Most drugs can irritate the bladder inducing chemical cystitis and a high fluid intake is recommended after the drug has been voided. Urinary frequency, urgency, and burning when passing urine are common following intravesical chemotherapy. Contact dermatitis may be experienced particularly with mitomycin C and this can be avoided by thorough washing of the hands and genitals immediately after instillation and subsequent voiding of urine. Sexually active patients should protect their partners from exposure to cytotoxic drugs by wearing a condom.

Few systemic side effects are experienced with mitomycin C and doxorubicin although allergic reactions have been reported with doxorubicin.

Intraperitoneal

The peritoneal cavity can act as a sanctuary site for tumour cells and cytotoxic drugs may be instilled to treat malignant ascites and control tumour growth. Intraperitoneal chemotherapy has been used primarily for treating ovarian cancer (📖 Ovarian cancer). Cytotoxic drugs can be delivered by a temporary suprapubic catheter, a Tenckhoff external catheter or an implantable port. Drugs are usually diluted in 2 litres of fluid, warmed and instilled by gravity.

Complications include catheter-related complications, abdominal pain, fatigue, haematological effects, metabolic abnormalities, and neuropathy. Respiratory distress, abdominal discomfort, and diarrhoea may also be experienced due to increased abdominal pressure. Infection is a further common problem and temperature should be monitored.

Subcutaneous and intramuscular routes

Few drugs are administered by these routes because of the potential for tissue damage, bleeding, discomfort and fibrosis. Drug absorption is also slow via these routes Drugs administered by these routes include: L-asparaginase and cytosine arabinoside.

The smallest needle size should be used and sites rotated to prevent side effects. For IM administration a large muscle and the Z track technique should be used to avoid leakage of the drug into the skin. Platelet counts should always be checked before administration to reduce the possibility of bruising and bleeding.

Intra-arterial

A high concentration of cytotoxic drug is delivered directly to the tumour by the artery that provides tumour blood supply. The concentration of drug to the tumour is increased while systemic circulation is decreased thus reducing the occurrence of side effects. Examples of use include cancers of the liver, pancreas, and colon.

Topical

Topical cytotoxic drugs may be used for skin lesions such as squamous cell carcinoma and T-cell lymphoma. 5% 5-fluorouracil cream is most commonly used. With repeated applications tissue necrosis and sloughing of dead tissue occurs. Normal tissue surrounding the lesion should be protected. Systemic effects are uncommon although slight nausea may occur.

Oral

(📖 Oral chemotherapy.)

Oral chemotherapy

Oral chemotherapy

The role of oral chemotherpy has markedly increased with the introduction of capecitabine in metastatic colorectal and breast cancer. Other examples of drugs given orally include etoposide, chlorambucil, and procarbazine. Many chemotherapy agents in development are also oral, so this trend towards oral chemotherapy is likely to continue.

Advantages of oral chemotherapy

There are many potential advantages:
• Most patients prefer it.
• Reduction of complications due to IV lines, pumps, e.g. spillage, infection.
• Shorter treatment time/reduction in patient–staff contact can free up nursing time for other service activities.
• Improved quality of life.
• Improved side effect profile.
• Cost effectiveness.

Potential risks

However, there are a number of important issues managing individuals receiving oral chemotherapy:
• Patients may think that oral chemotherapy is less serious or less dangerous than IV therapy.
• Patients have increased responsibly for administering their chemotherapy as well as monitoring and responding appropriately to adverse events.
• Patient compliance is difficult to assess. Patients need information about the importance of strict adherence to the prescribed drug regimen, the correct dosage, what to do if they miss a dose, and what to do if the have any side effects.

Note: it is essential to assess whether patients are able to safely manage an oral chemotherapy regime. Issues to consider include reading ability, manipulative abilities of elderly/frail patients, memory/concentration, support at home from family or other professionals.
• Patients have less contact time with staff. Patient education time may therefore be quite short, e.g. all initial vital information may need to be given at a one-off visit prior to treatment. Educational strategies and patient information material need to be well designed and evaluated.
• Oral drugs such as capecitabine have varied metabolism between patients, therefore dose modification and interruptions are a normal and essential part of therapy in response to any adverse events, i.e. hand and foot syndrome (HFS), diarrhoea, nausea and vomiting, mucositis. Absorption of oral drugs may also be affected by food, gastrointestinal problems e.g. nausea and vomiting or diarrhoea, and concurrent medications. In the presence of any of these factors patients may experience increased toxicity or a lower dose of drug than prescribed. These all raise important issues of education and compliance[1].

1 Chau I, Legge S, Fumoleau P. (2004). The vital role of education and information in patients receiving capecitabine (Xeloda®). *European Journal of Oncology Nursing*, **8**, Suppl 1, pp s41–53.

Patient compliance and education

To ensure that patients are safe in self-administering oral chemotherapy at home, effective patient education is essential. Pre-chemotherapy assessment clinics, dedicated oral chemotherapy clinics, and nurse-led follow-up (outpatient or telephone contact) are examples of developments that can support this process. Clear communication channels between primary and secondary care need to be developed. Well-designed information packs, treatment guides, and patient diaries will all help.

Patients may not wish to report adverse events if they think that dose reduction or interruption will reduce the efficacy of the drug. It is essential to inform patients that dose reductions up to 50% and short interruptions in treatment will not reduce the efficacy of their treatment.

Essential aspects of patient information and education include
• Correct dosage and administration schedule.
• Accurate and clear information about how to recognize, grade, and manage common side effects.
• Who to report to if any concerns.
• The role of dose reduction and interruptions.

Further reading

European Journal of Oncology Nursing (2004), **8**, Suppl 1.
Whole issue dedicated to issues of oral chemotherapy.

Administering vesicants and extravasation

Vesicant drugs have the potential to cause tissue damage and necrosis if extravasated. Extravasation is defined as infiltration of a drug into the subcutaneous tissues. The amount of damage usually correlates directly with the amount of drug infused. Damage may not be apparent immediately and it may be one or two days before evidence of progressive tissue damage occurs[1]. Damage can continue for several weeks after the extravasation. In severe cases extravasation can result in loss of function, or amputation. Surgical debridement or skin grafting may also be required. Prevention of extravasation is paramount when administering vesicant drugs. Extravasation is most frequently associated with peripheral cannulae but can also occur with the use of CVADs.

Table 17.4 Extravasation risk factors and prevention

Risk factors	Prevention
Previous chemotherapy as veins are often fragile and difficult to cannulate	Avoid small veins Avoid use of steel needles. Avoid veins adjacent to tendons, nerves, or arteries. Avoid sites distal to recent venepuncture or cannulation attempts
Previous radiotherapy	Avoid previously irradiated areas
Circulatory impairment e.g. lymphoedema, peripheral vascular disease, Raynauld's disease and comorbidity e.g. diabetes, superior vena cava syndrome	Administer vesicants first when vein integrity is greatest to reduce the risk of extravasation[2]. Administer bolus slowly into a fast running infusion. Check infusion flow quality, and cannula site regularly throughout infusion Never rush drug administration Never use infusion devices and pumps for vesicant drugs Use a PICC or central catheter for slow infusion of high risk drugs
No return blood flow from CVAD	Do not administer vesicant drugs before patency of CVAD is evaluated
Needle dislodgement with implanted ports	Monitor needle placement with continuous infusion of vesicants particularly during movement which increases the risk of dislodgement

---

1 Bertelli, G. (1995). Prevention and Management of Extravasation of Cytotoxic Drugs. *Drug Safety.* **12**(4): 245–255.

Table 17.5 NEIS Classification of cytotoxic drugs according to their potential to cause serious necrosis when extravasated (Reproduced with permission[2])

Group 1: neutral	Group 2: inflammitants	Group 3: irritants	Group 4: exfoliants	Group 5: vesicants
• Asparaginase.	• Etoposide. Phosphate.	• Carboplatin.	• Aclarubicin.	• Amsacrine.
• Bleomycin.	• Fluorouracil.	• Etoposide.	• Cisplatin.	• Carmustine.
• Cladribine.	• Methotrexate.	• Irinotecan.	• Daunorubicin. Liposomal.	• Dacarbazine.
• Cyclophosphamide.	• Raltitrexed.	• Teniposide.	• Docetaxel.	• Dactinomycin.
• Cytarabine.			• Doxorubicin. Liposomal.	• Daunorubicin.
• Edroclomab.			• Floxuridine.	• Doxorubicin.
• Fludarabine.			• Mitozanthrone.	• Epirubicin.
• Gemcitabine.			• Oxaliplatin.	• Idarubicin.
• Ifosfamide.			• Topotecan.	• Mitomycin.
• Melphalan.				• Mustine.
• Pentostatin.				• Paclitaxel.
• Rituximab.				• Streptozocin.
• Thiotepa.				• Treosulphan.
• Beta-interferons.				• Vinblastine.
• Aldesleukin (IL-2).				• Vincristine.
• Transtuzemab.				• Vindesine.
				• Vinoralbine.

There is some controversy about the vesicant nature of some drugs because of the difficulties in conducting extravasation research in human subjects. The National Extravasation Information Service[2], have classified drugs into five groups to help develop a grading system for extravasation risk. The higher the group number, the higher the risk of tissue damage if the drug extravasates.

Nurses administering chemotherapy should be knowledgeable about the vesicant properties of the drugs they are administering, observe the vein regularly during the administration procedure, recognize the signs and symptoms of extravasation, and be competent in managing such an emergency should it occur. Prompt recognition and management are imperative.

2 The National Extravasation Information Service. www.extravasation.org.uk updated October 2005. Accessed Feb 2006.

Recognizing extravasation

Signs of extravasation may initially be slight and neither nurses or patients may notice them. Patients should be asked to report any feelings of pain, burning or discomfort as they may quickly recognize if an injection feels different to previous experiences. Initially it may be difficult to differentiate between an extravasation and other reactions.

Table 17.6 Signs and symptoms of extravasation

Signs and symptoms	Other reactions complicating diagnosis
Erythema, discolouration, swelling, leakage, or a change in skin temperature	Flare reactions, common with drugs such as doxorubicin and epirubicin, often present as a red streak along the vein, blotchy skin, urticarial reactions, and pruritis. Flare reactions are temporary and subside within 30–90 minutes.
Burning stinging and pain	Venospasm may also result in pain on administration. Usually described as dull ache. Stinging and pain may occur with flare reaction.
Increased resistance to syringe or slowing of infusion rate	Patient position and kinking of administration set may also cause increased resistance
Lack of blood return	Can be misleading. The act of withdrawing blood can pull the cannula back into the vein and blood can be withdrawn. On recommencing administration extravasation occurs through the hole in the vessel wall exacerbating the injury.
	Vessel wall puncture can occur during venepuncture, the cannula remains in the vein and blood is returned but drugs can leak through the puncture hole into surrounding tissues[1].

Patient reports of pain, burning, or discomfort are particularly important for CVADs. Extravasation may not be immediately apparent. Signs and symptoms include:
• Difficulty withdrawing blood from CVAD.
• Shoulder pain—may be described as dull, aching, burning, or stinging sensation.
• Supraclavicular, chest wall or lower back pain can occur with extravasation from an implantable port.
• Pyrexia.
• Erythema, warmth and tenderness of chest wall or around port site.
• Pain and swelling along catheter tunnel or around port site.

---

1 The National Extravasation Information Service. www.extravasation.org.uk updated October 2005. Accessed Feb 2006.

Managing extravasation

Management of extravasation is controversial. Local protocols and procedures should be followed. Table 17.7 outlines generally accepted principles in the management of extravasation.

Table 17.7 Management of extravasation

Management	Rationale
Stop infusion immediately	Prevent further extravasation
Leave cannula in place	Allows aspiration of drug and administration of antidote
Inform doctor experienced in the management of extravasation injuries	Management of extravasation is controversial, an experienced person should always advise on management.
Mark affected area with a pen	Extravasated area is clearly marked
Aspirate as much of the drug as possible from the cannula. Subcutaneous injection of 0.9% sodium chloride may help to dilute the drug	Remove drug from tissues although it is recognized that little may be obtained
Remove the cannula For all drugs other than vinca alkaloids the principle of localize and neutralize is used. Ice packs should be applied regularly for 24–48 hours	Causes vasoconstriction and reduced local uptake of the drug
Topical dimethyl sulfoxide (DMSO) may be applied	Has been found to be particularly successful in the treatment of anthracycline extravasation
For vinca alkaloid extravasation administer subcutaneous hyaluronidase 1500 units as an antidote. Apply warm	The principle of spread and dilute is used for vinca alkaloid extravasation
Elevate the limb following the application of warm or cold packs.	To remove extravasated material while preserving the overlying skin
Some authorities advocate flushing the infiltrated area with 0.9% sodium chloride using multiple stab incisions in the subcutaneous tissue around the extravasated area.	
Accurately document the extravasation incident	

Side effects and complications

Common side effects and complications of chemotherapy are outlined in Table 17.8. Management of side effects and patient care are discussed in subsequent chapters.

Table 17.8 Short to medium side effects and complications

Short to medium side effects

Gastrointestinal
- Nausea and vomiting (can be delayed with some drugs e.g. cisplatin)
- Mucositis
- Constipation
- Diarrhoea
- Anorexia
- Taste changes
- Metallic taste (e.g. cyclophosphamide)

Skin and Nails
- Alopecia
- Plantar-palmar erythrodysaesthesis (hand/foot syndrome)
- Rash
- Erythema
- Hyperpigmentation
- Radiation recall
- Ridging of nails and Bowmans lines
- Nail loss

Bone marrow
- Myelosuppression, neutropenia, thrombocytopenia, and anaemia
- Is prolonged and delayed with some drugs e.g. carmustine, lomustine, melphalan, mitomycin C

General side effects
- Fatigue
- Flu-like symptoms
- Fluid retention and oedema (docetaxel, paclitaxel)

Reproductive system
- Amenorrhea/early menopause
- Infertility (particularly alkylating agents)

Cardiac
- Tachycardia and other rhythm disturbances
- Hypertension (mainly anthracyclines)

Neurological
- Peripheral neuropathy
- Autonomic neuropathy
- Cranial nerve neuropathy
- Ocular nerve toxicities

Renal and bladder
- Hyperuricaemia
- Coloured urine (doxorubicin, epirubicin, mitroxantrone)
- Haemorrhagic cystitis (cyclophosphamide, ifosfamide)

Complications
- Hypersensitivity reactions and anaphylaxis
- Tumour lysis syndrome
- Sepsis
- Pulmonary toxicity (e.g. pulmonary fibrosis with bleomycin, busulphan, chlorambucil, carmustine)
- Cardiomyopathy (anthracyclines)
- Neurotoxicity
- Ototoxicity (tinnitus and hearing loss with cisplatin)
- Nephrotoxicity
- Hepatotoxicity—l-asparaginase, amsacrine, carmustine, cisplatin, chlorambucil, dacarbazine, methotrexate) hepatic veno-occlusive disease (busulphan)
- Secondary cancers
- Cognitive dysfunction

Chemotherapy in the home setting

The use of chemotherapy in the home setting is likely to expand in the future with changes in the way health care is delivered (increasing move to outpatient care) and the increasing number of oral chemotherapy drugs available (📖 Oral chemotherapy). Nurses caring for patients at home need to be knowledgeable about the drugs the patient is receiving, potential side effects, safe handling, and who to contact if they need advice or support.

Before home administration is commenced it is vital that policies and procedures are developed for all aspects of cytotoxic drug administration including management of side effects and emergency situations e.g. spillage, extravasation, and hypersensitivity reactions. Safe handling guidelines and regulations should be adhered to at all times.

Considerations in home chemotherapy

- Drugs should be transported in a robust, tamper, and leak-proof contained, clearly marked cytotoxic.
- Drugs should be stored in the correct conditions in the patient's home and kept out of the reach of children and pets.
- Clear information on safely handling oral chemotherapy, e.g. hand washing, not crushing tablets.
- Disposal methods for cytotoxic drugs and waste should be clearly established.
- All necessary equipment should be available in the patient's home before drug administration including spillage and extravasation kits for IV chemotherapy.
- Administration and checking procedures should be adhered to.
- Clear communication pathways should be established between primary and secondary care.

New approaches in chemotherapy treatment

Targeted therapies

Cancer chemotherapy lacks specificity in its mechanism, targeting not only cancer cells, but any cells that happen to be dividing. Hence the wide range of toxicities, many of which are dose-limiting. In recent years the development of knowledge about cancer biology, combined with technological advances has enabled more effectively targeted therapies to be produced. New targets include cell signalling pathways, the cell cycle, metastatic spread, and angiogenesis. These drugs can be used alone or, more commonly, in conjunction with conventional therapies.
(📖 Biological therapies for more information).

Signal transductase inhibitors

Imatinib (Glivec®)

Cell growth is controlled by signalling pathways inside cells. Imatinib works by blocking faulty growth signalling pathways (in this case tyrosine kinase) within certain cancer cells. It has been used successfully to treat both chronic myeloid leukaemia (CML) and gastrointestinal stromal tumours (GIST). It also has the advantage of being given in tablet form. Side effects are generally mild, but include nausea, diarrhoea, leg aches or cramps, peripheral oedema, visual disturbances, and bone marrow suppression.

Epidermal growth factor receptor (EGFR) inhibitors

EGFR is a glycoprotein in the cell membrane. When a substance binds to the EGFR receptor, it causes activation of cell signals. EGFR is over-expressed in several cancers, eg breast cancer, and non-small cell lung cancer. Over expression of EGFR is associated with aggressive tumours, with a poor clinical outcome and resistance to chemotherapy.

Drugs which block EGFR could increase the sensitivity of chemo-resistant tumours to chemotherapy. Several EGFR inhibitors are currently under-going clinical trials to determine their place in therapy.

Cox-2 inhibitors

Cox-2 inhibitors are non-steroidal anti-inflammatory drugs (NSAIDs) which act by inhibition of an enzyme called cyclooxygenase-2 (COX-2). COX-2 expression is increased in cancer cells that are present in colon, breast, prostate, and lung cancer. COX-2 is also involved in angiogenesis. COX-2 inhibitors have been shown to have an anti-cancer effect in some of these tumours, but further trials are necessary before they become routine treatment.

New drug targets

Molecular biological targets of the future include further growth factor receptors, tyrosine kinases, angiogenesis, cyclo-oxygenase enzyme, onco-genes, telomerase enzyme, and immunological processes.

Research is being undertaken on how cancer cells detach from primary tumours to form metastases. At least one factor has been identified as a target for anti-metastatic agents. These agents would be administered after surgery to control any tumour that may be left behind.

Biological and targeted therapy will also be combined with traditional treatments such as chemotherapy and hormonal therapy for patients with metastatic disease, and may also have a role in cancer prevention in high-risk patients.

Overcoming resistance

New drug technologies are also being developed to overcome tumour resistance and drug toxicity. For example, Banoxantrone (AQ4N) is undergoing phase I and II clinical trials as a hypoxic cell-activated anti-tumour treatment. It uses the low oxygen conditions of cancer cells to convert it from an inactive form to its active, cytotoxic form. This methodology targets anti-cancer drugs to the tumour, minimising toxicity.

Further reading

Allwood M, Stanley A, Wright P (2001). *The Cytotoxics Handbook*, (4th edn), Oxford: Radcliffe Medical Press.

Barton-Burke M, Wilkes G M, Ingwerson K, (2001). *Cancer Chemotherapy: A Nursing Process Approach* (3rd edn). Boston: Jones & Bartlett.

Brighton D, Wood M, (eds) (2005). *The Royal Marsden Handbook of Cancer Chemotherapy*. Edinburgh: Elsevier.

Department of Health (2001). *National Guidelines on the Safe Administration of intrathecal chemotherapy*. London: DH.

Health and Safety Executive (1995). *Reporting Injuries, Diseases and Dangerous Occurrences Regulations* (RIDDOR). www.riddor.gov.uk (accessed Feb 2006).

Hormonal therapy

Background

Some tumours are hormone dependent, and their growth is stimulated by one of the sex hormones. These cancers can respond to hormonal therapy; they include breast, prostate, endometrium, renal cell, ovary, testis, and thyroid cancer.

Breast and prostate cancer treatment accounts for the vast majority of hormone therapy that is administered, and these are the main focus of this section.

Principles, uses, and therapeutic indications

The aim of hormonal therapy is to inhibit the production of the hormone influencing the cancer growth, or to block the effect of the hormone on the target organ. By inhibiting the action of the hormone, tumour cell growth can be slowed down, or the tumour volume can be shrunk. These treatments can often prolong survival for many years. However, hormone sensitive tumours can become resistant to hormonal therapy if the treatment fails to reduce the levels of hormones below the level needed for tumour cell growth.

The knowledge of how hormones or hormone antagonists act on cancer cells is the basis of hormone manipulation in cancer treatment. When a hormone enters a cell, it binds to a receptor. This receptor-hormone complex in turn stimulates the action of the hormone in the cell nucleus.

The strategies for hormonal therapy modifying tumour growth are:
- To reduce the overall amount of the stimulating hormone in the body.
- To prevent the hormone binding to a cell receptor by:
  - Competitive inhibition of the receptor site.
  - Reduction in receptor numbers.
- Blocking the hormone—receptor complex from activating the cell nucleus.

Key hormone targets in cancer therapy

Tumour type	Hormone to be blocked by treatment
Breast	Oestrogen
Endometrium	Oestrogen
Prostate	Testosterone

Oestrogen production

In pre-menopausal women the ovaries are the source of 90% of oestrogen production. This is regulated by the hypothalamus and the pituitary gland. If oestrogen levels are low the hypothalamus releases luteinizing hormone-releasing hormone (LHRH), also known as gonadotrophin hormone-releasing hormone (GHRH). This stimulates the release of the gonadotrophic hormones, luteinising hormone (LH) and follicle-stimulating hormone (FSH), by the pituitary. These stimulate the ovaries to produce oestrogen. Many tissues, including breast tissue, have specific receptors, which will be stimulated by oestrogen.

Around 10% of oestrogen is produced in subcutaneous fatty tissue under control of the adrenal glands. This continues after the menopause. The androgens that the adrenal gland produces are converted to oestrogen by the enzyme aromatase.

Testosterone production

Testosterone, an androgen hormone, is produced by the testes. A small amount is also produced by steroids released from the adrenal glands. Like ovarian production of oestrogen, it is under pituitary control, via LHRH and LH. Prostate tissue is dependent on androgens, mainly testosterone, for growth and function. Androgen receptors are found in the nucleus of prostate cells.

Hormonal therapy in prostate cancer aims to reduce testosterone production (LHRH analogues) or block the androgen receptors (anti-androgens).

Treatment decision making

There are now a number of different options involving hormone therapy for the treatment of breast and prostate cancer. Effective information on the impacts of these treatments on disease free and long term survival is starting to develop. However, information on the short and long-term quality of life impact of these treatments is currently scarce[1]. Patients need accurate and timely information and support to aid them in making decisions about the appropriate treatment approach (📖 Breast cancer: aromatase inhibitors).

Main hormone drugs

The mechanism of action, efficacy, and side effect profile for each medication is taken into account when deciding on the best hormonal therapy for a patient. In some cancers, notably breast cancer, it is possible to assess which hormone receptors are present in tumours. This ensures that the patient receives the most appropriate hormone treatment for the characteristics of their cancer.

The main classes of hormone treatments used in cancer include oestrogens, progestogens, and hormone antagonists. Examples of drugs in each of these classes and their use in treating different tumour types are shown in Table 18.1.

---

1 Fallowfield (2004). Evolution of breast cancer treatments: current options and quality-of-life considerations. *Eur J Oncol Nurs* **8**(2): 75–82.

Table 18.1 Commonly used hormonal therapies (more specific treatment information can be seen in chapters on breast cancer and prostate cancer)

Drug class	Mode of action	Tumour type	Drug
Oestrogen-receptor antagonist	Block oestrogen receptors	**Breast:** used as adjuvant in early breast cancer to reduce recurrence post-surgery. Can also be used as a neo-adjuvant, pre-surgery to shrink a tumour	• Tamoxifen
Aromatase inhibitors	Inhibit the conversion of androgens to oestrogens peripherally. This stops the stimulation of oestrogen-dependent tumours.	**Breast:** used first, second, or third line in post-menopausal breast cancer (📖 Breast cancer)	• Anastrozole • Exemestane • Letrozole • Fulvestrant • Toremifene
Progestogens	Directly reduce the adrenal and ovarian sex hormones and indirectly reduce pituitary gonadotrophin levels. Anti-oestrogen	**Endometrium Breast Prostate**	• Medroxyprogesterone acetate • Megestrol acetate
Luteinizing hormone-releasing hormone (LHRH) agonists	Treatment causes down-regulation of the pituitary, preventing luteinizing hormone (LH) release and causing a fall in testosterone serum levels in men and oestradiol serum levels in women	**Prostate:** used in a range of situations (see prostate caner) **Breast:** adjuvant treatment for pre-menopausal women with early disease. Also used in metasatatic diseae in pre-menopausal women. Initial treatment can cause a flare in symptoms by temporarily increasing hormone levels. Men can be treated with anti-androgens given immediately prior to and for the first few weeks of treatment. In women, these effects are managed symptomatically	• Buserelin • Goserelin • Leuprorelin • Triptorelin
Anti-androgens	Block testicular and adrenal androgens	**Prostate:** used alone or in combination with LHRH agonists	• Bicalutamide • Cyproterone acetate Flutamide
Oestrogens	Oppose the action of androgens. This suppresses the growth of androgen-dependent prostate cancer	**Prostate**	• Diethylstilbestrol • Ethinylestradiol

Assessment and management of side effects

As with any drug therapy, hormonal therapy can have side effects. Patients need to be assessed regularly for their response to treatment and any side effects they may be experiencing. The main side effects of the drugs are shown in Table 18.2.

The risks and benefits of treatment must be assessed if patients experience severe side effects. It is sometimes beneficial for patients to be prescribed another drug in the same class if they are experiencing severe side effects.

Management of menopausal symptoms

These can be severe and are generally worst in women who are initially pre-menopausal. Women with breast cancer are also currently advised not to take hormone replacement therapy (HRT), so are more likely to suffer from these symptoms.

Problems include
- Disruptions to the menstrual cycle, amenorrhoea.
- Hot flushes, night sweats, (can be severe).
- Difficulty sleeping, fatigue, depression.
- Joint pain, headaches.
- Vaginal dryness, painful intercourse.
- Psychological impact: ageing, body image, loss of fertility.

Patients need detailed and honest information about the whole potential impact of the menopause. An in-depth assessment is useful to plan with each individual what aspects of the menopause, if any, are major issues for her. A management package of pharmacological and non-pharmacological measures can then be planned.

Hot flushes (also occur with men having LHRH treatment)

Can range from frequent and severe, to mild. They can be very disruptive, may be accompanied by drenching sweats and can occur many times a day. They are generally more severe in those having cancer treatments rather than the natural menopause.

Pharmacological approaches
- Use of HRT is generally considered unsafe, due to oestrogen and the risk of breast cancer. However, there is controversy about whether HRT increases cancer recurrence.
- Gabapentin, SSRIs e.g. venlafaxine or paroxetine, clonidine. Many women find the side effect profile problematic (see *BNF* for further information).

Table 18.2 Common side effects of hormonal therapy

Drug	Common side effects
Tamoxifen	Increased risk of endometrial cancer, deep-vein thrombosis and stroke, mood swings, cataracts, hot flushes, fatigue, irregular menstrual cycles, vaginal discharge or bleeding, vaginal skin irritation, rashes, gastrointestinal disturbances, headache, visual disturbances
Anti-androgens	Loss of libido, impotence, damaged liver function, steroidal effects
Aromatase inhibitors	Hot flushes, osteoporosis, joint pains, drowsiness, fatigue, lethargy, rash, vaginal dryness, pain on intercourse
Progestogens	Nausea, fluid retention, weight gain, tremors, sweating, muscular cramps, Cushingoid features
Luteinizing hormone-releasing hormone (LHRH) analogues	Women: tumour flare, joint pains, loss of libido, fatigue Men: loss of libido, impotence, tumour flare, gynaecomastia
Oestrogens	Sodium retention with oedema, thromboembolism, jaundice, nausea, impotence, gynaecomastia (men)

Self-help/behavioural measures.

Many women will employ a range of self-help measures[1]:

- Behavioural modification, e.g. loose fitting layers of thin, absorbent clothes (cotton).
- Keeping diaries to identify patterns of flushing and exacerbating factors.
- Complementary therapies, e.g. evening primrose oil, black cohosh (limited evidence of effectiveness).

Cognitive strategies that have been effective include relaxation techniques. These may also improve other side effects and feelings of control in general[2] (📖 Progressive muscle relaxation therapy).

Osteoporosis

Dietary advice regarding increased calcium, exercise; improved fitness and muscle strength, monitoring for bone density. Dietary and exercise advice should also consider issues of weight gain.

Body image

(📖 Altered body image.)

Sexual health issues

(📖 Sexuality health and cancer.)

Further reading

Early Breast Cancer Trialists' Collaborative Group (2005). Effects of chemotherapy and hormonal therapy for early breast cancer on recurrence and 15 year survival: an overview of the randomized trials. *Lancet* **365,** 1687–717.

Erlichman C and Loprinzi C L (2001) Hormonal Therapies. In De Vita VT, Hellman S, Rosenberg S A, (eds). *Cancer Principles and Practice*, 6th edn, pp.478–88. Philadelphia Lippincott, Williams and Wilkins.

Souhami R L and Tobias J S (2005). *Cancer and Its Management*. 5th edn. Oxford: Blackwell.

National Institute for Clinical excellence (2006). Breast cancer (early)-hormonal treatments (appraisal consultation document). Accessed via www.nice.org.uk/page.aspx?o=318564

1 Fenlon D. (2005). Hormone Therapy. In Kearney N, Richardson A. (eds). *Nursing Patients with Cancer: Principles and Practice*, pp351–80. Edinburgh: Elsevier Churchill Livingstone.

2 Fenlon D. (1999). Relaxation therapy as an intervention for hot flushes in women with breast cancer. *European Journal of Oncology Nursing*, **3**, 223–31.

Biological therapy

Principles

Biological therapies aim to produce an anti-tumour effect, either by activating the patient's immune system, or by administering natural substances present in the immune system as treatments. These treatments cause an immune response in the patient that eliminates or delays tumour growth.

Increased knowledge of the molecular biology of cancer has led to the development of these treatments. Cancer biotherapy encompasses:

• Cytokines.
• Monoclonal antibodies.
• Vaccines.
• Cellular or humoral products.
• Gene therapy.

Biotherapies usually target the host cells that are involved in an immune response, rather than the tumour cells. Maximum tolerated doses of biotherapies may not be the ideal dose for modulating the immune system, and may be less effective than a lower dose. Higher doses may cause untoward side effects without increasing the desired biological effect. Lower doses of biotherapies may be more effective.

Most biological therapies produce similar side effects. These include acute side effects such as flu-like symptoms, i.e. fevers, chills, rigors, and myalgias. Other common side effects include fatigue, confusion, depression, and neurological side effects.

Further reading

Batchelor D (2005). Biological Therapy. In Kearney N and Richardson A (eds) *Nursing Patients with Cancer: Principles and Practice*, pp.303–28. Edinburgh: Elsevier Churchill Livingstone.

Battiato L A (2005). Biologic and targeted therapy. In Yarbro C H, Frogge M H, Goodman M (eds). *Cancer Nursing, Principles and practice*. 6th edn, pp.510–58. Massachusetts: Jones and Bartlett.

Hoffbrand A V, Pettit J E, Moss P A H (2001). *Essential haematology 4th ed.* Oxford: Blackwell Science.

Muehlbauer P M (2003). Antiangiogenesis in cancer therapy. *Seminars in Oncology Nursing*, **19**, 180–92.

Souhami R L and Tobias J S (2005). *Cancer and Its Management*, 5th edn. pp.105–7 Oxford: Blackwell.

Repetto L, Biganzoli L, Koehne G H et al. (2003). EORTC Cancer in the elderly taskforce guidelines for the use of colony-stimulating factors in elderly patients with caner. *European Journal of Cancer*, **39**, 2264–72.

Immunotherapy

Cytokines

Cytokines are soluble proteins, which have biological activity on several tissues, mainly on those originating from the immune system. The main cytokines that have therapeutic activity in cancer are:

- Interferons.
- Haemopoietic growth factors.

Interleukin-2 and tumour necrosis factor have also been used experimentally in some advanced cancers.

Interferons

Several types of interferon are produced by the immune system in response to viral infections. Interferon-alpha is the interferon used to treat a range of cancers (see box below).

Interferons have the following anti-tumour activity:
- They interfere with or directly stop tumour cell growth.
- They affect the expression of oncogenes.
- They make tumour cells more vulnerable to being killed by the immune system.
- They reduce the amount of blood vessels around the tumour.
- They promote tumour cells to change to less aggressive cells.

Cancers treated by cytokines

Interferon alpha
- Hairy-cell leukaemia
- Multiple myeloma
- Cutaneous T-cell lymphoma
- Malignant melanoma
- Carcinoid tumours
- Chronic myeloid leukaemia
- Non-Hodgkin's lymphoma
- Renal cell carcinoma
- Kaposi's sarcoma

Interelukin-2
- Renal cell
- Myeloid leukaemia
- Kaposi's sarcoma
- Metastatic malignant melanoma
- Non-Hodgkin's lymphoma

Tumourr necrosis factor
- Melanoma
- Sarcoma

The main *side effects* of interferons are: flu-like symptoms, anorexia, fatigue, rashes, gastrointestinal complaints, lethargy and thrombocytopenia. Flu-like symptoms can be treated with prophylactic paracetamol. Patients usually begin to tolerate the side effects of interferons after prolonged administration. The side effects are reversible once treatment stops. Slow release (pegylated) versions of interferons are now commercially available allowing less frequent administration than normal interferons.

Interleukins

Interleukins are cytokines produced by several immune system cells. They have an important role in mediating many immune responses. Interleukin-2 has been clinically evaluated and approved for the treatment of several advanced cancers: see box below.

Interleukin-2 is limited in clinical practice by its toxicity profile.

The main *side effects* are: flu-like symptoms, capillary leak syndrome, severe hypotension, angina, arrhythmias, respiratory distress, somnolence, anaemia, thrombocytopenia, and multi-organ failure.

Tumour necrosis factor (TNF)

TNF is a mediator of the inflammatory response. It is still an experimental treatment. The clinical use of TNF is limited by severe side effects, including acute fever, anaemia, thrombocytopenia, liver, renal, and central nervous system toxicity.

Haemopoietic growth factors

Haemopoietic growth factors are cytokines that have a role in controlling the formation and development of blood cells. Recombinant DNA technology has enabled synthetic production of naturally occurring growth factors for use in clinical practice[1]. They are primarily used to reduce the impact of bone marrow suppression caused by anti-cancer therapy. There are 3 main growth factors used in cancer care.

• Erythropoietin.
• Granulocyte colony-stimulating factor (G-CSF).
• Granulocyte-macrophage colony-stimulating factor (GM-CSF).

Erythropoietin (EPO)

EPO has a role in stimulating red blood cell production. In the cancer setting it is used to manage anaemia caused by chemotherapy (☐ Blood support).

Myeloid growth factors

Granulocyte colony stimulating factor (G-CSF) and granulocyte-macrophage colony stimulating factor (GM-CSF) are cytokines that regulate proliferation and differentiation of a range of haematopoietic cells. G-CSF. They can reduce the risk of neutropaenia, febrile neutropaenia, and infection in patients receiving myelosuppressive anti-cancer drugs. They are used with treatment where there is a high risk of febrile neutropaenia, e.g. high dose chemotherapy, blood and stem cell transplant settings. They can also be used to maintain the dose and schedule of drugs in standard chemotherapy regimes, e.g. testicular cancer, breast cancer. The EORTC[2] recommends their use in older patients receiving myelosuppressive chemotherapy, because of their higher risk of febrile neutropaenia and subsequent dose reduction. They are also used in mobilizing stem cells for stem cell harvest.

G-CSF has a short half-life and requires regular SC injections for each treatment. Pegylated G-CSF (pegfilgrastim) has an increased half-life and only one injection is required on each course of chemotherapy.

1 Gobel B H (2005). Hematopoietic Therapy. In Yarbro C H, Frogge M H, Goodman M (eds) Cancer Nursing, Principles and practice. 6th edn, pp.510–58. Massachusetts: Jones and Bartlett.
2 Repetto L, Biganzoli L, Koehne G H et al. (2003). EORTC Cancer in the elderly taskforce guidelines for the use of colony-stimulating factors in elderly patients with caner. *European Journal of Cancer*, **39**, 2264–72.

Monoclonal antibodies

Monoclonal antibody therapy is a new therapeutic modality that has been introduced into the treatment of some cancers. All cells have protein markers on their surface, known as antigens. Monoclonal antibodies are designed in the laboratory to recognize particular protein markers on the surface of some cancer cells. The monoclonal antibody then 'locks' onto this protein. Monoclonal antibodies have several mechanisms of action by which they destroy or prevent the replication of malignant cells, such as:

- Using tumour and natural immunology to kill the cell or to directly modulate tumour function.
- Carrying toxic therapy to specific cell targets by combining radionuclides, cytotoxic drugs, or cell toxins with the antibody.

Staff safety issues

Monoclonal antibodies are not infective, but as they are proteins, there is a theoretical risk of operator sensitization to non-human monoclonal antibodies on repeated exposure. However, there is little evidence to suggest this is a problem in practice. Ideally, the manipulation of mono-clonal antibody preparations should be undertaken in pharmacy aseptic facilities, to ensure operator protection from contamination, and patient protection from cross contamination.

- Vials should not be shaken to avoid prolonged foaming.
- It is important not to create aerosols when removing content from the vial.
- On addition of the vial's contents to an infusion bag, gently invert the bag to mix. Do not shake.

Hypersensitivity reactions

The most common side effects of monoclonal antibodies are infusion-related, including flu-like symptoms and a cytokine release syndrome. This is generally observed with the first or second dose, and the prob-ability of it occurring increases in patients with a large tumour burden or pulmonary insufficiency. The symptoms of this sort of reaction normally appear one or two hours after the infusion, and range from very mild to a severe and/or fatal anaphylactic reaction (☐ Anaphylaxis). It can also be associated with features of tumour lysis syndrome (☐ Tumour lysis syndrome). The risk of such reactions means that these drugs should be administered in areas where resuscitation equipment is available.

There are several examples of monoclonal antibodies, which have become standard treatments for some cancers:

Trastuzumab (Herceptin®)

Trastuzumab is a humanized monoclonal antibody used to treat breast cancer patients whose tumours over-express the HER-2 (human epidermal growth factor receptor-2) protein. The HER-2 protein is over-expressed in 20–30% of breast cancers and is a poor prognostic factor. Trastuzumab targets the HER-2 protein. Immunohistochemistry assays are required to assess whether patients are overexpressing the HER-2 protein. There is a standard scoring system (0, +1, +2, or +3). Patients with a HER-2 score of +3 are eligible for treatment with trastuzumab.

Trastuzumab works by:
- Down-regulating the HER-2 receptors.
- Inhibiting growth signal pathways.
- Engaging natural killer cells of the immune system to attack the tumour.
- Inducing cell lysis.
- Enhancing chemotherapy cytotoxicity.

Side effects:
- Fever or chills—can be prevented with prophylactic paracetamol.
- Hypersensitivity reactions (as above), can be delayed onset.
- Cardiotoxicity—patients' cardiac function must be monitored. (Echocardiography or MUGA scanning at baseline and then at three monthly intervals during treatment).

Rituximab

Rituximab is used for CD20-positive B-cell non-Hodgkin's lymphoma in combination with chemotherapy (usually CHOP). Rituximab binds the antigen CD20 on the cell surface, which is found in high levels on B-cell malignancies e.g. non-Hodgkin's lymphoma. This causes cell lysis.
- Infusion-related side effects of rituximab usually occur during the first infusion, and include fever, chills, and hypersensitivity reactions (see above).
- Patients should be pre-medicated with paracetamol and chlorphenamine to minimize these side effects.
- Patients at higher risk of this side effect include those with a high tumour burden, with pulmonary insufficiency, or tumour infiltration.
- Rituximab should be used with caution in patients receiving cardiotoxic chemotherapy, or in patients with cardiovascular disease.

Alemtuzumab (MabCampath®)

Alemtuzumab is a monoclonal antibody used for the treatment of B-cell chronic lymphocytic leukaemia. It has affinity for cells expressing the cell surface glycoprotein CD52. The CD52 glycoprotein is located on normal and malignant B and T lymphocytes, on natural killer cells, macrophages, monocytes, and male reproductive tissues. It binds to the antigen CD52 on the cell surface and causes the leukaemic cells to lyse via antibody-dependent cell-mediated cytotoxicity.

Alemtuzumab has a similar side effect profile to rituximab. Patients should be premedicated with paracetamol and chlorphenamine prior to the first dose, and any subsequent dose increases.

Bevacizumab (Avastin®)

Bevacizumab is a recombinant human monoclonal antibody against vascular endothelial growth factor (VEGF). VEGF is produced by most malignant cells, as it is required for the formation of blood vessels. In the UK it is licensed for treating metastatic colorectal cancer in combination with chemotherapy.

Cetuximab (Erbitux®)

Cetuximab is a monoclonal antibody against the epidermal growth factor receptor. In the UK it is licensed in combination with irinotecan chemotherapy for the treatment of metastatic colorectal cancer in patients with tumours expressing epidermal growth factor receptor that have failed on previous chemotherapy. It is also being trialled in locally advanced head and neck cancer.

Gemtuzumab (Mylotarg®)

Gemtuzumab is a monoclonal antibody targeted against CD33, which is found on the surface of myeloid cells. It is used in certain clinical trials to treat acute myeloid leukaemia. Gemtuzumab carries a chemotherapy drug, ozogamicin, directly to those targeted cells. Side effects include hypersensitivity reactions, nausea and vomiting, mucositis, bone marrow suppression, and abnormal liver function.

Other biological therapies

Vaccines

Tumour vaccines are a form of biological therapy. Trials are currently assessing the activity of vaccines for melanoma, lymphoma, kidney, ovarian, colorectal, breast, prostate, and lung cancers. Tumour vaccines are being developed in several different ways:

- Tumour vaccines are in development for cancers that are caused by a virus, such as the human papilloma virus (HPV) and the human retrovirus (HTLV).
- Vaccines are also in development for cancers that are not caused by a virus. Tumour cells or extracts of tumour cells can be used as cancer vaccines to enhance an immune response to the relevant tumours.
- Tumour vaccines using tumour-associated antigens are also being developed. These vaccines work by stimulating the immune system to recognize and destroy specific cancer cells.

Anti-angiogenesis agents

Angiogenesis is the formation of new blood vessels, which is essential for the growth and spread of a tumour beyond $1mm^3$. Therapeutic strategies for interfering with angiogenesis are being developed, and include the inhibition of substances that are involved in the angiogenic process. Anti-angiogenesis agents interfere with the angiogenesis process, and therefore prevent the growth of new blood vessels, halting the growth of the tumour.

Several agents may inhibit angiogenesis through several pathways, some of which are unknown. Some agents that have been shown to have anti-angiogenic activity in clinical trials include thalidomide (not a biological therapy), penicillamine, interleukin-12, captopril, taxanes, and matrix metalloproteinases inhibitors (MMPIs). MMPIs are undergoing trials to assess their efficacy in preventing tumour growth in breast, non-small cell lung cancer (NSCLC), gastric, pancreatic, colon, ovarian, and hormone-refractory prostate cancer.

Gene therapy

The development of genetically modified viruses, and advances in cloning and sequencing the human genome, has led to the development of gene therapy clinical trials for a wide variety of diseases, including cancer. The term 'gene therapy' applies to any clinical therapeutic procedure in which genes are intentionally introduced into human cells. Genes are delivered to the nucleus of target cells by vectors, in a process called gene transfer. Genetically modified (GM) viruses have proved to be the most efficient way of delivering DNA.

Currently, the majority of gene therapy clinical trials in cancer use a gene addition strategy, whereby a gene or genes may be 'added' to a cell to provide a new function, e.g. adding tumour suppressor genes to cancer cells. Gene therapy has been used in clinical trials for pancreas, lung, prostate, breast, and bladder cancer.

There are potential infectious hazards with gene therapy, which include possible transmission of infection to hospital personnel and the environment. Gene therapy products should therefore be manipulated in pharmacy aseptic units. A risk assessment should be made for each product, with input from the lead investigator or the trust's biological safety officer.

Cell based therapy

Cell based therapy is often a combination of a tumour vaccine and gene therapy.

- Tumour vaccines are being developed using tumour cells that are being genetically modified to induce an immune response in the patient to that tumour type.
- Cell based gene therapy uses the patient's host cells (often blood cells), which are incubated with a gene therapy vector containing a therapeutic gene. This results in engineered cells that contain the therapeutic gene. These engineered cells are injected back into the patient. This is called ex-vivo gene therapy.

Future advances

There will be a continuing increase in the knowledge of cancer and related biology, plus technological advances, which allow more accurate and quicker mapping of genes, more accurate diagnosis and delivery of drugs. These may lead to more individually tailored treatments. Vaccines to prevent cancer, or reduce risk may be just over the horizon. However, it is always difficult to predict the future. Gene therapy was hailed as the new breakthrough over 20 years ago and has yet to make a major impact. Yet few people foresaw the introduction of a tablet, imatinib, with few side effects that would fundamentally change the outlook for individuals with chronic myeloid leukaemia.

Management of common side effects of biological therapies

Chills and rigors

These begin after around 30 minutes, and can last for up to 90 minutes. Pre-medication with paracetamol and chlorphenamine. Medicating with pethidine is an option. Provide warmth (hot water bottles, blankets), reassurance (can be very frightening for both patient and carers)

Fever and sweating

Occurs after chills, often with headache, tachycardia and hypotension. Pre-medication with paracetamol. Encourage increased fluid and food intake.

Muscle and joint pains

Paracetamol, warmth, and comfort measures.

Side effects

Fatigue, hypersensitivity reactions, breathlessness, weight loss, nausea and vomiting, and diarrhoea are covered in the appropriate chapters under those headings).

High dose therapy (autologus transplant)

Principles and uses

Many haematological cancers are treated more effectively by higher doses of chemotherapy and radiotherapy than by lower doses. Continuing to escalate the dose given will theoretically increase the cure rate. However, the dose-limiting factor is the toxicity to normal tissues. The first tissue to be seriously affected is the bone marrow. Bone marrow suppression results in:

• Neutropenia—with increased risk of infection particularly by bacteria and fungi.
• Anaemia—with resulting dependence on red cell transfusions.
• Thrombocytopenia (low platelets)—with increased risk of bleeding and dependence on platelet concentrate transfusions.

High dose therapy (HDT) with autologous stem cell support, has been developed to overcome the problem posed by bone marrow toxicity (see Table 20.1). High doses of chemotherapy and/or radiotherapy are administered, followed by the infusion of haematopoietic (blood forming) stem cells. These have been previously collected from the patient and stored, in order to speed the recovery of the bone marrow and to minimize the risk of resulting marrow suppression. HDT is used routinely in a number of situations.

Note: high dose therapy should in theory improve survival for patients with solid tumours. However, results from clinical trials of HDT in solid tumours have been extremely disappointing.

Stem cell priming, collection, and storage

Prior to the HDT procedure, stem cells from the patient must be collected and stored. The most common way of collecting stem cells is peripheral blood stem cell (PBSC) collection.

Stem cell priming

Two approaches are used to increase the number of haematopoietic blood cells circulating in the peripheral blood of the patient (stem cell priming):

1. Chemotherapy is administered to the patient. The number of circulating stem cells increases as the bone marrow recovers from the suppression caused by the chemotherapy. About 10% of patients require admission for neutropenic fever as a result of the conditioning chemotherapy.

2. Growth factor (G-CSF) is administered. This appears to encourage the haematopoietic stem cells in the marrow to dislodge and enter the peripheral circulation. G-CSF is very safe and well tolerated, although it may produce bone pain which is usually responsive to simple analgesia.

The stem cell collection is usually scheduled for 8–10 days after the initial chemotherapy is given. In some centres, a specialized blood test can be used to determine the number of immature blood cells circulating in the blood stream, and therefore the best time to collect.

Table 20.1 Indications and outcome for HDT with autologous stem cell support (placing)

Indication	Intended outcome of HDT
Myeloma (front line therapy)	Increase survival by approximately one year
Relapsed Hodgkin's lymphoma responsive to chemotherapy	Potentially curative
Relapsed high grade non-Hodgkin's lymphoma responsive to chemotherapy	Potentially curative
Relapsed low grade non-Hodgkin's lymphoma responsive to chemotherapy	Induce a prolonged remission (unlikely to cure)

Stem cell collection

PBSC collection is achieved by an apheresis procedure. Blood from the patient is passed through an apheresis machine. The machine is programmed to collect white blood cells with a molecule on the surface called CD34. This marks out immature blood cells, and some of these cells will be haematopoietic stem cells. These are separated from the rest of the blood, and the remainder of the blood is returned to the patient.

To collect sufficient cells, the patient typically needs to spend 3–4 hours per day on the machine, for up to 2 or 3 consecutive days. The most common complication is citrate toxicity, which occurs because citrate is used in the machine tubing to prevent the blood from clotting. This can reduce blood calcium, which is managed by taking oral calcium. Other complications include reduced platelet count and venous damage.

Special rigid lines or large bore peripheral cannulae are required for apheresis due to the high rate of blood withdrawal and return.

Bone marrow harvest is a less common way of collecting stem cells directly from the patient. This involves a general anaesthetic, and multiple punctures of the posterior portion of the iliac crest, with a bone marrow aspirate needle. The main side effects are post-operative pain, anaemia requiring a blood transfusion, and complications of the anaesthetic.

Stem cell storage

Stem cells are stored in liquid nitrogen. A chemical called DMSO is added to the cells before freezing, to protect them from the freezing process. Stem cells can be stored for as long as is needed, although if they have been stored for many years, a check on their viability may be performed before they are re-infused into the patient.

Conditioning

Chemotherapy and/or radiotherapy administered prior to stem cell infusion is called conditioning chemotherapy. The role of conditioning therapy in autologous transplantation is simply to kill the cancer. The type of chemotherapy depends upon the condition being treated. Regimens commonly used in the UK are outlined in Table 20.2.

Note: by convention, the day of stem cell infusion is termed day zero (D0).

Stem cell administration

On the day of stem cell infusion (D0), the frozen bags containing the cells are brought to the ward. They are placed in a water bath to thaw them, prior to being administered to the patient. The usual means of infusion is via a central venous catheter, although a peripheral cannula can also be used.

The most common complication of a stem cell infusion is an allergic-type reaction to the DMSO. The patient may complain of an itch or a wheeze or they may develop an urticarial rash. Before the stem cells are given, the patient receives a pre-med of chlorpheniramine 4mg orally or 10mg IV and hydrocortisone 100mg IV. In severe cases, anaphylaxis may occur with severe bronchospasm, tachycardia, and hypotension.

The patient is carefully and frequently monitored during and shortly after the stem cell infusion, which is carried out according to local ward protocols. A mild reaction may be treated with:
• Slowing the infusion.
• Hydrocortisone 100mg IV.

A more severe reaction should be treated as an anaphylactic episode (□ Anaphylaxis).

Patients are also pre- and post-hydrated to counter the dehydrating effects of the DMSO. Urine output is carefully monitored throughout. Nausea and sometimes vomiting are also side effects of the DMSO; this should be managed preventatively, with anti-emetics. The number of bags of stem cells given depends upon the dose of stem cells per bag. This is highly variable and depends upon how well the stem cells were mobilized during the harvest. If many bags are given, the patient may develop a headache, lethargy, and possible renal or liver impairment as a result of DMSO toxicity.

Table 20.2 Common conditioning regimens in the UK

Name of regimen	Drugs administered	Condition
BEAM	• Bleomycin • Etoposide • Cytarabine (Ara-C) • Melphalan	• Relapsed Hodgkin's lymphoma • Relapsed high or low grade NHL
High dose melphalan	• Melphalan	• Myeloma
Cy/TBI	• High dose cyclophosphamide • Total body irradiation	• Lymphoblastic lymphoma • Relapsed acute leukaemia

Nursing issues of high dose therapy

Patients who have had high dose therapy are prone to similar side effects to those who have had standard chemotherapy regimes. However, these are often more severe, prolonged, and patients may face a range of concurrent side effects. The specific side effects are dependent on the drug regimens.

Bone marrow suppression

Neutropenia: the more prolonged a neutropenia, the greater the risk of severe and overwhelming infection, with patients at risk of septic shock and becoming extremely unwell very quickly (⊞ Neutropaenic sepsis). Continued immunosuppression post-transplant can increase risk of fungal infections and pneumocytis carinii pneumonia. Patients are often supported with G-CSF to ensure rapid maturation of newly forming neutrophils (⊞ Biological therapy). This can reduce neutropenia from near 21 days, to around 10–14 days. Patients need to be informed about signs and symptoms of longer-term infections as well as the need to immediately contact their GP or the hematology centre about any potential signs of infection.

Anaemia and thrombocytopenia (⊞ Bone marrow suppression)
Nursing assessment includes: daily weight, regular observations, and observation for any signs and symptoms of infection, including daily line site dressings.

Mucositis

This can be severe. Patients may require opioids to relieve pain and IV fluid support due to inability to take oral fluids. Nutritional support is normally in the form of supplements (⊞ Oral mucositis).

Diarrhoea

Often develops at the same time as oral mucositis. This should be actively managed with IV fluids and loperamide (as indicated) to prevent dehydration (⊞ Diarrhoea).

Alteration in taste

This often occurs because of the high dose of the drugs used and because of the mucositis. It can be a troubling symptom and can take many months to resolve.

Veno occlusive disease (VOD)

(⊞ Haematopoietic stem cell transplant)

Late side effects

Late side effects of high dose therapy are also regimen dependent. For those receiving radiotherapy, cataracts and long-term infertility are common. Cataracts are unusual in chemotherapy only regimens. The risk of infertility is more variable in chemotherapy only regimens. It is more common in older women (⊞ Sexual health and cancer).

Patients receiving high dose therapy can require intensive nursing support, involving:

• Administering IV fluids, a range of anti-microbial agents and nutritional support.
• Regular vital signs and blood count monitoring, daily weights.
• Administering blood and platelet support.
• Managing the infection risk and severe pain from mucositis.
• Limiting the psychological effects of isolation and boredom, and separation from family.
• Psychological support for both the patient and the family facing a life threatening illness and rigorous treatment regimen. For some this may be their first hospital experience, or their first experience away from their usual haematology centre.

Such intensive nursing is rewarding but can also be extremely stressful. Nurses in such areas should have access to support networks such as clinical supervision.

Further reading

Atkinson J and Richardson C (2006). Blood and Marrow Transplantation. In Grundy M. (ed) *Nursing in haematological oncology* 2nd ed. pp265–92. Edinburgh: Elsevier, Baillière Tindall.

Gaston-Johansson F, Lachica E M, Fall-Dickson J M, *et al.* (2004). Psychological distress, fatigue, burden of care, and quality of life in primary caregivers of patients with breast cancer undergoing autologous bone marrow transplantation. *Oncology Nursing Forum*, **31**(6), 1161–9.

Hoffbrand A V, Pettit J E, Moss P A H (2001). *Essential haematology 4th ed.* Oxford: Blackwell Science.

Larsen J, Nordstrom G, Ljungman P, and Gardulf A (2004). Symptom occurrence, symptom intensity, and symptom distress in patients undergoing high-dose chemotherapy with stem-cell transplantation. *Cancer Nursing*, **27**(1), 55–64.

Lewis A (2005). Autologous stem cells derived from the peripheral blood compared to standard bone marrow transplant; time to engraftment: a systematic review. *International Journal of Nursing Studies*, **42**(5), 589–96.

National Institute for Clinical excellence (2003). *Guidance on Cancer Services- Improving Outcomes in Haematological Cancers: The Manual.* London: NICE.

Quinn B. and Stephens M. (2005). Bone Marrow Transplantation. In Kearney N. and Richardson A. (eds) (2005). *Nursing Patients with Cancer: Principles and Practice.* Edinburgh: Elsevier Churchill Livingstone.

Souhami R L and Tobias J S (2005). *Cancer and Its Management.* 5th edn. Oxford: Blackwell.

Yarbro CH, Frogge MH, Goodman M (eds) (2005). *Cancer Nursing, Principles and practice.* 6th edn. Massachusetts: Jones and Bartlett.

Allogeneic haemopoietic stem cell transplantation

Principles

An allogeneic stem cell transplant is where the source of haemopoietic (blood forming) stem cells is from someone other than the patient. There are a number of reasons why an allogeneic stem cell transplant may be useful:

- It enables high doses of chemotherapy to be given, while minimizing the time spent with low blood counts, due to bone marrow suppression. The high doses of chemotherapy are given to increase the chance of eradicating the underlying cancer.
- Autologous stem cells (☐ High dose therapy) used in people with haematological malignancies may well be contaminated with cancer cells. An allogeneic source of stem cells prevents this.
- The main benefit is thought to be due to the graft-versus-malignancy (GvM) effect (see below).

Graft versus malignancy (GvM)

Haemopoietic stem cells produce all of the cellular components of blood, including the lymphocytes. Lymphocytes are designed to recognize anything that is not of the host (i.e. non-self) and attack it. Lymphocytes made from a stem cell that is not from the patient (i.e. is *not* derived from an allogeneic donor) will recognize the patient as non-self. This has the beneficial effect of seeing the patient's cancer cells as non-self and attacking them—the so-called GvM effect. On the other hand, the lymphocytes will also recognize the patient's normal tissues as non-self and attack them. This causes the potentially serious side effect of allogeneic stem cell transplantation called graft-versus-host disease (GvHD)—see Fig. 21.1 and below.

Uses

The main indications for allogeneic stem cell transplantation are:

- Poor risk acute myeloid leukaemia in first remission.
- Relapsed acute myeloid leukaemia in second remission.
- Poor risk (especially Philadelphia chromosome positive) acute lymphoblastic leukaemia in first remission.
- Chronic myeloid leukaemia (although the introduction of imatinib is changing the initial management of this condition).
- Aplastic anaemia.

Less common indications include chronic lymphocytic leukaemia, myelodysplasia, relapsed high or low-grade non-Hodgkin's lymphoma, myeloma, myelofibrosis.

Donor source

There are two main sources of donor:

- Matched sibling (brother or sister): this is normally the preferred type of donor. Matching is done using the human leukocyte antigen (HLA) system (see box over page).
- Matched unrelated donor (MUD)—also known as voluntary unrelated donor (VUD). The complication rate is higher using this sort of donor.

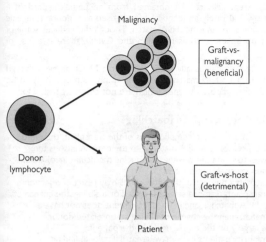

Fig. 21.1 Mechanism of graft-versus-malignancy and graft-versus-host effect.

Occasionally, stem cells can be obtained from an umbilical cord of a newborn baby, and rarely an identical twin is used as a donor (syngenic transplant). These are an exact HLA match. Though this reduces some of the risks of transplant, such as rejection and GvHD, there is a loss of GvM effect.

Note: a sibling donor is usually preferred over a MUD, as even though both donors may be fully matched, a sibling donor is more likely to be matched for other important genes, which are not currently tested for.

Human leukocyte antigen matching

- In order to minimize the complications of the transplant, the donor should be a reasonable HLA match with the patient. HLA is the name given to a number of genes producing molecules involved in the immune recognition process.
- A mismatch in a number of the HLA genes may result in rejection of the transplant, or more severe GvHD. For a sibling, the chance of being an HLA match is one in four. If a patient does not have a sibling match, then the chance of finding an unrelated donor depends largely on the ethnic origin of the patient.
- Ethnic minority patients often have great difficulty in finding a match due to the relatively low number of donors from a similar group (and therefore of a similar genetic make-up) on the transplant registers.

Stem cell collection

Collection of stem cells from the donor is similar to that used for the collection of autologous stem cells from a patient (📖 High dose therapy). The main difference is that priming only involves the use of growth factor injections, and no chemotherapy is used. Some concerns have been raised over the potential long-term effects of using G-CSF in a healthy donor, but there is currently no evidence to support these.

Complications of allogeneic transplant

This section will deal with complications specific to allogeneic stem cell transplantation. High dose chemotherapy and radiotherapy used in the conditioning process also have their own associated complications (⊞ High dose therapy).

Graft-vs-Host Disease (GvHD)

GvHD is caused by donor T lymphocytes recognizing and attacking the recipient's normal tissues. If this occurs within 100 days of the transplant, it is called acute GvHD; if it persists or develops after 100 days it is called chronic GvHD. Whilst a small amount of GVHD is thought to be a positive development, enhancing the GvM effect, extensive GVHD can be a life threatening complication.

Predisposing factors include:
- HLA mismatched transplant.
- CMV seropositive patient.
- Increasing age of the patient and donor.
- Sex mismatched transplant.

Clinical features

Acute GvHD frequently involves:
- Skin—erythema which may progress to blistering and desquamation.
- Gut—diarrhoea which may progress to abdominal pain, ileus formation and perforation.
- Liver—mild alteration in LFTs, jaundice which may progress to fulminant hepatic failure.

Chronic GvHD may affect any organ. It may result in thickened, fibrotic skin; sore, dry mouth; dry vagina; photosensitive or dry eyes; hepatitis; lung involvement with an obliterative bronchiolitis.

Prevention

A number of measures are taken to reduce the risk of GvHD:
- Donor selection: a good HLA match (see above) reduces the risk of GvHD.
- Immunosuppression—various immunosuppressive agents which damp down T-lymphocyte activity are used, e.g. ciclosporine.
- Low dose methotrexate boluses are often used in the early post-transplant period to prevent GvHD.
- T-cell depletion of the transplant. Although this is effective in reducing GvHD, it is also thought to reduce the GvM effect, leading to higher rates of relapse.

Management

Severe, acute GvHD requires intensive medical and nursing input.
- Accurate measurement of stool volumes should be attempted, as this determines the severity of gut GvHD and guides treatment. Attention is required to the skin around the anus as this may become excoriated and a site for infection. Strict fluid balance and fluid replacement. Gut biopsy may be indicated.

- Regular fluid balance assessment including daily or twice daily weight.
- Careful attention to pressure areas.
- Regular temperature, pulse, blood pressure, respiratory rate, saturations.
- Daily urea & electrolyte, magnesium, calcium and phosphate with replacement of depleted electrolytes.
- Patients with GvHD are immunosuppressed, so that frequent septic screens are needed (blood cultures, CMV, urine cultures, chest X-ray, stool cultures).
- Symptomatic treatment involves:
  - Diarrhoea: loperamide and possibly octreotide. Barrier creams to prevent excoriation, sudocrem or metanium with olive oil to clean. Ensure ciclopsorin and other drugs are given IV so as to ensure absorption.
  - Liver failure: avoidance of sedatives, monitoring of electrolytes, and blood glucose. Reviewing of all IV drugs so as to reduce toxicity on the liver.
  - Pain: paracetamol initially, but opioids are often necessary. Involvement of the acute pain team or palliative care team may be indicated if difficult to manage.
  - Skin: pressure area care needs to be managed extremely carefully, with regular turning and special mattresses essential.
- Specific treatment involves:
  - Continuing GvHD prophylaxis usually with ciclosporin or tacrolimus. Ciclosporin levels are monitored frequently to ensure correct dosing and minimize toxicity.
  - IV high dose steroids (methylprednisolone).

Note: if the GvHD is steroid resistant, the outlook is extremely poor, with a very high mortality rate. Other immunosuppressant options exist.

GvHD nursing

Nursing a patient with severe GvHD is extremely complex and stressful. The symptoms are difficult to manage. The effect on the patient's body image and self-esteem can be dramatic. In the worst-case scenario, a patient may have a combination of skin desquamation, severe liver failure, and continuous uncontrollable diarrhoea. They may be confused and in severe pain. Intensive physical and psychological support is required for both the patient and their family. These patients need at least one-to-one nursing care, possibly even more at times. Involvement of palliative care specialists can support effective symptom management and work with the emotional distress of the family and other carers.

Veno-occlusive disease (VOD)

Hepatic VOD is due to the obstruction of small blood vessels within the liver, which causes damage to the surrounding liver cells. It usually occurs due to the chemotherapy and/or radiotherapy given during an allogeneic stem cell transplant. Increasing age, previous hepatic disease or dysfunction and prior intensive chemotherapy are risk factors for developing VOD. Although approximately half of all cases resolve, the mortality rate can be over 90% in severe cases.

Clinical features
The following occur within 21 days of the transplant:
- Enlarged liver.
- Ascites.
- Weight gain >5% from baseline.
- Raised bilirubin.

Prevention
A continuous infusion of low-dose unfractionated heparin is often used during the transplant period to reduce the risk of VOD.

Treatment
- Supportive care:
  - Ascites: low salt diet, avoid saline infusions, cautious use of loop diuretics such as furosemide.
  - Confusion (hepatic encephalopathy): avoid sedatives and opiate analgesia, correct known causative factors such as constipation, electrolyte imbalance, and infection.
  - Avoid drugs which damage the liver and ensure ciclosporin level is not too high as the kidneys are at risk of damage.
- Specific treatment:
  - IV defibrotide infusion.

VOD nursing

Continuous assessment of fluid balance, and abdominal girth and weight is essential. It allows assessment of the distribution of the patient's body fluids, guiding appropriate therapy. Patients can be confused, requiring psychological support and maintenance of a safe environment. They may also develop respiratory symptoms due to hepato/splenomegaly and pleural effusion. If liver damage is severe then pain management can be problematic and may require support from the specialist palliative care team.

Cytomegalovirus (CMV) reactivation and CMV disease

CMV is a common infection in children and young adults. After the acute infection, the virus persists in the body without causing disease (a state called latency). If that person then becomes profoundly immunosuppressed, the virus can reactivate. They may be initially asymptomatic (see Fig. 21.2), but continued reactivation leads to CMV disease, which can be very serious.

In the past, CMV disease was a major killer of stem cell transplant patients, but with improved detection of reactivation *before* it can cause disease, along with treatment at this stage (called pre-emptive treatment), death from CMV disease is now rare.

CMV management
The patient and their donor are tested for CMV immunoglobulin prior to the transplant. If the patient or the donor were CMV positive, then the patient is tested regularly for CMV reactivation. If 2 consecutive tests are positive then treatment with ganciclovir is commenced. Foscarnet is used for ganciclovir-resistant cases.

Prevention of CMV
- Aciclovir prophylaxis is often given to transplant patients where the donor or the recipient is sero-positive.
- If the patient and donor were CMV sero-negative, patients receive CMV negative blood products before and after the transplant.

Note: the risk of transmission of the virus in leucodepleted blood products (which are now routinely used) is very low, and in an emergency CMV unscreened products can be used.

CMV disease
CMV may manifest in a variety of ways but it most commonly causes colitis (with bloody diarrhea) or pneumonitis (with cough and breathlessness). Treatment is as for CMV reactivation, i.e. ganciclovir and foscarnet for ganciclovir-resistant cases. IV immunoglobulin can also be used.

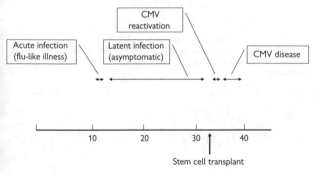

Fig. 21.2 Stages of CMV infection in a patient who has an allogeneic stem cell transplant aged 32.

Other infections

Stem cell transplant patients are susceptible to a wide variety of infections, due to profound immunosuppression. The most common are bacterial, causing line infections, pneumonias, urinary tract infections, and septicaemia.

The exact treatment depends on the type of infection and the time elapsed since the transplant. A patient who has recently had a transplant should be treated urgently with broad spectrum antibiotics, even if they are not neutropenic, as they remain profoundly immunosuppressed (see Table 21.1).

Interstitial pneumonia syndrome (IPS)

IPS may occur anytime, from a few days to several months after treatment when the patient has returned home. High-dose chemotherapy/radiotherapy can directly damage the cells of the lungs. A dry non-productive cough or shortness of breath are early manifestations of IPS. Any patient experiencing these symptoms after high dose therapy should be seen by a haematology doctor immediately, since this can be a fatal complication. It is essential that patients, carers, and their GPs are fully informed about this risk.

Long-term survival

Allogeneic stem cell transplantation is a high-risk procedure. The mortality rate from the procedure varies greatly according to:
- Age.
- Disease being transplanted.
- Remission status at time of transplant.
- Type of transplant (sibling versus MUD).
- CMV status of donor and recipient.

For conventional transplantation in a young person, the usual mortality rate of the procedure is in the region of 15–20% for a matched sibling transplant.

Table 21.1 Relatively common oinfections in allogeneic stem-cell transplant patients

Infection	Clinical problem	Treatment
Invasive fungal infection e.g. *Aspergillus*	Pneumonia (common), abscesses e.g. liver, brain	Antifungals e.g. amphotericin, voricaonazole, caspofungin
Pneumocystis carinii pneumonia (PCP)	Pneumonia (may cause pneumothorax)	High dose co-trimoxazole
Respiratory syncytial virus (RSV)	Pneumonitis	Nebulized ribavirin

Reduced intensity conditioning (RIC) transplants

The high mortality rate of a conventional transplant means that it is only suitable for patients up to their mid 40s. This is due to the intensity of the conditioning chemotherapy, which typically involves high dose cyclophosphamide and total body irradiation.

In an attempt to reduce the mortality rate and extend the age limit, RIC transplants have been developed. These use more gentle conditioning regimens with the aim of preventing graft rejection by the patient.

Once the transplant has engrafted, more reliance is placed on the graft-versus-malignancy effect to eradicate any residual disease. Various protocols have been developed with more or less intense conditioning regimens. In the UK, a typical conditioning regimen involves fludarabine and melphalan or cyclophosphamide with or without alemtuzumab to deplete T-cells.

Although regarded as experimental, RIC transplants are increasing in popularity. The indications are as for conventional transplantation (see above) but the age and fitness of the patient are less of a consideration. RIC's are now commonly performed in patients into their 60s. The mortality is around 10% and it is still too early to predict their long-term efficacy for cure.

Donor lymphocyte infusions (DLI)

In the event of a relapse after an allogeneic stem cell transplant, one treatment option available is DLI. Lymphocytes are collected from the original donor—this usually requires just one additional apheresis session (with no priming required).

The lymphocytes are then infused into the patient at a given dose, according to the patient's weight. The T-lymphocytes in the infusion then recognize the patient's cancer cells as non-self and attack them.

The lymphocytes themselves would normally be rejected by the patient, but they are not, due to the previous stem cell transplant. The main disadvantage of DLIs is that they can induce graft-versus-host disease.

Further reading

Atkinson J and Richardson C (2006). Blood and Marrow Transplantation. In Grundy M (ed) *Nursing in haematological oncology* 2nd ed. pp.265–92. Edinburgh: Elsevier Baillière Tindall.

Childs R W (2001). Allogeneic stem cell transplantation. In De Vita V T, Hellman S, Rosenberg S A, (eds) *Cancer Principles and Practice.* 6th edn, pp.2779–98. Philadelphia: Lippincott, Williams and Wilkins.

Chiodi S, Spinelli S, Ravera G *et al.* (2000). Quality of life in 244 recipients of allogeneic bone marrow transplantation. *Br J Haematol* **110**; 614–19.

Devine H, and DeMeyer E (2003). Hematopoietic cell transplantation in the treatment of leukemia. *Seminars in Oncology,* **19**(2), 118–32.

Hoffbrand A V, Pettit J E, Moss P A H (2001). *Essential haematology 4th ed.* Oxford: Blackwell Science.

National Institute for Clinical excellence (2003). *Guidance on Cancer Services. Improving Outcomes in Haematological Cancers-The Manual,* London: NICE.

Quinn B and Stephens M (2005). Bone Marrow Transplantation. In Kearney N Richardson A (eds) *Nursing Patients with Cancer: Principles and Practice.* Edinburgh: Elsevier Churchill Livingstone.

Souhami R L and Tobias J S (2005). *Cancer and Its Management,* 5th edn. Oxford: Blackwell.

Yarbro C H, Frogge M H, Goodman M (eds) (2005). *Cancer Nursing, Principles and practice.* 6th edn, pp.458–509. Massachusetts: Jones and Bartlett.

Clinical trials

Clinical trials in the cancer setting

Research governance and research guidelines in a clinical setting

Historically, medical experiments were conducted with only the ethics and morality of individual researchers and some local agreements guiding the conduct of the study. However following the horrific medical experiments conducted during World War II, there has been international and national guidelines and legislation developed to regulate trial conduct. These include.

- *Nuremberg Code*—this set out to protect human subjects and introduced voluntary consent to research participation.
- *The Declaration of Helsinki*—the World Medical Association's interpretation of the Nuremberg Code which aims to safeguard research participants by ensuring that the well-being of human subjects takes precedence over the interests of science or society.
- *International Conference of Harmonisation Tripartite Guidelines for Good Clinical Practice* (ICHGCP)—sets out responsibilities for researchers and underpins current research practice. It is a requirement that researchers in the UK are trained in ICHGCP.
- *EU Clinical Trials Directive 2001*—aims to ensure that all European countries are operating clinical trials to a uniform standard, while ensuring safety, efficacy, and quality. It aims to allow agents trialled and licensed in one European country to be adopted in another without further research being required.
- *Research Governance Framework for Health and Social Care*— ensures that research which involves NHS patients, data, staff, or equipment, complies with all professional, ethical, and scientific standards. It ensures legal requirements are met and quality standards are implemented.

Before a clinical trial can proceed within the UK, it needs to have approvals from multiple bodies:

Ethics approval. All clinical trials conducted in partnership with the NHS, must be submitted to the Central Office for Research Ethics Committees (COREC). Submissions will then be reviewed by a designated Ethics Committee. The Ethics Committee will have representation from the health care and lay communities and may include a statistician. The committees will ensure that the dignity, rights, safety, and well-being of participants are key considerations when granting approval for a clinical trial.

Medicines and Health care Products Regulatory Authority (MHRA). Where medicinal products are involved in the clinical trial, approval for use of the product must be sought from the MHRA. Following review of the preclinical and clinical data, if the product is deemed to be safe then Clinical Trial Authorisation will be granted.

Research and Development Department. This is needed where clinical trials involve utilising NHS staff, patients, data, or equipment. Where their Trust is involved in a clinical trial, the Chief Executive need grant approval.

In order to gain approval from the regulatory bodies, clinical trials must have undergone expert independent scientific review. All research staff participating in clinical trial activity must be qualified by education, training, or experience and must have appropriate supervision, support, and training. The training needs of research staff are not clearly described however in practice bi-annual evidence of ICHGCP training is considered acceptable in many hospital settings.

The Research Governance Framework outlines the responsibilities of the main people and organizations involved in health and social care research. Among the many responsibilities of the clinical trial sponsor, is the role of monitor. This involves checking that the data being collected is accurate which will positively impact on the quality of results and subsequent analysis of trial data. The sponsor must ensure that any suspected unexpected serious adverse events are reported promptly, promoting safety for trial participants.

Further information on the conduct of Clinical Trials can be found at: www.corec.org.uk and www.dh.gov.uk

With increased regulation, and standardization across Europe, more time and personnel are required to conduct clinical trials. There is additional pressure with the introduction of the government target of 10% of newly diagnosed cancer patients being recruited into clinical trials. The introduction of more research staff into clinical areas through the National Cancer Research Network has ensured that many Networks are achieving this target.

Phases of clinical trials

The initial phase of all new drug development is the pre-clinical stage, where new agents or combinations are investigated by performing pharmacological, pharmacokinetic, and toxicology testing in animal and in-vitro models. Once an agent or combination has been found to be of potential benefit it is moved from the laboratory to clinical testing.

Clinical trials are then conducted using human volunteers. In most cancer treatment trials, patients with cancer are most likely to be the participants in the trial rather than the more common use of healthy volunteers. This is due to the toxic nature of many of the agents being tested. The trials are conducted in four phases:

Phase I: is it safe?

This is the first use in humans and in cancer treatments are usually offered to patients for whom there is no other available treatment. The primary aim is to determine the maximum tolerated dose.

They may be offered to patients from a variety of tumour types. The exceptions to this are trials of gene therapies, and vaccines which are specifically designed for individual tumour types and therefore will only be tested on patients with an appropriate diagnosis.

The dose of drug initially is very small but increases in stages until the toxicity is considered unacceptable. Three to six patients are treated at each dose level and the level is only increased once the toxicity has been assessed at the lower dose and it is considered safe to increase. Pharmacokinetic and pharmacodynamic testing is conducted as part of the phase I trial, which will determine the potential treatment schedules for further trials.

Phase II: does it work?

The aims are to assess the activity of the drug in designated tumour types and the toxicity at a given dose and treatment schedule. These trials are normally offered to patients with metastatic disease and activity is measured by assessing tumour response. Multiple studies of the same drug may be conducted in different tumour types at the same time. The number of patients participating in each phase II study varies, but often start recruiting up to 25 then may increase if found to be effective.

Phase III: is it better than what is already being used?

This is the first time a new agent or combination will be directly compared with the current standard treatment in terms of efficacy and safety, usually in the form of a randomized controlled trial. Quality of life is normally assessed during this type of trial as there may be little difference in terms of efficacy but significant differences in terms of tolerability and impact on patient well-being.

Phase IV: what are the long-term effects?

The aim is to assess the long-term effects of the agents and combinations. Phase IV trials in cancer treatments are uncommon as many of the phase III trials have an end point of evaluating survival and therefore follow patients up for life rendering the phase IV trial superfluous.

While this linear approach to treatment development appears straight-forward, not all trials will follow this path, with some drugs being tested in phase I and phase III simultaneously. This can occur when a drug has progressed through phases I and II in one disease pathway and then is found to be potentially useful in a different disease pathway, such as the use of methotrexate in both cancers and rheumatoid diseases. Equally, further testing in early phases may be required when an agent or combination is to be administered on a different schedule, e.g. weekly rather than three weekly, or by a different route, e.g. IV or IM.

Nurses' responsibilities

The key responsibility for nurses caring for patients participating in clinical trials is safety by minimizing risk and maximizing benefit. The role and responsibilities for nurses working in clinical trials are multi-faceted and include education, advocacy, coordination, care giving, and paperwork/administration.

Education
- *Clinical staff:* educating clinical staff about the trial protocol, specific study requirements, and treatment plan. Where new agents or combinations are being used, education on expected and potential side effects is needed.
- *Patients and families:* all information required for informed consent which will include randomization and registration process, explanation of the treatment, its mode of action, treatment goals, study requirements e.g. how frequent hospital/clinic visits occur, potential side effects and complications.

Patient advocate
- Assess patient understanding of clinical trial and participant rights.
- Assess patient ability to adhere to the demands of the trial protocol.
- Communicate assessments of specific issues and concerns to study personnel and the patient's clinician.
- Support patient withdrawal from the trial—it is important that patients understand their right to withdraw from the study at any point without affecting their future care.

Coordination of trial
- Ensure necessary regulatory approval is in place.
- Ensure patients are suitable and eligible for trial entry.
- Ensure trial protocol is adhered to by patients and clinicians.
- Day-to-day organization of participant pathways—patient and researcher in the right place at the right time, treatment available when needed, registration of patient and, where appropriate, randomization.
- Liaison with other agencies such as drug companies.

Care giver
- Support with diagnosis and prognosis.
- Administration of trial agent(s).
- Assessment of side effects and toxicity.
- Collecting blood and urine samples, recording observations, further tests such as ECGs as required by study protocol.

Paperwork/administration

It is essential to keep complete documented records of all trial information. Source data must be available and every trial record must be completed in full. Data is transferred from medical notes or a specifically designed data capture record onto case report forms. Essentials include:

• Case report form completion.
• Adverse Event Reporting.
• Management of investigator and study files.
• Production of data collection tools, e.g. brief study guide or patient diary card, specific for each clinical trial and suitable for use in their own area.

See Medical Research Council website[1] for further guidance.

Research nurses may have the greatest working knowledge of the protocol, and as such may be utilized in a consultancy role for the duration of patient recruitment and treatment.

Ward, clinic, and day unit nurses

The responsibilities of department nurses are very similar to those of the research nurse. The challenge for these nurses is that trial activity is only a limited aspect of their role, yet they need to understand the trial protocol, treatment schedule and intent, possible side effects, and trial risks and benefits. Each clinical area is likely to be caring for patients entering a broad spectrum of trials and therefore the nurses need to have enough knowledge of each trial to ensure patient safety.

Vulnerable patients

Vulnerable patients can be defined as those who may suffer harm, abuse, or maltreatment as a result of decreased capacity, disempowerment, or minority grouping.

Vulnerability may be due to:
- Physical or mental illness including incurable disease.
- Low education level.
- Position in health-care hierarchy.
- Physical surroundings, e.g. hospital environment.
- Age—both elderly and children.
- Ethnic minorities.
- Homeless.

Anyone currently in receipt of health care may be considered to be vulnerable, by the nature of their dependence on professional support. In addition to this, no clinical trial is free from risk, and every clinical research patient may therefore be considered to be vulnerable. It is the responsibility of both researchers and ethics committees to reduce levels of vulnerability by ensuring that the principles of minimizing risk while maximizing benefit are adhered to.

Reasons for trial participation

Willingness to participate in clinical trials may be due to many factors, which include:
- Financial gain—many healthy volunteers are paid for participating in clinical trials.
- Expectation of benefit associated with participation.
- To please health care professionals or family.
- To gain access to medicinal agents which may otherwise not be available.
- To participate in development of future treatments.

Reducing risk

These factors may increase vulnerability, particularly their desire to please clinicians in charge of their care and expected benefits associated with participation. Patients may fear rejection by clinicians if they do not agree to participate in trials or may see participation as a means of thanking clinicians for previous care. Other patients may agree to take part as they believe they will receive the best treatment and may have unrealistic expectations of the impact treatment may have on their disease.

Gaining valid informed consent attempts to minimize vulnerability and ensure that clinical trial participants are fully aware of what they are agreeing to. Information regarding study participation should be given to the potential recruit at least 24 hours before they consent to take part, except in emergency situations, though these are rare in cancer clinical trials. Information should be both written and verbal, giving the patient the opportunity to ask questions and they should be encouraged to discuss their participation with family or friends, or health care professionals not associated with the research, e.g. GP, district nurse, clinical nurse specialist.

The researcher must ensure that, prior to participation in the trial, the patient understands what taking part will involve. Participation may include not only exposure to novel agents, but additional investigations and tests, extra hospital and clinic visits, or prolonged hospital admissions. The researcher must also ensure that participants are free from duress, This may be due to a sense of obligation to clinicians or because of a limited availability of potential treatments outside of a clinical trial. This is often relevant in randomized controlled trials where a new treatment has been found to be effective but is not yet licensed for general use. Patients need to clearly understand the randomization process as they may be randomized to an arm of the trial, which does not include the new treatment.

Informed consent is an ongoing process and is a means of continuing to protect vulnerable patients. The responsibility for ensuring valid consent rests with each individual engaged in the research process. It is also essential that patients understand that they can withdraw from clinical trials at any time without giving a reason and that this decision will not negatively impact on their future care.

Researchers have a duty of care towards research participants and in most cancer trials this relationship is complicated by the fact that the researcher is also the clinician in charge of the patient's treatment. Awareness of issues influencing vulnerability, and adherence to clinical trials guidelines and legislation, will minimize risk of harm, abuse, or maltreatment.

Further reading

Department of Health (2005). *Research Governance Framework for Health and Social Care.* 2nd edn. London: HMSO.

Earl-Slater A. (2002). *The Handbook of Clinical Trials and Other Research.* Abingdon: Radcliffe Medical Press.

Girling D, Parmar M, Stenning S et al. (2003). *Clinical trials in cancer, principles and practice.* Oxford: Oxford University Press.

Medical Research Council (1998). *MRC guidelines for good clinical practice in clinical trials.* London: MRC.

Section 6

Management of major cancers

Bone cancer

Bone sarcomas

Bone sarcomas are extremely rare, with less than 550 new cases per annum in the UK. They account for only 0.2% of all new cancers, but 5% of childhood cancers. The main types of bone sarcoma/tumour are:

- Osteosarcoma.
- Chondrosarcoma.
- Ewings sarcoma.
- Malignant fibrous histiocytoma of bone.

Osteosarcoma is the commonest primary bone tumour, accounting for 20% of all cases.

Risk factors

Most patients have no known risk factors. Bone sarcomas are occasionally associated with genetically inherited disease, e.g. Li–Fraumeni syndrome or hereditary retinoblastoma (osteosarcoma).

Presentation

- Painful bony swelling, with warm and red overlying tissues—can be associated with local trauma.
- Axial lesions may cause pain—with compression of abdominal organs, urinary tract, or nerve.
- 10% of Ewing's sarcomas develop fever and a hot swollen limb—mimicking osteomyelitis.

Diagnosis

- Plain X-ray and isotope bone scan.
- CT chest and abdomen. MRI scan of primary lesions and hot spots.
- Trephine or core biopsy.
- In Ewing's sarcoma, a bone marrow aspirate (x2) and trephine from sites distant from known disease.
- Staging is through TNM, (□ Diagnosis and staging) plus whether or not the tumour is confined within or beyond the cortex. The cell type (pathological grade) is also important.
- Poor prognostic factors include tumours in the axial skeleton, poor initial response to chemotherapy, high grade, and local recurrence.

Note: patients with suspected bone malignancy must be referred to an orthopaedic oncologist for biopsy—inappropriate biopsy siting can result in tumour spillage and unnecessary requirement for limb amputation.

Osteosarcoma

This occurs predominantly in adolescence—its peak incidence coincides with the growth spurt. Vascular invasion is common and it typically spreads to the lung and bone. Overall, five-year survival rate is 55–70%.

Management of patients with osteosarcoma

- 2–3 cycles of chemotherapy usually delivered, followed by limb sparing surgery, followed by a further 3–4 cycles of chemotherapy. The most active agents are doxorubicin, cisplatin, high-dose methotrexate, and ifosfamide.

- Approximately 80% of osteosarcomas are treated successfully with limb-sparing techniques. A wide variety of endo-prosthetic devices are available, including extendable prostheses for growing children.
- The use of radiotherapy is limited to non-resectable axial osteosarcomas—for those who refuse surgery, or who have poor excision margins—and palliative treatment of bone metastases.
- Around 15% of new cases have metastatic disease at presentation. Combined with treatment as above, a subset of these patients can benefit from resection of the metastatic disease, enabling long-term survival in around 20–30% of cases.

Risk versus benefit of limb sparing surgery

In large, poorly differentiated tumours, the quality of life benefits of limb-sparing surgery need to be carefully weighed against the risk of local recurrence

Ewing's sarcoma

This is a highly malignant rare primary bone tumour, with peak age of 10–20 years. It may affect any bone with 55% arising in the axial skeleton. Blood borne spread to the lung and bone is common.

Management of Ewing's tumours

Management consists of six cycles of preoperative chemotherapy followed by limb-sparing surgery ± adjuvant radiotherapy. Further chemotherapy is continued—up to another eight cycles of conventional chemotherapy or high-dose therapy with peripheral blood stem cell support.

Note: the intensification of chemotherapy regimens has led to significant improvement in the outcome of treatment, but at the cost of significant toxicities, such as severe myelosuppression, a risk of neutropaenic sepsis, mucositis, and a risk of graft versus host reaction. Late effects of treatment include cardiomyopathy, nephrotoxicity, infertility, and second malignancy (e.g. leukaemia, osteosarcoma).

Management of metastatic disease

Metastatic disease is initially managed as above, with induction chemotherapy followed by local therapy to the primary tumour.

- Patients with lung metastases may then be treated with conventional chemotherapy and whole-lung irradiation or high-dose chemotherapy with peripheral blood stem cell support (📖 High dose therapy).
- Patients with bone or marrow metastases have a poorer prognosis and high-dose chemotherapy may be considered for many of them.

Chondrosarcoma

- This is a cartilage forming malignancy of middle to late age. It is the second most common primary bone tumour accounting for 15% of the incidence.
- Chondrosarcoma typically presents with a painful enlarging mass in the pelvis, proximal femur, humerus, shoulders, or ribs. It is unusual in the distal bones.

Management of chondrosarcoma

Treatment is surgical resection with limb conservation if possible. There is no proven role for adjuvant chemotherapy. Radiotherapy is used after incomplete resection or palliation of advanced disease. The tumour grade is the best prognostic indicator. Grade 1 has a 90% 5-year survival. Grade 3 has a 40% 5-year survival.

Soft tissue sarcomas

Epidemiology and aetiology

- These are rare tumours, with around 1200 cases per annum in the UK. They account for about 1% of adult cancers and 6% of childhood cancers.
- There are over 70 different histological subtypes.
- Soft tissue sarcomas are occasionally associated with genetically inherited disease or previous radiation exposure.

Presenting symptoms and signs

Most patients present with a painless soft tissue mass, 45% of these are on the lower limb, 15% on the upper limb, 10% on the head and neck, and 15% are retroperitoneal. Up to 30% of soft tissue sarcomas are subcutaneous.

Staging system

A combination of grading, tumour size, and evidence of metastatic spread is used. Histological grading and tumour size are crucial. Low-grade sarcomas rarely metastasize, and may be dealt with successfully by surgery alone. High-grade sarcomas are locally invasive and typically metastasize via blood supply to the lung.

Pathological classification of soft tissue sarcomas

- Liposarcoma
- Malignant fibrous histiocytoma
- Leiomyosarcoma
- Extra osseous Ewing's tumour
- Epithelioid sarcoma
- Alveolar soft part sarcoma
- Malignant peripheral nerve sheath tumour
- Fibrosarcoma
- Rhabdomyosarcoma
- Angiosarcoma
- Synovial sarcoma
- Clear cell sarcoma
- GI stromal tumour

Investigations: see Bone Sarcomas.

Management

Surgery

- Ideally, localized sarcomas are managed by complete excision, with clear excision margins, together with removal of any biopsy tract.
- A radical excision—dissection of the tumour and muscular compartment as one unit reduces the risk of local recurrence, but it may lead to unacceptable loss of function. Post-operative radiotherapy may enhance the oppurtunity for limb preservation. If the disease cannot be completely excised with the conservation of a functional limb, amputation is infrequently indicated.
- For the majority of soft tissue sarcomas, surgery is the main local treatment. Surgery may also be appropriate for local recurrence and for metastatic disease, in particular solitary pulmonary metastasis.

- Locally advanced disease not amenable to primary surgery may be treated with preoperative radiotherapy or chemotherapy in order to facilitate resection.

Chemotherapy

The majority of adult sarcomas are only moderately chemo-sensitive. The most active agents are doxorubicin and ifosfamide, with response rates of 10–30% in advanced disease.

The role of adjuvant chemotherapy remains controversial. For some disease, e.g. extra osseous Ewing's, chemotherapy has a major impact on survival. The benefits of chemotherapy in other adult sarcomas are less clear—it reduces the risk of disease recurrence but has no impact on overall survival.

Radiotherapy

Most adult soft tissue sarcomas are only moderately radiosensitive. The most important role for radiotherapy is in the postoperative adjuvant setting, particularly for high-grade sarcomas that have been treated by wide excision, as microscopic tumours may still be present within the muscle compartment.

Treatment outcome and prognostic factors

Overall, the five-year survival rate is around 70%; it is nearer 20% for those with metastatic disease at presentation. Treatment outcomes are worse with high-grade disease, large tumours, deep tumours, visceral/retroperitoneal, and metastatic disease at presentation.

Surgical treatments

The main treatments for bone and soft tissue sarcomas are surgery, radiotherapy, and chemotherapy. Support of individuals receiving radiotherapy and chemotherapy are covered in Chapters 16 and 17. This section will look at the surgical treatment and nursing care of these patients.

Types of surgery

Endoprosthesis: removal of diseased bone, usually close to a joint, and insertion of a prosthesis into the body, for example, to replace part of the femur. An endoprosthesis tends to be very much like a custom made joint replacement with a longer stem inserted into the remaining bone left after excision of the diseased bone.

Wide excision: this surgical procedure is used to completely excise the tumour including a clear margin of normal tissue. This is the most common procedure used in the removal of soft tissue sarcomas. It allows the clear removal of the tumour. Wide excision surgery is not always undertaken, for example if the tumour involves nerves or blood vessels that cannot be removed without serious loss of function to the patient. If a wide excision is not an option, it usually means the only option for surgery is an amputation.

Amputation: removal of a limb in order to completely excise the tumour and disease. Not commonly used, but it may be necessary if the tumour cannot be fully excised with other surgical procedures.

Plastic surgery: the use of plastic surgery is very important in cases where patients have had major soft tissue surgery to remove a tumour. Some patients have flaps moved from other parts of the body to fill the gap left by the tumour removal.

Preoperative care

If an amputation is being performed it is important for the patient to have been seen by a specialist from the prosthetics service. The prosthetics specialist will deal with the patient's concerns, and answer questions relating to prosthetics options following surgery.

Issues that will be covered include:
• The exact nature of the surgery.
• Prosthetic options.
• Phantom limb pain due to nerve damage.
• Altered body image.

Having an amputation does not automatically mean that a prosthesis will be available. It depends on the nature of the surgery and how much bone and tissue are left.

It is important to ensure issues of altered body image have been addressed with the patient. Patients can be concerned about how friends and family will react. Sometimes it can be useful to get them to talk to patients who have gone through similar surgery (□ Altered body image).

Preoperative exercises are also very important. It can be useful to build up the muscles that are going to be used significantly after amputation, e.g. building up arm muscles if using crutches to mobilise.

Postoperative care

The immediate postoperative care for patients who have undergone limb surgery is largely the same for any postoperative patient (📖 Surgery). However, with limb surgery, it is very important to:

- Observe the limb and the surgical site.
- Ensure that blood flow and nerve conduction has not been compromised by the surgery.
- For patients who have undergone plastic reconstruction with flap surgery, it is **vital** that flap observations, including temperature, dopplar, and capillary refill are done regularly, beginning with ¼ hourly observations.
- If flaps are going to fail it can happen very quickly. Plastic surgeons need contacted directly about any concerns with the flap.

Upper limb surgery

Patients who have undergone upper limb surgery are encouraged to mobilize as soon as possible as to reduce the risk of DVT. Nursing care of these patients may include assistance with all activities of daily living. It is important to remember that having upper arm surgery may mean the patient is unable to do even simple things like drinking from a cup, it is therefore important to ensure that all aids are in place to help the patient.

Lower limb surgery

Patients who have had lower limb surgery will require a longer period of bed rest. Lower limbs support body weight (unlike upper limbs), and support will be required to recover full walking function.

Infection

It is very important to prevent wound infection if at all possible, as the consequences can be severe and disabling. If a patient's endoprosthesis gets infected it could mean the prosthesis will need to be removed. Revision of an endoprosthesis is difficult since:

- More bone may need removing reducing its function and stability.
- If a patient has undergone radiotherapy they are less able to heal effectively post surgery.
- Patients receiving chemotherapy may be neutropaenic or immuno-suppressed.

Psychological care

As with all cancers, psychological care of patients and their families is of utmost importance. For patients who have had amputation, it is important to remember they may well need counselling to help with problems such as altered body image, and loss of the limb.

Patients who have undergone proximal femoral endoprosthetic replacement, for example, may need support in terms of sexual health. They may need advice about other ways of enjoying their sex lives as intercourse may not be possible for a number of weeks. This is because the implant needs time to become completely stable (📖 Sexual health and cancer).

Rehabilitation

Rehabilitation of patients who have had surgery for bone and soft tissue tumours depends on the extent and type of surgery performed. Some patients who have surgery to remove a soft tissue tumour from a fore-arm, for example, may be back to normal activities in a number of days. Patients having had femoral endoprosthesis insertion may be unable to walk without aids for a number of weeks, and unable to drive for at least 4–6 weeks. Physiotherapy and occupational therapy are very important as well as the nursing care of these patients.

Post-amputation rehabilitation can last for a matter of months or years. For an amputation of the leg, patients may require fitting of a prosthesis. Limb swelling must have gone in order for the prosthesis to fit correctly. Once fitted, a number of sessions with both physiotherapists and occupa-tional therapists are undertaken to get full and safe use of the prosthesis.

With an upper limb amputation physiotherapy and occupational therapy are important as it may be the patient's dominant arm that is missing. Some patients may spend years learning to do everyday routines in a completely different way to what they were used to preoperatively.

There are many makes and models of prosthetic limbs around on the market and patients need to have guidance as to which would be best for them. It is also seen in practice that many patients who have prostheses made actually find them hard work and manage very well without them.

It is also important for the patients to have contact details of someone, for example, the CNS. This allows them to feel that they are still being cared for. It gives them a contact for any questions or enquiries that they may have.

Further reading

Agarwal M and Puri A (2003). Limb salvage for malignant primary bone tumours: Current status with a review of the literature. *Indian Journal of Surgery*. **65**,(4), 354–60.

Department of Health (2000). *The NHS Cancer Plan: A plan for investment, a plan reform*. London: DH.

National Institute for Clinical excellence (2006) *Guidelines for improving outcomes for people with Sarcoma*. NICE, London.

Patterson, A J and Harmon, D C. (2001). Bone tumours and soft tissue sarcomas. Cited in Spence RAJ, and Johnston, PG. (ed) pp.359–383. *Oncology*. Oxford: Oxford University Press.

Shidham V (2004). Benign and malignant soft tissue tumors. Available at www.emedicine.com/orthoped/topic377.htm

Souhami R and Tobias J (2005). Bone and soft tissue sarcomas. *Cancer and its Management*. 5th edn, pp.386–404. Oxford: Blackwell.

Websites

▦ Sarcoma UK: www.sarcoma-uk.org

▦ Pathology Outlines.com: http://pathologyoutlines.com/bone.html

Metastatic bone disease (MBD)

Bone is the third most common site of metastases after liver and lung. MBD is actually far more common than primary bone cancer. The most common sites of MBD are: vertebrae, pelvis, ribs, femur, and skull. MBD is particularly common in the following cancers:

- Breast.
- Prostate.
- Lung.
- Kidney.
- Thyroid.
- Myeloma.

Aetiology

Bone destruction due to metastatic cancer is a complex process involving:

- Tumour produced osteoclast (cells that break down bone) factors.
- Direct destruction by the tumour cells.
- Increased osteoblast (bone forming cells) activity, producing unstable bone matrix.

Presenting symptoms

- Pain (most common presentation).
- Impaired mobility.
- Hypercalcaemia (📖 Hypercalcaemia).
- Pathological fracture.
- Spinal cord compression (📖 Spinal cord compression).
- Bone marrow suppression (📖 Bone marrow suppression).

Diagnosis

- History, physical examination.
- X-rays—can miss small lesions.
- MRI or CT scan.
- Bone scans.

Management of bone metastases

Bone metastases are a sign of progressive and advanced disease. Management is therefore based around principles of effective symptom management and palliative care. Effective pain and mobility management can lead to an improvement in quality of life.

Treatment of the underlying disease

This may improve the symptoms of bone metastases. Approaches include chemotherapy, hormonal manipulation, or radiotherapy.

Bisphosphonate therapy

For people with known metastatic bone cancer, bisphosphonates have been shown to reduce bone pain, reduce the incidence and rate of skeletal events (e.g. lytic lesions, pathological fractures), and to improve the quality of life in a number of different cancers.

Options include IV pamidronate, zolendronate, or ibandronate. O
options include clodronate or ibandronate. The specific drug, the rout.
and the dose will depend on the specific disease as well as the patient's
health status and wishes.

Side effects

- Infusional related reactions are rare, but include high temperature
  and chills, headache, and a temporary increase in bone pain.
- Other side effects are usually mild. They include renal toxicity
  (zolendronate), stomach upset, nausea, vomiting, and diarrhoea.

Bone pain

This usually develops progressively over weeks and months. It is often
described as dull and unremitting, is generally worse at night and on
weight bearing. It can include a nerve pain component, and can be difficult
to fully resolve.

Analgesic management includes:

- NSAIDs and opioids, often used in conjunction.
- Localized short doses of radiotherapy—can be completely effective
  in around one third of patients and give some relief in up to 80% of
  patients. Strontium-89, a radionuclide which is given IV, is also used to
  treat multifocal bone pain in prostate cancer. The main side effect is
  mild bone marrow suppression.
- Bispohosphonate therapy (see above) can reduce bone pain as an
  adjunct to other pain management.
- Pain on weight bearing may require the support of mobility aids
  such as walking sticks or walking frames. Adapting the individual's
  home environment with physiotherapy and OT involvement may
  also be required.

The nurse's role in assessing the individual's functional ability, including
their mobility is essential to plan effective care. Maintaining the maximum
independence and level of desired mobility is an important goal.

Pathological fractures

Bone integrity can be severely reduced due to MBD, leading to bone
fractures. Pathological fractures in long bones can cause severe pain and
disability. Untreated pathological fractures rarely heal. Rib fractures and
vertebral collapse are the most common. Implications of these are pain,
restricted breathing, reduced mobility, and risk of spinal cord compression
(Spinal cord compression).

Management

- Orthopaedic surgical stabilization of long bones and pelvic/shoulder
  area can be successful in reducing pain and re-establishing
  mobility/function. The aim should be to stabilize the bone for the
  lifespan of the patient. Careful patient selection is required due
  to the potential morbidity of such procedures.
- A single dose of postoperative radiotherapy can be given to the
  site of the fracture.
- Some patients with MBD may be candidates for prophylactic
  fixation, if they are at high risk of pathological fracture.

ality of life issues

one metastases can have a huge impact on patient and family quality of ife. Pain and reduced mobility can impact on personal role function, body image, and self-concept, and are also risk factors for anxiety and depression. Individuals can become housebound and isolated. Psychological assessment and support are key elements of care.

Nurses have an important role in discussing the risks of pathological fractures and the possible treatment options with patients and their families. Nurses also need to liaise with other health professionals, such as occupational therapists and physiotherapists, to assist with fracture prevention, e.g. walking aids, education and environment adaptations.

Spinal cord compression and hypercalcaemia are potential emergency consequences of bone metastases. Nurses have a key role in educating patients and their families about the signs and symptoms of both, and the need to urgently contact a health professional if any of these signs and symptoms develop.

Further reading

McQuay H J, Collins S L, Carroll D et al. (1999) Radiotherapy for the palliation of painful bone metastases. *The Cochrane database of systematic reviews*, issue 3. Art No.: CD001793.

Wong R, Wiffen P J (2002). Bisphosphonates for the relief of pain secondary to bone metastases. *The Cochrane database of systematic reviews*, issue 2. Art No.: CD002068.

The Prostate Cancer Charity www.prostate-cancer.org.uk/pdf/BAUS_Guidelines.pdf Accessed 6th June 2006.

Breast cancer

ntroduction

Epidemiology
- Breast cancer is the most common cancer in females in the UK and Europe—accounting for almost 1 in 3 of cancers in females in the UK.
- 42,000 cases of breast cancer are diagnosed in the UK per year; its incidence is increasing by about 1% per year.
- Currently there are 13,000 breast cancer deaths per year in the UK.
- UK breast cancer mortality has fallen by over 25% since the 1980s.
- Male breast cancer is rare, with about 300 cases per annum in UK.

Risk factors
- Age—the incidence of breast cancer doubles every 10 years until the menopause. After 50 years of age, the rate of increase slows.
- Early menarche and late menopause.
- Having had no children or late age at first pregnancy.
- Genetic predisposition accounts for around 10% of female and 20% of male breast cancers.
- Hormone replacement therapy.
- Diet—associations have been shown with obesity and alcohol consumption.

Hereditary breast cancer
5–10% of female breast cancer is due to inheritance of a mutated copy of either the *BRCA1* or *BRCA2* gene. This brings with it an increased risk of breast cancer at an early age and an elevated lifetime risk of breast cancer—from 36% up to 87% by the age of 70 years. There is an associated risk of ovarian cancer (greater with *BRCA1*). Male carriers of either *BRCA1* or 2 are at increased risk of prostate cancer and for *BRCA2* carriers, breast cancer.

Note; the management of hereditary breast cancer is essentially the same as that of non-hereditary disease, though *BRCA1* cancers may be more aggressive.

Pathology
- 85% of breast carcinomas arise in the ducts of the breast. Over 80% of these are invasive.
- Ductal carcinoma in situ (DCIS) remains within the confines of the ductal basement membrane.
- Lobular carcinomas account for 15% of breast cancers. About 20% of these develop contralateral breast cancer.
- Oestrogen and progesterone receptor status varies between cancers and impacts on prognosis and treatment options.
- High levels of HER2 can be associated with oestrogen receptor (ER) and progesterone receptor (PR) negativity and poorer prognosis.

Routes of spread

- Lymphatic regional nodes—most commonly the axillary, less often, the internal mammary.
- Systemic spread—most commonly bone, lung or pleura, liver, skin, and CNS.

Prognostic factors

The most important independent prognostic factors are:
- Tumour size.
- Number of histologically positive axillary lymph nodes.
- Tumour grade (a lower grade tumour has a better prognosis).
- Other prognostic factors include:
  - Hormone receptor status (oestrogen and progesterone receptors).
  - HER2*neu* over-expression.
  - Histological subtype.
  - Lymphovascular invasion.
  - Proliferative index (rate of cell division in the tumour).

Nottingham prognostic index (NPI) calculation

NPI = (0.2 × pathological tumour size (cm) + grade (1–3) + axillary node score)

Axillary node status	Score
No lymph nodes positive	1
1–3 lymph nodes positive	2
>3 lymph nodes positive	3
NPI	**Prognosis**
<3.41	Good
3.41–5.4	Intermediate
>5.4	Poor

Further reading

Chapman D D (2005). Breast Cancer. In Yarbro C H, Frogge M H, Goodman M. (eds). *Cancer Nursing, Principles and practice.* 6th edn, pp.1022–1088. Massachusetts: Jones and Bartlett.

Dixon J M (2005). *ABC of Breast Diseases,* 3rd ed. *BMJ* publishing group, Oxford.

Early Breast Cancer Trialists' Collaborative Group. (2000) Favourable and unfavourable effect on long-term survival of radiotherapy for early breast cancer: an overview of the randomized trials. *Lancet* **355**, 1757–70.

Early Breast Cancer Trialists' Collaborative Group (2005). Effects of chemotherapy and hormonal therapy for early breast cancer on recurrence and 15 year survival: an overview of the randomized trials. *Lancet* **365**, 1687–1717.

Harcourt D and Rumsey N (2001). Psychological aspects of breast reconstruction: a review of the literature. *J Adv Nurs,* **35**(4), 477–87.

agnosis and staging

resentation

- Abnormal screening mammogram (at least 25% of cases and increasing due to increase in screening up to 70 years of age).
- Breast lump or thickening.
- Axillary tumour.
- Breast skin changes such as dimpling, puckering, or erythema.
- Nipple changes such as inversion or discharge.
- Persistent breast tenderness or pain.

Note: less commonly, there may be symptoms from metastatic disease such as bone pain, pathological fracture or spinal cord compression. See Table 24.1 for criteria to refer urgently to a breast clinic.

Diagnosis

The diagnosis of breast cancer is made by a 'triple assessment' including:
- A full clinical examination.
- A bilateral mammography, often combined with ultrasound.
- Fine needle aspiration (FNA) cytology and/or core biopsy.

In a few cases where there is still uncertainty, excision biopsy of the breast lesion may be required. The axilla is staged surgically in patients with invasive disease. A chest X-ray and blood tests are done pre-operatively, bone scan or CT scan may be done if there is advanced local disease or signs/symptoms of metastatic spread.

Breast cancer is staged using the tumour node metastasis (TNM) staging system (💷 Diagnosis and classification). See Table 24.2 for prognostic relevance of different stages.

Table 24.1 Indications for referral to breast clinic

Screen-detected breast cancer

Breast lump:

- Any new discrete lump.
- New lump in pre-existing nodularity.
- Asymmetrical nodularity persisting after menstruation.
- Abscess/inflammation which does not settle after one course of antibiotics.
- Persistent or recurrent cyst.

Pain:

- Associated with a lump.
- Intractable pain which interferes with the patient's life and fails to respond to simple measures (well-supporting bra, simple analgesics, abstinence from caffeine, trial of evening primrose oil).
- Unilateral persistent pain in post-menopausal women.

Nipple discharge:

- In any women age >50 years.
- In younger women if blood-stained, persistent single duct or bilateral, sufficient to stain clothes.

Nipple retraction, distortion, or eczema

Change in breast skin contour

Axillary lump and strong family history

Table 24.2 Breast Cancer Survival Rates—based on stage of disease

Stage	10 year survival
0	> 95%
I	75–95%
IIA	45–85%
IIB	40–80%
IIIA	10–60%
IIIB	0–35%
IIIC	0–30%
IV	<5%

...agement of non-invasive ...east cancer

...uctal carcinoma *in situ* (DCIS)

Treatment options

Surgery/radiotherapy

- Options are a simple mastectomy or lumpectomy and breast irradiation.
- Mastectomy remains the standard treatment for large in situ cancers, for multifocal disease and recurrence of DCIS.
- The risk of recurrence is less than 10% at 5-years for either treatment.

Adjuvant hormone therapy

Half of local recurrences are invasive. Clinical trials with aromatase inhibitors are underway to assess their role in preventing recurrence.

Lobular carcinoma *in situ* (LCIS) (also referred to as lobular neoplasia)

The management of LCIS is controversial. Strictly speaking it is not a pre-malignant condition, but it does identify women at increased risk of developing invasive breast cancer, in either breast. Most subsequent cancers are ductal, not lobular.[1]

- Many cases are managed by wide local excision and regular mammogram surveillance.
- Problems include:
  - LCIS is commonly missed on mammograms.
  - There is a risk of multifocal disease in the same breast (ipsilateral).
  - There is a risk of disease in the other breast (contralateral).

For all patients with breast cancer, the key to selecting the optimum treatment is multidisciplinary discussion including radiology, pathology, surgery, oncology, and clinical nurse specialist input. Appropriate treatment options can then be presented to the patient to help them choose according to their individual circumstances and preferences.

1 National Cancer Institute (2007). www.cancer.gov/cancertopics/types/breast

Management of early breast cancer

Introduction
Early breast cancer is defined as disease that can be completely removed by surgery, that is T1–3, and N0–1 tumours. The management of early breast cancer involves:
- Surgical treatment of the breast and axilla.
- Pathological assessment and staging to direct adjuvant therapy including, chemotherapy, radiotherapy, and endocrine therapy.

Breast surgery
The options are:
- Wide local excision followed by breast irradiation.
- Mastectomy.
- The local recurrence rate for each is less than 10% after 10 years follow up.
- The preferred treatment for the majority of T1-2 breast cancers is wide local excision followed by breast irradiation.
- Breast conservation may not always be appropriate, e.g.:
  - Multifocal disease.
  - Large tumour in a small breast.
  - Where breast irradiation would be contraindicated.
  - Some patients prefer mastectomy, not least because of the possible avoidance of radiotherapy.

Breast reconstruction can be offered after surgery, either at the time of primary surgery or at a later date (📖 Breast reconstruction).

Axillary surgery
Total axillary clearance
This offers good regional control, but has a high risk of lymphoedema, and arm pain, both of which can be disabling. It also leads to the over-treatment of some women, i.e. after clearance they will be found to be node negative and therefore will have had this procedure unnecessarily.

Axillary sampling
- A minimum of four lymph nodes are sampled from the lower axilla.
- If positive, they are treated by axillary clearance or more commonly, by axillary radiotherapy.
- There is less morbidity for node negative patients with equivalent local control rates and survival to total axillary clearance.

Sentinel node biopsy
This is being offered in a trial setting and is standard practice in some units. The aim is to identify node negative patients and to spare them axillary clearance by providing more effectively targeted treatment.

Loco-regional radiotherapy
Breast irradiation
Whole breast radiotherapy reduces the risk of local recurrence after breast-conserving surgery to less than 10% at 10 years. Care must be taken to minimize the volume of lung and heart irradiated.

Post-mastectomy radiotherapy to the chest wall increases survival in patients at high risk of relapse, and is recommended for patients with at least 2 of the following:
- Size >4cm.
- Grade 3.
- Lymph node positive.
- Vascular invasion.

Axillary radiotherapy
This is indicated after positive lymph node sampling. It is generally avoided after axillary clearance because of the high risk of lymphoedema and brachial plexopathy.

Radiotherapy timing
In general, radiotherapy should begin as soon as possible after surgery. However enhanced normal tissue damage can result when radiotherapy and adjuvant chemotherapy are given together, and radiotherapy is often postponed until chemotherapy is completed.

djuvant treatment of early breast cancer

Adjuvant systemic therapy

- Many women have occult micro-metastases at diagnosis. If untreated, these can cause metastatic disease.
- Effective systemic treatment at the time of the breast cancer diagnosis produces a significant survival benefit in the majority of women.
- The risk of micro-metastatic disease correlates well with the prognostic factors summarized by the Nottingham Prognostic Index (📖 Breast cancer: Introduction).

Estimates of the potential benefit from adjuvant chemotherapy may be calculated for individual patients via www.adjuvantonline.com.

Adjuvant chemotherapy

Combination chemotherapy reduces recurrence and mortality in most groups of women and should be considered in:
- All but very good prognosis pre-menopausal breast cancer. Almost always recommended in women under age 35.
- Post-menopausal women with intermediate or poor prognosis breast cancer.
- Current practice is 6 cycles of FEC chemotherapy, unless contraindicated by cardiac problems.
- Ongoing trials are exploring taxane-based regimens, epirubicin/CMF, the use of capecitabine and also the use of G-CSF to reduce dose intervals.
- Promising preliminary results of adjuvant chemotherapy followed by trastuzumab (Herceptin®), have arisen in trials from the USA. Herceptin was licensed in 2006 in the adjuvant setting in the UK after NICE approved its use in early breast cancer.

Adjuvant endocrine therapy

- 60% of breast cancers are oestrogen receptor (ER) positive.
- Adjuvant hormone therapy confers survival benefits in these patients, in some cases greater than with chemotherapy.
- Toxicity is less than chemotherapy, although menopausal symptoms can be distressing for some.

Tamoxifen

- 20 mg daily for 5 years improves survival in both pre- and post-menopausal women. It reduces the risk of contralateral breast cancer and osteoporosis.
- Tamoxifen offers no benefit in ER negative breast cancer.
- It increases the risk of thromboembolic disease and endometrial cancer (x 2.5).

Note: tamoxifen should only be commenced after completion of chemotherapy, as it reduces the effectiveness of chemotherapy.

Aromatase inhibitors (AIs) and breast cancer

Evidence is accumulating that the AIs are more effective than tamoxifen alone in reducing recurrence. and have a reduced risk of thromboembolic disease and endometrial cancer. The optimum duration of therapy remains uncertain. They can cause fatigue, joint pain, and reduction in bone density. At time of writing recommendations[1] are that:

- The AIs anastrozole, exemestane, and letrozole, are options for the adjuvant treatment of early oestrogen-receptor-positive invasive breast cancer in post-menopausal women.
- The choice of treatment strategies include
  - Primary adjuvant treatment with an aromatase inhibitor.
  - Switching from tamoxifen to an aromatase inhibitor.
  - Use of an aromatase inhibitor after completion of 5 years of tamoxifen treatment.

There is a need to consider
- Whether the patient has already received tamoxifen.
- The side effect profiles of the individual drugs.
- The assessed risk of recurrence.

Women with questions about their use should currently be referred to their breast care clinician and CNS.

The role of AIs in preventing breast cancer is also being studied in women at high risk of the disease[2].

Breast cancer treatment guidelines

Exact treatment guidelines for breast cancer are changing frequently as new research comes through into clinical practice. Practice in individual centres may vary and may change as new guidelines are updated/ published etc.

You can check for the latest national guidelines on The National Institute for Health and Clinical Excellence website. www.nice.org.uk and check for local guidelines from your local cancer network.

Ovarian oblation

For pre-menopausal women, ovarian ablation provides a 10.6% improvement in 10 year survival.

Neo-adjuvant therapy (preoperative treatment)

Preoperative treatment downstages the primary tumour and, in some women, it facilitates breast-conserving surgery where mastectomy would otherwise be required. No difference in survival has been shown between people given pre- or post-operative chemotherapy.

1 NICE (2006). www.nice.org.uk
2 CRUK website. Accessed May 24th 2006. www.cancerhelp.org.uk/help/default.asp?page=3269

Management of locally advanced breast cancer

- Locally advanced disease is defined by the presence of infiltration of the skin or the chest wall or fixed axillary nodes e.g. T4 or N2–3.
- The risk of metastatic disease is more than 70%. Long-term survival is possible and the median survival of these patients exceeds two years.
- Staging investigations should assess possible metastatic disease and include:
  - A chest X-ray.
  - An isotope bone scan.
  - A liver ultrasound or CT scan.
- Local control of the tumour and the prevention of tumour fungation are of major importance to the quality of life of these women, irrespective of the presence of metastases.
- A combination of primary systemic treatment and radiotherapy is commonly used.

Older patients and those with ER positive disease

- First-line therapy in this group should be with one of the AIs (anastrozole, letrozole, or exemestane), which may downstage disease to make it operable.
- Radiotherapy is reserved to control bleeding or other uncontrolled symptoms such as lymphoedema.

Younger patients and those with ER negative disease

- First line therapy is primary chemotherapy, usually an anthracycline based combination.
- Surgery may be feasible in some patients with a good response to systemic treatment, followed by loco-regional radiotherapy.
- Hormone therapy is started after chemotherapy for ER positive tumours:
  - Pre-menopausal—tamoxifen and add in ovarian suppression (LHRH agonist) for poor prognosis patients. May also use bisphosphonates (📖 Bisphosphonate)
  - Post-menopausal—aromatase inhibitor.

Management of metastatic breast cancer

~5% of patients with metastatic breast cancer survive for at least 5 years. ER positive disease and bone metastases have the best prognosis. Visceral metastatic disease generally has a poor prognosis, and the aim of treatment with these patients is palliation.

Endocrine therapy

This is preferred over chemotherapy in older patients, and for non-visceral metastatic disease.

First-line treatment should be as follows:

- Pre-menopausal women—ovarian suppression (LHRH agonist) plus tamoxifen.
- Post-menopausal women—AI (anastrozole, letrozole, or exemestane).
- Subsequent further therapy with agents to which the patient has not previously been exposed can be of benefit.

Chemotherapy

- Combination chemotherapy is the preferred treatment for patients with visceral disease and ER negative tumours.
- Despite the toxicity of chemotherapy, the quality of life of women improves as they respond to treatment. Around 50% of women will respond, with median time 8 months to further disease progression.
- Following disease progression 2nd or 3rd line chemotherapy can be offered, although tumour responses will reduce and fewer patients will remain fit to tolerate such regimes.

Immunotherapy

- 25–30% of breast cancers overexpress HER2, a growth factor receptor, associated with poor prognosis disease
- Trastuzumab (Herceptin®) is a monoclonal antibody targeted against HER2, which is administered once weekly or three-weekly intravenously.

  It has shown improved response rates over chemotherapy alone in HER2 positive breast cancer. However, long-term benefits have not yet been established. It can be given alone or in combination with chemotherapy (it is contraindicated with anthracyclines due to cardiotoxicity) (📖 Biological therapy).

Radiotherapy

Low-dose radiotherapy (e.g. 20Gy/5#) provides effective palliation for

- Painful bone metastases.
- Soft tissue disease.
- Spread to brain or choroid.

Bisphosphonates (e.g. Pamidronate or Zoledronate)
- These drugs have an important role for patients with bone metastases from breast cancer. This includes:
  - Treatment and prevention of malignant hypercalcaemia.
  - Healing of osteolytic metastases.
  - Reducing bone pain.
  - Reducing progression of bone disease.
- Prolonged treatment is recommended, starting from the time of diagnosis of bone metastases, and continuing even in the face of progressive disease.
- Recent trials are exploring prophylactic treatment with these agents, e.g., preventing bone metastases in women with high-risk early breast cancer.

Breast reconstruction

- Breast reconstruction should be made available to all suitable patients as part of their cancer treatment.
- It may be done immediately post-mastectomy/partial mastectomy or as a delayed procedure after adjuvant therapies, such as chemotherapy/radiotherapy, are completed.
- It is also available for women having prophylactic surgery either to reduce risk of developing familial breast cancer or of contralateral disease.
- There is no evidence to show that reconstruction delays the identification of local recurrence, and it can reduce the psychological and emotional impact of a mastectomy.

Aims

- Replace breast tissue volume.
- Provide women with a breast mound (does not recreate their breast).
- Provide symmetry in volume and projection and sometimes ptosis (sagging) leading to a more natural appearance.
- Removes the need for an external prosthesis.
- Reduce impact of a mastectomy on the patient's body image.
- Provide an oncologically safe operation.

Immediate versus delayed reconstruction

Reconstruction can provide immediate psychological benefit. However, without tumour histopathology it is not known what adjuvant therapies are required. Radiotherapy is contra-indicated with certain types of reconstruction.

In delayed reconstruction, patients will have completed all of their adjuvant therapies. There can be a long recovery period post-reconstruction, which can be exacerbated by adjuvant therapies. Some patients prefer to complete the cancer side of their treatment first.

Types of surgery

- Implants—most commonly tissue expanders.
- LD (latissimus dorsi) muscle flap reconstruction.
- TRAM (transverse rectus abdominis muscle) flap reconstruction.
- DIEP—deep inferior epigastric perforator flap.
- SGAP—superior gluteal artery perforator flap.

Tissue expanders

Part silicone and part saline implant is placed under pectoralis major muscle in a deflated state. Once the incision has healed the implant is gradually inflated over a number of weeks with saline. This can be done as an outpatient procedure. In order to produce a more natural, supple contour the implant is over-inflated for 2–3 months and then deflated to achieve symmetry in volume. The inflation procedure can be uncomfortable. It can sometimes be done as a 2-stage procedure, where expander implant is replaced with a fixed volume implant. It is the simplest type of reconstructive surgery with no additional scarring. Suitable for smaller breasted patients and bi-lateral surgery.

Disadvantages
Formation of scar tissue around the implant can cause it to become misshapen and uncomfortable for the patient. Not suitable post radio-therapy due to lack of elasticity of skin and muscle. It is less suitable for fuller breasted women as difficult to provide symmetry.

Latissimus dorsi Flap (LD Flap)
This involves movement of skin, fat, and muscle to replace breast tissue. The flap is rotated onto the mastectomy site. The muscle remains attached to its original blood supply in the axilla. It takes 3–4 hours and produces additional scarring. This can provide a more natural shape and is very suitable post partial mastectomy. It offers the possibility of avoiding an implant, though an implant may be required to provide addition volume and projection.

Disadvantages
Flap necrosis, though rare, can occur. Seroma formation under the donor site may require repeated aspirations. It may not be suitable for patients who enjoy certain activities such as rock climbing or surfing.

TRAM flap
The movement of the transverse rectus abdominus muscle with overlying fat and skin to re-create breast volume. The blood supply to the muscle is attached to the infra mammary vein and artery with microsurgery. This produces the most natural cosmetic result as no implant is required—can achieve more ptosis and greater symmetry for fuller breasted women. Suitable procedure for immediate bi-lateral reconstruction.

Disadvantages
Can take up to 8 hours, with lower abdominal scarring and longer recovery period of 2–3 months. Flap necrosis is more frequent than with LD flap. Can get abdominal hernia. Synthetic mesh can be used to strengthen abdominal wall. Not suitable for smokers or women with a body mass index over 30.

DIEP and SGAP flaps
These involve moving fat and skin from the lower abdomen or buttocks. There is no abdominal weakness from procedure. There is a higher risk of flap necrosis due to the need to surgically establish new microvascular blood supply. It is not widely available.

Nipple preservation
Some patients wish to preserve the nipple. This is not recommended if the nipple is inverted due to the cancer, if there is evidence of disease in the ducts behind the nipple, or evidence of Pagets disease of the nipple. Patients should be made aware that nipple preservation increases the risk of disease recurrence by 5–10%

Nipple reconstruction
This is often done as a delayed procedure once the new breast has set-tled in volume and shape. Skin may be grafted from other nipple/areola or from inner thigh where skin is naturally darker. The areola may be tattooed to enhance cosmetic effect.

Prosthetic nipples

A cast can be taken of the remaining nipple to make a silicon replica. This can be colour-matched with the remaining nipple. The nipple is attached to the breast with surgical glue.

Surgery to contralateral breast

Women can be offered surgery on the contralateral breast, e.g. mastopexy—breast lift or mammoplasty—breast reduction. This can be offered during initial surgery, preventing the need for surgery at a later date.

Patient education issues

Patient education and support from a breast care nurse and the rest of the clinical team is essential in preparing women for any possible reconstructive surgery. Key issues to cover include:

- The individual's expectations and beliefs about the outcome.
- Potential risks of surgery, including failure of flaps, or possible need for further surgery.
- Altered sensation and prolonged post-operative neuropathic pain.
- The relationship between surgery and further anti-cancer treatment.

Nursing management issues

Nursing management issues

Nursing people with breast cancer can be challenging in many different ways. Due to the improving prognosis, women, even with locally advanced or metastatic disease may survive for many years with the disease. Breast cancer has been likened to a chronic disease trajectory for some, with periods of relapse and intensive treatment followed by long remission or more benign treatment.

Women will need different levels and types of support throughout this process. Supporting women to set and achieve realistic goals at different stages requires skilled and knowledgeable nursing care.

Treatment decision-making

Women face difficult decisions about treatment at diagnosis, after surgery or at disease recurrence. This may include what type of surgery to have, choices of chemotherapy or endocrine therapy. The potential benefit of treatments may be slight, and they all include some risk. Anxiety and fear may also reduce a woman's ability to make effective decisions.

- Good information and emotional support can aid decision-making. Nurses can help clarify the differences between treatment options, explain why these options exist, and give women access to information.
- Acting as a liaison between patients and medical staff can also be a supportive role for the nurse.
- Many women will appreciate a shared approach to decisions, reducing the burden on them at a difficult time.
- Good emotional support can aid decision-making. A specialist palliative care team referral may be helpful for those with advanced disease.
- Excellent breast cancer charities such as Breast Cancer Care offer specific support to younger women with breast cancer and partners of breast cancer patients (Partner Volunteer service).
- Breast cancer has a very high media profile and nurses can help patients to work through the plethora of information available through the various media.

Surgery

After surgery, the nurse can offer advice on appropriate exercises to prevent shoulder stiffness and lymphoedema, as well as assess for complications such as seroma or infection.

Note: Early referral to a lymphoedema specialist is important to establish the most effective management of lymphoedema (Lymphoedema).

Adjuvant treatment

Chemotherapy and radiotherapy treatment often lasts for six months or more and can be exhausting. For many women, this is followed by years of endocrine therapy. Preparing women for what to expect is essential.

- Common side effects of chemotherapy are: fatigue, hair loss, risk of infection, nausea and vomiting, and mucositis (Chemotherapy and specific symptom management chapters).

- Radiotherapy side effects include fatigue and sore skin. Axillary radiotherapy can also contribute to lymphoedema and brachial plexopathy (📖 Radiotherapy).
- Hormonal therapy such as tamoxifen can give severe menopausal side effects. Aromatase inhibitors can cause fatigue, nausea, headaches, and joint pains (📖 Hormonal therapy).
- Both chemotherapy and hormonal therapy can affect fertility. All breast cancer patients should have access to a fertility expert to discuss treatment options if required. (📖 Sexual health and cancer).

Psychosocial issues

These can be prominent throughout the disease process. Early and continuous assessment of potential psychological problems is essential. Referral to psychological support services may be appropriate for further advice or support (📖 Psychological support).

- Surgery, hair loss, and weight change all impact on an individual's body image and sexuality (📖 Altered body image).
- Depression and anxiety are not uncommon and are often under-diagnosed (📖 Anxiety; Depression).
- Recurrence of the disease is a particularly difficult time, with all the implications it holds and the impact of advanced cancer.
- A significant group of patients will be young or have young children.
  - The potentially hereditary nature of breast cancer may add to fears women have for their children.
  - Support from genetic counsellors or specialists can help clarify issues around genetic cancer links (📖 Genetic screening).

Advanced cancer symptom issues

Common problems experienced with advanced breast cancer include:

- Fungating breast tumours. Radiotherapy can be helpful in reducing bleeding. Topical antibiotics, e.g. metronidazole and regular dressings can help maintain dignity. Use of deodorizers may also reduce smell.
- Lung metastases can cause breathlessness and cough (📖 Breathlessness).
- Liver metastases can cause capsular pain, which responds to NSAIDs and steroids. Also nausea and vomiting, reduced appetite and ascites.
- Brain metastases: can cause a range of problems including confusion and change of personality (📖 Acute confusional states).
- Bone metastases: these cause a range of problems including.
  - Bone pain: radiotherapy, bisphosphonates, NSAIDs, and opioids can all be effective (📖 Metastatic bone disease).
  - Pathological fractures: these may need treatment with radiotherapy or orthopaedic surgical intervention (📖 Metastatic bone disease).
  - Hypercalcaemia: treatment with hydration and bisphosphonates can be helpful (📖 Hypercalcaemia).
  - Spinal cord compression: it is essential to diagnose this early to try and prevent major morbidity (📖 Spinal cord compression).

Central nervous system cancer

Introduction

Primary malignancies of the central nervous system are uncommon, but are difficult to treat when they occur. They are often characterized by a marked deterioration in the patient's functional ability and mental state. As a result, they can be devastating and life changing for the patient and their family.

There are many types of CNS malignancy, and the most common tumours have a poor prognosis. Recent advances in cancer treatment, imaging and surgical modalities have so far failed to improve overall survival for this group of patients.

The management of brain tumours presents a considerable challenge for the multidisciplinary team, both in the hospital and in the community. An integrated approach is essential.

Note: management of metastatic brain tumours and leptomeningeal carcinomatosis are also covered briefly within the chapter.

Epidemiology
- CNS cancers account for 2% of all cancers diagnosed.
- CNS cancers account for 20% of cancers diagnosed in children under the age of 15.
- The incidence of CNS cancers peaks in childhood, falls, and then rises exponentially until the age of 75.
- The incidence and age profile of CNS cancer is consistent across the world.
- The 5-year survival rate for all brain tumours is 15–20% across Europe.

Risk factors
- Age—children and those over 50 years.
- No clear environmental factors have been proven—apart from a rising incidence with exposure to ionizing radiation, particularly in early life.
- The increasing incidence is likely to be due to better detection and imaging and an aging population.

Common presenting symptoms
- Change in personality.
- Depression (often misdiagnosed as psychological in origin).
- Seizures.
- Changes to, or loss of, sensation in limbs.
- Headache.
- Collapse.
- Tiredness and fatigue.

Investigations

- Neurological assessment and medical interpretation of signs and symptoms.
- Preferably MRI scan of the head or spine, otherwise cranial or spinal CT scan.
- Tissue diagnosis may be required in order to determine the exact nature of the tumour—for example whether it is a primary or a metastatic tumour and to assess histology.
- Most brain tumours do not metastasize, apart from, very rarely, to the spinal cord.

Biopsy

The following should be considered before making a decision to obtain a tissue sample:

- Should the tumour be excised, a biopsy taken, or neither?
- Is the patient fit for either, or one of these procedures?
- Is the tumour safely accessible by surgery?

These decisions are complex, and are ideally made within a multi-disciplinary setting, with the involvement of the patient and carers. They should include specialist neurological and neurosurgical input.

Stereotactic biopsy is the approach of choice. It is a minimally invasive technique that utilizes imaging in order to obtain a tissue sample. It may be used where a tumour is likely to be malignant, and is in a functionally important or inaccessible area. It is normally followed by radiotherapy.

Classification of primary CNS tumours

The pathophysiological classification of CNS tumours is complex. It is based on the type of cell from which the tumour originates. Only the most common CNS malignancies are covered here (see Table 25.1). By far the most common primary CNS malignancy is the brain tumour, with spinal cord tumours accounting for only 10–15% of primary tumours.

Gliomas

Gliomas—including astrocytomas, oligodendrogliomas and ependymomas—are the most common brain tumours. They arise from neuroepithelial (or glial) cells within the brain. These are one of the few groups of neural cells that divide. Gliomas are further classified by the malignancy of the cells within the tumour, and their ability to cause necrosis. Grade 1 is the least malignant, and grade 4 the most.)

Astrocytomas

Astrocytomas account for around 70% of all brain tumours. They generally arise within the cerebral hemispheres, but can occur in the spinal cord. Grade 1 and 2 tumours are typically well differentiated, whilst grade 3 and 4 tumours show far higher levels of necrosis and vascular changes.

The most malignant form of astrocytoma (grade 4)—is also called a glioblastoma multiforme. It is the most common astrocytoma, and accounts for 60% of all adult primary brain tumours. These tumours are resistant to surgical and non-surgical treatment, and are associated with a particularly poor prognosis.

Oligodendroglioma

These gliomas are typically slow growing tumours that occur within the frontal lobes. They account for around 5% of primary brain tumours, and tend to be more chemosensitive than other gliomas.

Ependymoma

These gliomas arise from ependymal glial cells, and account for around 6% of all brain tumours. They can occur in adults, but are more common in children. They are unusual in that they can spread (via the CSF) to the spinal cord. Patients may present with a cerebral ependymoma and lesions in the spinal cord. Spinal ependymomas account for more than 50% of all primary spinal tumours.

Non–glioma tumours

Meningioma

These tumours arise from the cells of the meninges—the inner lining of the brain. They tend to be slow growing, low-grade tumours. They can often be successfully excised surgically, because of their more superficial nature.

Table 25.1 Survival chart for different tumour types

Tumour group	Treatment	5-year survival
Low grade astrocytoma (grade 1 and 2)	Surgery radiotherapy	50–60%
High grade astrocytoma (grade 3 and 4)	All treatments	<5%
Oligodendroglioma	Surgery + radiotherapy	35%
Ependymoma	Surgery + radiotherapy	56–80%
Meningioma	Surgery	45–80%
CNS lymphoma	All treatments	3%

Primary CNS lymphoma

These account for less than 1% of primary brain tumours. They are much more common in immunosupressed patients, e.g. after an organ transplant or people with long-term HIV disease (📖 HIV related malignancies). Primary treatment is generally chemotherapy, with radiotherapy held in reserve as a second line treatment. Primary CNS lymphoma is associated with a poor long-term prognosis.

Spinal tumours

80% of spinal tumours are metastatic in origin with the sites of origin being myeloma, breast, lung, or lymphoma. The remainder are typically as a result of ependymoma, meningioma, or more rarely, astrocytoma. Diagnosis of spinal tumors is determined by clinical examination followed by MRI scan. The recognition and swift treatment of metastatic spinal tumours is important, as they can result in spinal cord compression, an oncological emergency (📖 Spinal cord compression).

Management of primary CNS malignancy

Treatment modalities

Surgery

Surgery can be used as a primary treatment (full or partial resection) or used to facilitate non-surgical treatments (debulking or stereotactic biopsy). Surgery is often the primary treatment of choice for patients with a CNS malignancy, and it offers the best chance of long-term survival.

The aim is to excise the tumour with as wide a margin as possible to avoid an incomplete excision. The extent to which this is possible depends on:

- The type of tumour and the degree to which it is encapsulated.
- The location of the tumour and its proximity to key functional areas within the brain and/or CNS.
- The general fitness of the patient.

The extent to which the margins of a tumour can be excised in neuro-surgery, is limited by the possible damage to healthy brain tissue, and the resulting possible long-term neurological damage inflicted on the patient. Where a complete resection is not possible, a tumour may be excised as much as possible, or debulked and then followed up with post-operative radiotherapy.

With any neurosurgery, the main postoperative risks are cerebral oedema, intercranial bleeding, and infection. All of these can be life threatening or may leave the patient with neurological deficits and a disability. Patients should therefore be cared for in a specialist neurosurgical unit in the immediate post-operative period, as their condition can deteriorate rapidly.

The degree to which surgery is successful in improving survival depends largely on the tumour type. 80% of meningiomas are successfully treated with surgery alone, whereas grade 4 astrocytomas (glioblastoma multiforme) will almost certainly recur.

Chemotherapy

The success of chemotherapeutic agents has been very limited in the treatment of CNS malignancy. Therapy is limited by the presence of the blood–brain barrier and many tumours are not chemo-sensitive.

Most cytotoxic agents do not pass through the blood–brain barrier and are therefore rendered ineffective. Procarbazine and Lomustine (CCNU?) are exceptions to this general rule—they can bypass the blood–brain barrier and are frequently employed in treating brain tumours, together with Vincristine (see box opposite).

Recently, Temozolamide has been developed. This drug has shown promise in clinical trials, particularly when combined with radiotherapy. Another development is intracavity chemotherapy. Wafers containing slow-release carmustine (BCNU) are placed in the tumour bed following excision of the tumour. The cytotoxic agent is released over the next few days, reducing the incidence of local recurrence. The wafers then break down harmlessly.

The blood–brain barrier

The blood–brain barrier consists of the tightly joined linings of cells surrounding cerebral capillaries. These prevent the exchange of water-soluble ions, proteins, and drugs between the vessel and the surrounding neural tissues. Smaller molecules and fat-soluble ions diffuse more readily. The blood–brain barrier protects the sensitive neural tissue from potentially damaging fluctuations in the biochemical environment.

The blood–brain barrier can also be bypassed by administering chemotherapy directly into or around a brain tumour—using a reservoir system, usually an Ommaya reservoir. This is placed under the scalp, and has a fine tube that passes into the CSF or into a cystic tumour. It can also be used as a drainage device to prevent a build up of fluid within a cystic tumour. These devices should only be used by specially trained staff.

Radiotherapy

For the most common types of CNS malignancy, the main role of radiotherapy is as an adjunct to surgical resection, rather than as a primary treatment. Exceeding the maximum tolerance of nerve tissue can cause tissue necrosis, with accompanying loss of brain tissue and neurological damage.

Steroids

Steroids have a vital role in the management of CNS tumours, particularly brain tumours, as they can stabilize a patient's condition at many stages throughout their illness. Dexamethasone is generally used.

Steroids are powerful anti-inflammatory agents, and can dramatically improve a patients overall condition by reducing cerebral oedema.

Steroids have a wide range of side effects—the guiding principle is to keep steroid dosage down to the minimal level, and to reduce the dose of steroids once the patient's condition has stabilized. (See Table 25.2).

Table 25.2 Common steroid side effects and their management

Side effect	Management strategies
Gastric ulceration	Administer regular omeprazole/ranitidine
Sleep disturbance	Administer steroids in morning rather than afternoon
Diabetes	Monitor urine daily for sugar, and treat diabetes if necessary
Weight gain	Monitor dietary intake and provide guidance
Confusional state 'Steroid psychosis'	Reduce steroid dose if acute and distressing and treat with benzodiazepines or haloperidol if severe
Addisonian crisis	Reduce steroids gradually, rather than stopping them

Note: it should also be remembered that steroids can mask pyrexia, making a potential infection more difficult to assess.

Metastatic brain disease

Aetiology

- 10 times more common than primary malignant CNS tumours. However, many patients are asymptomatic (found only on autopsy).
- Most occur in cerebral hemispheres, with minority in the cerebellum or brain stem. Over half have multiple lesions.
- Caused by haematological spread from primary cancer. Most commonly lung and breast primaries. Also melanoma, kidney, and colon cancer.

Presenting symptoms

- Focal neurological disturbances: hemiparesis, dysphasia, cranial nerve palsies.
- Raised ICP, headache, nausea and vomiting, lethargy.
- Epileptic seizures.
- Cognitive behavior change.

Management

Surgery

In a small group of patients with single lesions surgery may be appropriate, particularly if it is a radiotherapy resistant tumour. A specialist neurosurgeon can assess the risks and potential benefit of surgery.

Radiotherapy

For most patients surgery is not an option due to multifocal brain lesions, tumour inaccessibility, widespread systemic disease, performance status, and comorbidity.

Options include:

- Whole brain radiotherapy and steroid therapy is the standard treatment. This provides a symptomatic improvement in about 70% of patients.
- Stereotactic radiotherapy—fractionated treatment which accurately targets the tumours, reducing the impact on healthy tissue.
- Radiosurgery (single high does stereotactic radiotherapy) can be used to treat small lesions.

Note: stereotactic treatment is not available in all treatment centres.

Symptoms of radiotherapy include somnolence and long-term memory/cognitive impairment (not always relevant due to the short life expectancy) of many of these patients.

Chemotherapy

Adjuvant chemotherapy can be considered in chemotherapy sensitive disease, e.g. germ-cell, haematological, or small cell lung cancers.

Leptomeningeal carcinomatosis

This is diffuse seeding of cancer cells throughout the cerebrospinal (CSF) and the meninges. It is generally caused by progressive system cancers, most commonly haematological disease such as leukaemia and lymphoma. It can also occur in, breast, lung, and gastrointestinal cancer.

Common presenting symptoms

Cranial nerve problems, headache, back pain, leg weakness.

Diagnosis

- Lumbar puncture with cytology of CSF.
- MRI scan.

Management

- Leptomeningeal carcinomatosis can be treated with intrathecal chemotherapy as well as localized radiotherapy to deal with specific symptoms.
- Median survival is very poor, other than a few curative haematological cancer patients.

sing management issues

rsing patients with tumours of the CNS can be extremely challenging ue to invasive treatments, complex symptom management, and often, a poor prognosis. The long-term changes in an individual's behaviour and personality can be very distressing for family members.

Common nursing challenges include:
- Hemiparesis or other neurological deficit.
- Aphasia or dysphasia.
- Depression (📖 Depression).
- Confusional state (📖 Acute confusional states).
- Fluctuating level of awareness.
- Swallowing difficulties and aspiration.
- Cerebral oedema (caused by disease, surgery, or radiotherapy).

Management of cerebral oedema

Cerebral oedema is swelling of the brain caused by a build up of fluid within the brain tissue. It occurs as a result of irritation to the brain, either by the effects of the tumour itself, by invasive surgery and other procedures, or by radiotherapy.

If allowed to proceed unchecked, cerebral oedema can damage brain tissue, causing deterioration in the patient's condition, and ultimately proving fatal.

The key aspects in managing this problem are:
- Patient assessment—noting that the patient's condition has changed either by formal assessment (neurological observations) or more informally, by knowing your patient and the significance of any change.
- High dose steroid treatment (up to 16mg of dexamethasone per day) and reduce once patient's condition has stabilized.
- Management of steroid side effects (see Table 25.2).
- Occasionally high dose diuretics e.g. mannitol.

MDT working and team approach

It is vital that care for a person with a CNS tumour is planned and coordinated in a holistic and consistent way, and that carers are supported. This is best managed via a responsive and regularly reviewed multidisciplinary plan of care.

The role of the key worker is vital in coordinating the plan and referring to other specialists as the patient's condition changes.

Key referrals for individuals with CNS tumours

- Speech therapy (swallowing and dysphasia).
- Dieticians (poor oral intake, steroid induced diabetes).
- Occupational therapists (functional assessment and forward planning).
- Social services (care management).
- District nurses (community support and care).
- Palliative care teams (acute, trust, and community).
- Psychological services—(advice on management of acute confusional states).

Ethical issues (📖 Ethics in cancer care)

The treatment of patients with CNS tumours is an area where ethical issues are often brought into sharp focus. This is because:

- It is often not clear whether a patient can consent to treatment or not.
- Patients are often treated with long, and potentially taxing, regimens of chemotherapy or radiotherapy with an overall poor prognosis.
- The perception of the patient may differ widely from that of the carers or health care professionals.
- Because swallowing can often be impaired, there may be issues around supported feeding and hydration (via NG or PEG) for patients with severe disabilities.

Many of these issues do not have an overall right or wrong answer. What is in the best interest of a patient may vary with time and circumstance, and may not be applicable to another patient. What is crucial is involving the patient, and where possible, the carers, in decision-making and raising the issues in an open and inclusive manner (📖 Patient and family involvement in decision making).

Further reading

Graham C A and Cloughesy T F (2004). Brain tumor treatment: chemotherapy and other new developments. *Seminars in Oncology Nursing*, **20**(4), 260–72.

Guerrero D (1998). *Neuro-Oncology For Nurses*. West Sussex: Whurr Publishers.

Kaye A H and Laws E R Jr (eds) (2001). *Brain Tumours: An Encyclopaedic Approach* (2nd Edn). London: Churchill Livingstone.

Lovely MP (2004). Symptom management of brain tumor patients. *Seminars in Oncology Nursing*, **20**(4), pp273–83.

National Institute for Clinical Excellence (2006). *Service guidance for improving outcomes for people with brain and other central nervous system tumours*. London: NICE.

Colorectal cancer

Introduction

Incidence

- Colorectal cancer is the third commonest cancer in UK (fourth worldwide) with over 34,000 UK cases diagnosed annually.
- It affects men and women almost equally.
- It is rare under 40 years of age. Over half of deaths are in the over 75s.
- Most cases are lower colon and rectum.
- Approx 30% of individuals present with advanced disease. A further 35% will go on to develop advanced disease.

Risk factors

- Approx 7% of cases are associated with genetic predisposition syndromes such as familial adenomatous polyposis (FAP) and hereditary non polyposis colon cancer (HNPCC).
- Other risk factors include a fat rich diet and inflammatory bowel disease.

Presenting symptoms

These are partly dependent on where the tumour occurs in the bowel
- **Early:** rectal bleeding, persisting change in bowel habit, and anaemia.
- **Late:** weight loss, nausea, anorexia, and abdominal pain.

Common sites of spread

- Liver, lungs, and peritoneum.
- Local recurrence at anastomosis site or pre-sacral.
- Liver metastases are the most common because the colon's venous drainage is mainly via the portal system.

Staging and diagnosis

Commonly staged using TNM classification (traditionally Dukes is used as well) (📖 Diagnosis and classification).

Useful investigations include:
- Full colonoscopy or proctosigmoidoscopy + barium enema.
- Liver CT and/or ultrasound.
- CT scan of colon, chest, abdomen, and pelvis.
- MRI and ultrasound of the pelvis for rectal cancers.

Treatment approaches to colorectal cancer

Surgery
- Surgery is the main curative therapy for colorectal cancer. Curative resection requires the excision of the primary tumour and its lymphatic drainage with an enveloping margin of normal tissue.
- Minimally invasive colon surgery is becoming more common, but there is concern over adequacy of clearance in patients with more advanced cancers.

Rectal cancer
- Total excision of the mesorectum is considered essential. This has been shown to effectively reduce local relapse rates.
- About 5% of rectal cancers may be removed by non-radical transanal surgery.

Hepatic metastases
- Metastasis confined to one lobe of the liver or less than four in both lobes may warrant resection, as there is up to a 30% chance of cure.

Complications of surgery
- Infection and intra abdominal abscesses.
- Anastamotic leak and GU tract injury—both require immediate surgical intervention.
- Large bowel obstruction—may respond to conservative management (📖 Bowel obstruction).
- Sexual dysfunction—abdominoperineal resection can cause impotence due to surgical nerve damage (📖 Sexual health and cancer).

Stoma formation
About 15% of patients diagnosed with colorectal cancer end up with a permanent colostomy. Many others will require a temporary colostomy or ileostomy whilst they recover from their surgery (📖 Stoma care).

Non-surgical
Adjuvant therapy of colorectal cancer
50% of patients who undergo apparently curative resection of bowel cancer will have residual micro-metastases that are invisible at the time of surgery. These eventually lead to locally recurrent or distant metastatic disease. Adjuvant chemotherapy aims to eradicate these micro-metastases and thereby prevent future relapse.

Indications
It is normally offered to those with stage 3 disease cancers. Adjuvant therapy for rectal cancer may include both radiotherapy and chemotherapy, aimed at local and systemic micro-metastases respectively.

Chemotherapy used in adjuvant setting

5-fluorouracil (5FU) ± oxaliplatin remains standard therapy. Tar⌐
therapies are also being investigated, e.g.
• Cetuximab—targeting epidermal growth factor receptor.
• Bevacizumab—angiogenesis inhibitor.

Chemo-irradiation

For patients with rectal cancer, preoperative pelvic radiotherapy can be
given concurrently with chemotherapy. This may be followed by a more
prolonged course of standard adjuvant chemotherapy aimed at distant
micrometastases.

Side effects of treatment

The side effects vary considerably from patient to patient and depend on
the dose and the schedules used. Side effects should be tolerable for
most patients and chemotherapy can normally be given to the elderly.

Common side effects

• Nausea and vomiting.
• Oral mucositis.
• Diarrhoea.
• Red, painful palms and soles (palmar planter syndrome).
• Peripheral neuropathy (when oxaliplatin is included).

Chemotherapy in advanced colorectal cancer

• The median survival time for such patients without further therapy
  is 6 months.
• In most cases the aim of therapy is palliation.
• Survival has been modestly prolonged by using modern
  chemotherapy agents.
• A few patients have advanced disease, which could be made
  resectable by volume reduction (down-staging) using chemotherapy.

First line chemotherapy

• Infusional 5-fluorouracil (5FU) with either oxalipatin (FOLFOX) or
  irinotecan (FOLFIRI).
• Survival improvements of about 6 months over best supportive
  care alone.
• Other options include capecitabine, which is orally administered.
  This is being used more frequently now. The convenience of oral
  treatment can be an important factor in advanced disease (🕮 Oral
  chemotherapy).
• The following are still unclear:
  • Which combination is best.
  • The optimum duration of therapy.
  • If continuous or intermittent exposure to treatment is best.

...ne chemotherapy

...tecan is standard second line therapy in patients who relapse
...lowing 5FU or progress whilst on this therapy.
Oxaliplatin has not been tested so extensively as a single agent in
second line, but has shown some promise.

Novel cytotoxic agents

- Erbitux® (cetuximab) is a monoclonal antibody which targets the
  epithelial growth factor receptor:
  - It has shown activity both as a single agent and in combination
    with cytotoxic drugs, particularly Irinotecan.
- Avastin® (bevacizumab) is an anti-angiogenic compound:
  - Full integration of this agent awaits further clinical trials in
    various combinations and schedules.

Radiotherapy in colorectal cancer

- Preoperative radiotherapy is becoming standard practice in rectal
  cancer to reduce the risk of recurrence. It can increase the chance of
  complete surgical resection in some patients with large tumours that
  have not yet metastasized.
- Pelvic chemoradiotherapy reduces the risk of relapse for patients
  with stage II and III rectal cancer.
- Radiotherapy is also used within palliative situations, for example
  recurrent rectal cancer.

e of the patient with a stoma

.toma is the result of a surgical intervention in which the stream of
.eces or urine is diverted away from its normal route.

There are three main types of stoma.
- Ileostomy: loop or end ileostomy, sited on the right side of the
  abdomen. Can be temporary or permanent. Output from an
  ileostomy is primarily liquid.
- Colostomy: loop or end colostomy, sited on the left side of the
  abdomen. Can be permanent or temporary. Output is generally solid.
- Urostomy: always permanent and sited on right side of abdomen.
  Output is urine.

Uses of different stomas

Temporary ileostomy
- To protect an anastomosis (join in the bowel) following removal of
  low rectal cancer.
- As a palliative procedure to relieve obstruction in inoperable tumours.
- To relieve obstructive symptoms during long course down-staging
  chemotherapy or radiotherapy.

Permanent ileostomy
When the patient has multiple tumours or hereditary polyposis and the
entire large bowel has to be removed.

Temporary colostomy
- When the patient has presented as an emergency and tumour has
  been removed but bowel not rejoined (Hartmann's procedure).
- To relieve obstructive symptoms during long course down-staging
  chemotherapy/radiotherapy.

Permanent colostomy
- When low rectal tumour cannot be removed leaving disease free
  margins. To enable bowel to be joined (anastomosis). This operation
  would be an abdo-perineal excision of rectum.
- As a palliative procedure to alleviate symptoms of obstruction.

Urostomy
Used when the bladder cannot be preserved either because of trauma or
disease, e.g. bladder cancer.

Nursing management

Pre-operatively
It is essential that all patients are referred to a stomatherapy clinical
nurse specialist, for pre- and post-operative information, and for a clear
discussion about the potential impact of the stoma on a patient's lifestyle.
This prepares the patient and their family and allows the nurse to assess
the patient prior to surgery for any potential difficulties they may have,
both physically and psychologically, adjusting to life with a stoma.

Post-operatively

Surgical complications. A range of surgical problems can occur with stoma formation. If the stoma does not have adequate blood supply it can become necrotic and appears a maroon or black colour. This may require further surgery. It is important to observe the stoma for colour, which should be a dark pink and have a wet appearance similar to the inside of the mouth.

Other complications include:
- Stenosing (narrowing) due to extensive scar tissue, which may require further surgery or use of dilatation.
- Prolapsing due to herniation of the stoma. This can be caused by over exertion and may need surgical repair.
- Para-stomal hernia due to herniation around the stoma—may need surgery to correct.
- Retraction of the stoma, where it recedes back into the abdomen. It becomes difficult to seal appliances and it may need surgical repair.

Stoma care

Sore skin is a common problem if the appliance is incorrectly applied and has been leaking; this in turn creates further problems with appliance adherence. Teaching patients management and application of pouches, the importance of maintaining skin care, and a high level of personal hygiene is essential. The aim is for independence in stoma care upon discharge.

Note: patients should be assessed by a stomatherapy clinical nurse specialist prior to discharge to ensure that they are independent in stoma management.

It is important to observe stoma output for amount, colour, and consistency. For colostomies this should be faecal brown colour and formed stool. Ileostomies should produce loose stool, faecal coloured and the appliance should be emptied 5/6 times in 24 hours. Urostomies should drain straw colored urine, approx 3 litres volume a day. Whenever these stomas drain blood, this needs to be reported and investigated.

Patients with an ileostomy can become dehydrated, caused by stoma over activity, leading to readmission for intravenous fluids. Patients are encouraged to have a higher intake of salt in their diet or take 1 litre of isotonic drink daily.

Note: constipation and diarrhoea can still be a problem for patients with stomas and should be treated in the usual way.

Dietary advice

- Colostomy patients should be encouraged to have a normal diet including high-fibre foods.
- Ileostomy patients should take a low-fibre diet and caution with some fruit and vegetables, to reduce bowel action.
- Urostomy patients are encouraged to drink 3 litres of fluid a day (to include a mixture of drinks not just water). Some patients are encouraged to drink 1 x glass of cranberry juice a day (to alter the pH of the urine and reduce the incidence of stone formation and infection), although evidence for the effectiveness of this is limited.

Exercise

Exercise (including driving) should not be undertaken for at least one month if the patient has a large abdominal wound and heavy lifting should not begin until after three months. This is to avoid rupture of internal repairs and for the patient's long-term recovery and comfort. If key-hole surgery has been performed, driving may commence after 2 weeks and lifting after 6 weeks.

Psychological issues

Having to cope with a stoma can be very difficult for some patients. A stoma can impact on body image, social and sexual functioning and feelings of disgust, anger, embarrassment, or shame can occur. Allow patients time to express and talk about their feelings include partners/ relatives. Remember that the patient will be watching you for your response whilst you are undertaking stoma care. Patients can be reassured that these feelings, although new to them, are normal following stoma surgery. The cancer site-specific clinical nurse specialist or stoma specialist are excellent sources of support both for the patients and their families.

Sexual function

Ensure that the patient is informed preoperatively that sexual function may be affected following surgery.

- Explain that following surgery, chemotherapy or radiotherapy, sexual function can take weeks or months to regain.
- Encourage patients to discuss any fears and anxieties that they may have by giving them time and privacy to discuss sexuality issues.
- Advise them when referral to a psychosexual counsellor is an option.
- Men who have urostomies will be impotent and will therefore need advice re use of medication and penile implants.

Practical advice can include:
- Empty appliance before sex.
- Use of underwear/lingerie to cover appliance.
- Reassure that stoma won't be damaged during sex.
(📖 Sexual health & cancer.)

Further reading

Fillingham S and Douglas A (2003). *Urological Nursing* 3rd edn. London, Bailliere Tindall.
Porrett T and Daniel N (1999). *Essential coloproctology for nurses*. Bognor Regis: Wiley.
Swan E (2005). *Colorectal Cancer* Bognor Regis: Wiley.

Nursing management issues

A number of specific challenges face nurses supporting individuals with colorectal cancer. Body image and psychosexual issues often emerge both from the nature of the disease and from treatment side effects, Those patients with advanced cancer may also have complex and difficult symptoms such as bowel obstruction, pain, and bowel fistulae. Effective multidisciplinary management is crucial to support these patients effectively (Ⅲ For detailed exploration of specific issues see the appropriate chapters in sections 4 and 7).

Treatment issues

Post-surgical

Many men will suffer a level of impotence and/or ejaculatory problems after colorectal surgery. Women may also suffer urinary problems such as dysuria and incontinence. Patients requiring stoma formation also report many problems with body image and sexuality issues. Faecal incontinence or increased bowel movements are also a problem (Ⅲ Care of patient with a stoma).

- Patients can become socially isolated and face periods of depression. Many of these difficulties can occur months after surgery.
- It is essential to assess patients' social and psychosexual well-being regularly, to pick up issues early and to offer support both in hospital and in the community.
- Nurses can play an important part in offering advice on lifestyle changes, coordinating care, and referring to appropriate specialist services.

Radiotherapy

Radiotherapy can be debilitating. Common problems include:
- Diarrhoea.
- Fatigue.
- Sore skin.
- Perineal wound infection if used pre-surgery.

Chemotherapy

Chemotherapy regimens are generally well tolerated. Particular issues are
- Severe diarrhoea (irinotecan/capecitabine based regimes).
- Nausea, infection, and fatigue.

Pain

Liver metastases can cause capsular pain, which responds to NSAIDs and steroids.

Local rectal recurrence

- Can cause severe neuropathic perineal and pelvic pain as well as tenesmus (painful sensation of rectal fullness).
- Each can be difficult to manage successfully and only partially responds to opioids.
- Management options include, analgesics, anti-convulsants, radiotherapy, and local nerve blocks.

- Skilled nursing pain management is required to support these patients effectively (📖 Pain management). Specialist palliative care teams can be invaluable for these symptoms.

Altered bowel habit

Diarrhoea and constipation
- Patients can suffer from diarrhoea and/or constipation on a regular basis.
- For patients with diarrhoea, it is important to rule out faecal impaction.
- Alternating diarrhoea and constipation could be a warning of developing bowel obstruction.

Bowel obstruction
- Can be a major problem after surgery (where it normally responds to conservative approaches) and in advanced cancer.
- Nurses have a key role in early diagnosis by assessing patients for signs of obstruction.

Nutritional issues
- Many colorectal patients will suffer from weight loss, anorexia, and malnutrition, with associated fatigue and weakness.
- It is important that the multidisciplinary team, especially the dietitian and the patient's family are fully involved in managing nutritional disorders.

Further reading

Fillingham S and Douglas A (2003). *Urological Nursing* 3rd edn. London: Bailliere Tindall.

National Institute for Clinical excellence (2004). *Guidance on Cancer Services-Improving Outcomes in Colorectal Cancers: The Manual*. London: NICE.

Porrett T and Daniel N (1999). *Essential coloproctology for nurses*. Bognor Regis: Wiley.

Swan E (2005). *Colorectal Cancer for nurses*. Bognor Regis: Wiley & Sons.

Wilkes G. (2005). Colon, rectal and anal cancers. In Yarbro C H, Frogge M H, Goodman M (eds) *Cancer Nursing, Principles and practice*. 6th edn, pp.1155–1214. Massachusetts: Jones and Bartlett.

Cancer of unknown primary (CUP)

Introduction and prognosis

Introduction
- Common oncological problem representing up to 15% of all referrals.
- The primary site of a carcinoma remains undetected even after postmortem examination in around 20–25% of these cases.
- Normally arises due to the unusual metastatic potential of the tumour but occasionally there has been regression of the primary (well recognized in melanoma).
- Carcinoma of the lung and pancreas are the most common primary carcinomas that initially present as CUP. Others include colorectal, breast, prostate cancer and head and neck cancer.
- The majority are adenocarcinoma (60–70%) and poorly differentiated carcinoma (20–30%).

Prognosis
- Overall prognosis is poor, with a median survival of around 4 months, with less than 25% of patients surviving 1 year.
- About 5% of head and neck cancers present as a cervical neck node, with unknown primary. Radical treatment can lead to 5 year survival of over 30%.
- It is important to exclude potentially curable malignancies e.g. germ cells, lymphomas, thyroid cancer, but to also only carry out investigations that may change clinical outcome. There is a danger of exhausting the patient with extensive but futile investigations.
- Favourable prognostic factors include female sex, fewer sites of metastatic disease, and a good performance status. Discussion at an appropriate MDT is essential.

Treatment and nursing management

Treatment is dependent on:
- Tumour characteristics (chemo-responsiveness).
- Patient characteristics including organ function, performance status, and quality of life issues.
- Appropriate patients can be selected who may benefit from chemotherapy with palliative intent.
- Local treatment for symptomatic metastases should be considered e.g. radiotherapy for painful bone metastases or for brain metastases.
- Occasionally a single metastatic site of disease is identified which can be successfully treated with resection. However, other metastatic sites normally appear despite this treatment.

These will require sensitive discussion with the patient and their family. Involvement of palliative care services is usually appropriate for all patients.

Nursing management

The lack of certainty around diagnosis means that it is difficult to give the patient and their family adequate information about potential outcomes of the disease or treatment. It is essential to remain honest about the uncertainties and the general poor prognosis. This uncertainty may cause high levels of anxiety, distress, and anger both for the patient and their family (☐ Psychological reactions to cancer).

Information giving issues will include:
- Clarifying reasons for a particular treatment approach.
- Potential further approaches if initial treatment is unsuccessful.
- The balance between full investigations and the potentially futile nature of such investigations.

Further reading

Hainsworth J D, Greco F A (2000). Management of patients with cancer of unknown primary site. *Oncology*, **12**, 563–7.

Lindeman, G J and Tattershall, M (1995). Tumours of unknown primary site. In Peckham M, Pinedo H and Veronesi (eds). *Oxford Textbook of Oncology*, pp.2155–65. Oxford: Oxford University Press.

Endocrine cancers

Introduction and types of endocrine cancers

Endocrine tumours arise from glands that secrete endocrine hormones. This includes the pituitary, thyroid, parathyroid, and adrenal glands as well as the gonads and the islets of Langerhans in the pancreas.

Endocrine tumours are rare, and are benign in most cases. Benign tumours can still cause significant morbidity, but they are not covered in this book (see Further reading below).

The causes of most cases of endocrine cancer are unknown. There is an autosomal dominant inheritance called multiple endocrine neoplasia (MEN), in which several endocrine malignancies occur at once, generally earlier in life, with multicentric and bilateral presentation.

Nursing people with these cancers requires knowledge of the hormones secreted, and their effects on body systems. Nursing management needs to focus on the symptoms caused by these hormones.

Thyroid cancer

Thyroid cancer accounts for 90% of endocrine tumours. The most common is papillary carcinoma, which has a 10-year survival rate of over 90%. Anaplastic thyroid cancer is rarer, and has a very poor prognosis of 4–7 months median survival.

The commonest clinical presentation for thyroid cancer is with a painless lump in the neck—a solitary thyroid nodule. Anaplastic cancer generally presents with a rapidly enlarging neck mass and enlarged lymph nodes.

Surgery is the commonest treatment, involving partial or total thyroidectomy. Potential complications of this include hypoparathyroidism and laryngeal nerve injury. Radio-iodine therapy can be used post surgery. External beam radiotherapy may be used to downstage some tumours and for palliation of symptoms from metastatic disease.

Anaplastic carcinoma is generally too advanced at diagnosis for surgery. Anaplastic thyroid cancer is not responsive to iodine therapy.

Adrenal cancer

Adrenal tumours are rare, with an incidence of about 1–1.5 per 1,000,000 in the adult population. Almost all patients with benign disease are cured by surgery.

Prognosis is poor for patients with malignant disease. Untreated, the median survival is 3–9 months. Even if the carcinoma is apparently confined to the adrenal gland, survival following surgery may be as little as 2–3 years.

Further reading

Current Opinions in Oncology. Both January 2005, vol 17(1), and January 2004, vol 16(1) explore endocrine tumours.

Chapter 29

Upper gastrointestinal cancers

Introduction

The cancers of the upper gastrointestinal (GI) tract are a diverse group of cancers accounting for around one fifth of all cancers diagnosed in the UK. Improved surgical treatment of early stage disease can offer excellent survival rates, but most patients will present with regional or advanced spread of the disease. The symptoms of many of the upper GI cancers are vague and non-specific and often occur late in the course of the disease. Combined with poor overall responses to chemotherapy and radiotherapy, this makes them difficult to treat; as a result long-term survival rates tend to be low.

For some diseases such as pancreatic cancer, the outcome may be bleak, with a short life expectancy and rapid physical deterioration not unusual.

Individuals and their families will need a lot of support coping throughout the whole period of the illness. Treatment morbidity, and common symptoms of dysphagia, severe weight loss, and malnutrition amongst others can create high levels of physical and psychological distress.

Multidisciplinary team involvement, including surgeons, oncologists, site-specific CNS, palliative care specialists, and dietitians, is crucial to the effective management of these patients. The following covers the key treatment approaches for each cancer. Key nursing issues and cross references for relevant symptom management are highlighted at the end of the section.

Oesophageal cancer

Incidence
- Approximately 7,500 people in the UK are diagnosed with oesophageal cancer each year.
- It is at least twice as common in males than females.
- The incidence increases with age eight-fold between 45–54 and 65–74 years.
- Most people present with advanced disease. Less than 30% survive for 5 years or more.

Risk factors
- Alcohol and smoking: heavy smokers and drinkers have a 100-fold increased risk.
- Barrett's oesophagus (dysplastic changes in the lower oesophagus).
- Obesity: may increase oesophageal reflux and incidence of Barrett's oesophagus.

Presenting symptoms
- Dysphagia.
- Dyspepsia.
- Weight loss.
- Chest pain.

Diagnosis and staging
- Endoscopy and tissue biopsy.
- Endoluminal ultrasound—shows extent of local invasion and lymph node involvement.
- CT scan—to assess further nodal involvement and distant metastases.
- Further staging is done with laparoscopy and less commonly barium swallow.

Common sites of spread
- Early lymphatic spread is common before symptoms occur.
- Distant metastases to liver, adrenal glands, lung, bone, and brain are common in advanced disease.

Treatment

A multidisciplinary approach is strongly advised for optimum patient management. This should involve the surgeon, gastroenterologist, radiologist, oncologist, and dietitian.

Resectable tumours

- Surgical resection is the treatment of choice for early stage disease. Fit patients treated with resection alone have expected five-year survival rates of 68–85%.
- For patients with regional spread there is no definite evidence that surgery is superior to chemo-irradiation and carries greater morbidity. Five-year survival is between 15–28%.
- Pre-operative chemo-irradiation is being investigated to downstage these tumours (🕮 Chemotherapy). Drugs used include 5-fluorouracil (5FU) cisplatin, mitomycin, paclitaxel, and methotrexate.

Adjuvant chemotherapy

Has not been shown to improve survival and is difficult to deliver after major oesophageal surgery. Post-resection irradiation can improve the loco-regional control but not if there is nodal involvement.

Unresectable tumours

The majority of patients are in this group. Combined chemo-irradiation is more effective than radiotherapy alone in treating locally advanced oeso-phageal cancer. It is also an alternative to surgery for patients with poor performance status. Side effects can be severe, particularly oesophagitis and pneumonitis; as a result both chemotherapy and radiotherapy doses may need to be reduced.

Palliative support

The median survival for stage IV disease remains around 8 months. Progressive dysphagia is the most distressing symptom in most cases. The inability to swallow even liquids or saliva can be extremely distressing and debilitating. Platinum based chemotherapy regimes may palliate symptoms in patients who are fit. Otherwise endoscopic stenting can provide excellent palliation.

Gastrostomy or jejunostomy tubes can also be used to provide nutritional support but do not relieve other symptoms related to poor swallowing.

Gastric cancer

Epidemiology
- This is the second most common cancer worldwide and the sixth most common in the UK.
- It is rare prior to the sixth decade with the incidence rising steeply thereafter.
- In most countries, the incidence of stomach cancer is declining due to improved refrigeration.
- In the UK, an increase in cancers of the oesophageal gastric junction (OGJ) has been detected.

Risk factors
- *Helicobacter pylori*: 3–6-fold increase in risk and causes chronic gastritis
- Diet high in salted meat/fish.
- Smoking.
- Barrett's oesophagus: associated with increase in gastro-oesophageal cancer.
- Pernicious anaemia: 3-fold increase.
- Lower social class.

Presenting signs and symptoms
- Anaemia.
- Weight loss.
- Dyspepsia.
- Appetite disturbance.
- Nausea and vomiting.

Diagnosis and staging
- History and examination.
- Endoscopy and biopsy.
- Barium swallow—demonstrates extent of tumour length.
- Endoluminal ultrasound—shows the extent of local invasion and lymph node involvement.
- CT scan— assesses further nodal involvement and distant metastases.
- Laparoscopy may be indicated to assess peritoneal disease if surgery is being considered.

Common sites of spread
- Usually advanced at diagnosis.
- Local extension—to pancreas, liver, oesophagus.
- Local and distant nodes—left side of neck.
- Distant spread—to liver, peritoneal cavity, adrenals, lung, and bone.

Treatment

Resectable disease

Surgery remains the only curative option for early disease. The type of operation will depend on the site and extent of the tumour.

Partial or total gastrectomy and regional lymphadonectomy are most commonly used. Oesophagogastrectomy may be required for cancers of the OGJ and proximal stomach.

Note: patients with distal tumours do better overall than those with proximally located tumours.

Complications of surgery

- Infection, anastamotic leak, hemorrhage, and reflux aspiration are common complications.
- Large bowel obstruction (📖 Bowel obstruction).
- Sexual dysfunction: abdominoperineal resection can cause impotence due to surgical nerve damage. Now rarely seen due to improvements in surgical technique (📖 Sexual health and cancer).

Chemotherapy and radiotherapy

There is currently no clear evidence of any benefit from adjuvant chemotherapy or radiotherapy for those with resectable disease. Patients should be entered into current trials of chemotherapy or chemo-irradiation, which are slightly more encouraging.

Advanced disease

- *Surgical resection* to relieve bleeding, pain or obstruction may be offered for those fit enough.
- *Radiotherapy* can also be used for managing bleeding tumours.
- *Chemotherapy* has shown convincing palliative benefits for patients with locally advanced or distant disease. It may also provide an increase in survival of a few months.

mall intestine and carcinoid tumours

introduction

- These are rare tumours with an incidence peak between 50–60 years.
- They make up less than 10% of all gastrointestinal tumours.
- They include adenocarcinomas, lymphoma, and sarcomas.
- Carcinoid tumours are neuroendocrine tumours of the gastrointestinal tract and represent 30% of all small bowel malignancies.

Pathology

- Tumours can derive from all cell types originating in the small intestine.
- There is increased risk of the development of a second malignant tumour, frequently in the colon.

Presenting features

These tend to be vague and late in the course of the disease:

- Abdominal pain and jaundice (obstruction).
- Anaemia—due to occult bleeding.
- Small bowel obstruction (carcinoid).
- Weight loss.
- Carcinoid syndrome (flushing, diarrhoea, bronchial constriction, right-sided valvular heart disease).

Diagnosis

- Barium studies.
- Endoscopy.
- Laparoscopy/laparotomy.

Carcinoid tumours

The majority of these patients have liver metastases, elevated urinary 5-HIAA levels and plasma chromogranin A and tachykinins (neurokinin A and substance-P). These tumours and metastases can be seen on somatostatin receptor scintigraphy (octreoscan). This is a specialized scanning technique using a radionuclide. A CT or MRI scan can detect lymph node and liver metastases.

For carcinoid tumours with local disease, five-year survival is 75–95%; with regional lymph node involvement, 40–60%; with liver metastases and the carcinoid syndrome, 20–30%.

Treatment

Surgery

Surgical resection is the most important therapy for all small bowel tumours. All benign tumours can be cured by adequate segmental resections with clear margins. The same holds true for the malignant tumours, although surgery should include lymph node resection.

Chemotherapy

Chemotherapy for most malignant small bowel tumours is based around 5FU. Sarcomas are treated with doxorubicin-based regimens. Five-year survival in patients with small bowel adenocarcinoma or sarcoma is only 20–30%. Lymphomas are commonly treated with regimens such as CHOP. (📖 Heamatological cancers: Non Hodgkins lymphoma).

Radiotherapy

Tumour-targeted radiotherapy can be applied to carcinoid tumour either radio-labelled octreotide or 131MIBG. Response rates of 3(have been reported.

Other treatments

Cytokine treatment using α-interferon can be used alone or with chemotherapy for adenocarcinomas and carcinoids of the small bowel.

Somatostatin analogues, e.g. octreotide or lanreotide, are useful for managing clinical symptoms such as diarrhoea and flushing related to carcinoid tumours, with some anti-tumour effect. This can be given by long-acting depot injections.

Further reading

Souhami R and Tobias J (2005). *Cancer and its management*. Blackwell, Oxford.

Cancer of the liver (hepatocellular cancer)

Epidemiology
- There is a low incidence of liver cancer in the UK and Europe.
- It is commonest where hepatitis B is endemic, e.g. in sub-saharan Africa, southeast Asia and China.
- The majority of cases of liver cancer are under the age of 50.
- Males are affected more frequently than females.

Risk factors
- Chronic hepatitis B or C infection.
- Cirrhosis secondary to alcohol-induced liver injury or haemochromatosis.

Symptoms
- Right upper-quadrant abdominal pain.
- Abdominal distension.
- Fatigue.
- Anorexia and weight loss.
- Jaundice is uncommon.
- Para-neoplastic effects include: hypoglycaemia, erythrocytosis, hypercalcaemia and hypercholesterolaemia.

Diagnosis and staging
- History.
- CT scan.
- Laparoscopy and US.
- Biopsy.
- Angiography.
- CXR and CT chest to exclude metastases.
- α fetoprotein—useful for diagnosis and monitoring recurrence.
- Liver function tests—to assess functional reserve.

Treatment options
Surgical resection
Surgery offers the only hope of a cure of hepatocellular cancer (HCC). However resection is not possible in many patients due to multifocal disease and liver failure associated with cirrhosis.

Liver transplantation
This is appropriate for some cirrhotic patients with HCC less than 3cm. It is preferred in the treatment of HCC arising from hepatitis C because of the high likelihood of further tumour development in these patients.

Systemic chemotherapy
Systemic chemotherapy has been used for unresectable tumours, but response rates have been poor.

Transarterial chemo-embolization
- Chemotherapy is administered directly to the tumour through a radologically placed catheter in the hepatic artery.
- Repeat embolization is performed at 2–3 month intervals. This may render some tumours resectable.
- Can be complicated by acute abdominal pain and fever (self-limiting) and liver failure (uncommon).

Prognosis

Overall survival is poor, with less than 10% of patients alive at three years. Survival for unresectable disease is about 2–6 months.

...er of the gall bladder and ...e ducts

...pidemiology and aetiology

These are rare cancers in the UK. Women are affected twice as often as men because of their increased predisposition to gallstones—this is the most important aetiological factor.

Clinical presentation

There are two modes of presentation

1. A tumour is found during routine cholecystectomy for gallstones. It is often early stage and there is a high rate of cure. More than 80% of people with early stage tumours survive for 5 years.
2. People present with obstructive jaundice. This is the most common presentation. There is a poor prognosis, with less than 15% surviving for 5 years.

Routes of spread

- Infiltrates the muscular wall of the gall bladder and the neighbouring liver tissue, and spreads to regional lymph nodes and to the liver.
- Distant metastases occur late.

Signs and symptoms

Jaundice, abdominal pain, fever, pruritis (itch).

Diagnosis

- Liver function tests may be abnormal.
- CEA, CA19–9 may be increased.
- Ultrasound may reveal:
  - Tumour.
  - Invasion of ducts.
  - Nodes.
  - Liver secondaries.
- CT scan.
- Angiogram—may show vessel invasion.

Treatment

Resectable tumours

Radical surgery involving removal of gallbladder, resection of liver segments 4 and 5, bile duct, and regional lymphatics.

Unresectable tumours

Surgical or radiological biliary drainage is performed.

~eatic cancer

~niology
- ~e incidence of pancreatic cancer is 9–12 per 100,000.
- ~ is the seventh most common cause of cancer death in the UK. 90% are adenocarcinomas. 75% arise in the head of the organ, 15% in the body, and 10% in the tail.
- 40% of cases present before the age of 75 years.

Risk factors
- Smoking is the highest risk factor.
- Diets high in saturated fats may be important.
- Chronic pancreatitis.
- Diabetes mellitus.

Common sites of spread
- Most patients will present with advanced disease.
- The spread is mainly to retroperitoneal tissue, the liver, and the peritoneum. Distant metastases to the liver, lung, and the bone.

Presentation
- Insidious onset of symptoms.
- Classical signs are painless jaundice, weight loss, and back pain.

Investigations
- Tumour markers CA19–9, elevated in most, but poor sensitivity.
- Endoluminal ultrasound—90% accuracy.
- Endoscopic retrograde cholangiopancreatography (ERCP)—positive cytology in 60%.
- Fine-needle aspiration—percutaneous.
- CT, MRI scan—chest, abdomen, and pelvis.
- Laparoscopy—assess peritoneal involvement.

Treatment options

Surgery
Less than 20% present with surgically resectable disease. Even then, 5-year survival is less than 30%. A pancreaticduodenectomy (Whipple's procedure) is the operation of choice. The surgical mortality rate is approaching 10%. Post-operative complications include bronchopneumonia, pancreatic fistulae, sepsis, abscess, and haemorrhage. Oral pancreatic enzyme supplements may be required for pancreatic exocrine insufficiency.

Palliative surgical bypass procedures
These procedures may be possible for some patients. Generally non-surgical relief of jaundice is indicated. Endoscopic or percutaneously inserted stents have relatively low morbidity rates.

Chemotherapy

Gemcitabine has shown both palliative benefit and a small survival incre
in unresectable disease. Trials of adjuvant chemotherapy are ongoing.

Radiotherapy

Patients with good performance status and localized resectable tumour
may be considered for radiotherapy, with or without chemotherapy.
Both external-beam radiotherapy (EBRT) and intraoperative radiotherapy
(IORT) have been used in the adjuvant settings.

Prognosis

The median survival rate in advanced disease is poor—between 3 and 6
months; the overall 5-year survival rate is 0.5%.

Nursing management issues

Complex nursing care is required to support patients with upper GI tumours and their families. Complications from the disease and its treatment are many and varied. Managing symptoms can be difficult from diagnosis, throughout treatment, and for patients with advanced disease. The physical and psychosocial impact can be severe.

Accurate assessment and coordination of care is required for the effective support of patients and their families. A multidisciplinary approach is essential throughout, with the early involvement of specialist palliative care services recommended for many patients.

Specific issues that affect these patients are discussed below with cross-referencing to where they are covered elsewhere. Other symptoms that may be experienced are covered in Sections 4 and 7 of this handbook.

Nutritional issues

This is probably the biggest single management issue for individuals with upper GI cancer. Dysphagia, severe weight loss, anorexia, and malnutrition—due to a range of enzyme deficiencies—are all common. The impact on the patient, their family, and their quality of life can be enormous. Social activities may be curtailed, body image is affected, and fatigue and weakness may be severe. It is important that the multidisciplinary team, especially the dietitian and the patient's family are fully involved in managing nutritional disorders (☐ Nutritional support).

Pain

Patients with upper GI cancers face a range of different pain due to their disease. Liver pain caused by stretching of the liver capsule, due to primary liver disease or liver metastases is common. This pain is only partially responsive to opioids, but responds well to NSAIDs and oral steroids.

Coeliac plexus involvement occurs in some upper GI cancers, including pancreatic cancer. This can create abdominal and mid back pain, which is often difficult to control. Anaesthetic nerve blocks can be useful (☐ Pain management).

Bleeding

Liver involvement may cause clotting abnormalities. Locally advanced tumours can also occasionally cause bleeding, which can be severe or even life threatening. This can often be reduced by local treatment such as endoscopic laser treatment or localized radiotherapy (☐ Haemorrhage).

Liver failure

Patients may have ascites (☐ Malignant effusions), peripheral oedema, and in advanced stages encephalopathy (☐ Acute confusional states).

Further reading

Souhami R L and Tobias J S (2005). *Cancer and Its Management.* 5th edn. Oxford: Blackwell.

Yarbro C H, Frogge M H Goodman M (eds) (2005). *Cancer Nursing, Principles and practice.* 6th edn. Massachusetts: Jones and Bartlett.

Thompson A M and Wells M (2005). Surgery. In Kearney N and Richardson A (2005). *Nursing Patients with Cancer: Principles and Practice* pp.247–53. Edinburgh: Churchill Livingstone.

Genitourinary cancers

cancer

emiology and aetiology
- here are 6000 cases annually in the UK.
- It is 1.5 times more common in men than women.
- Frequency increases with age—most patients are 60+ years old.
- Smoking doubles relative risk.
- Inherited predisposition causes 2% of renal cancer—often multifocal/ bilateral.

Pathology
- 85% of renal cancers are adenocarcinomas and arise from renal tubular epithelium.
- Approximately one-third of patients have metastatic spread at diagnosis. Common sites are lungs, soft tissues, bones, and liver.
- Transitional cell carcinomas can arise within the urothelium of the renal pelvis and represent the majority of the remaining tumours.

Presenting symptoms and signs
- Haematuria.
- General malaise.
- Night sweats.
- Loin pain.
- Anaemia.
- Weight loss.
- Pyrexia.
- Syndromes of hypertension, hypercalcaemia, polycythaemia.

Up to 30% of renal cancers are asymptomatic and are discovered during imaging for other reasons.

Investigations
- US scan or IVU.
- Contrast CT scan of the abdomen and chest.
- FBC, biochemical profile.

Staging/prognosis
The Robson staging system is simple and commonly used. See Table 30.1.

Resectable disease
- For patients who are fit for surgery, complete surgical resection is the only potentially curative treatment.
- Patients with metastatic disease but good Performance Status (0–1) (🕮 Performance status) and resectable primary tumour may benefit from nephrectomy as a palliative procedure to provide:
  - Control of local symptoms.
  - Modest survival benefit combined with immunotherapy.

- Regression of metastases following nephrectomy is reported extremely rare (<1%).
- In some elderly asymptomatic patients, conservative management appropriate as tumour growth may be slow.

Note: Adjuvant immunotherapy in resectable disease has not yet show clear evidence of improved disease survival.

Advanced disease

The management of patients with advanced and/or metastatic renal cancer is palliative.

Systemic therapy

Renal cancer rarely responds to chemotherapy or radiotherapy. Palliative radiotherapy is appropriate for:
- Painful or bleeding primary tumour.
- Non-resectable metastatic disease e.g. bone, brain, or soft tissue.

Biological therapy

Use of interferon alpha or interleukin can occasionally create a long-term response. Prognostic factors that predict higher response rates include:
- Long disease-free interval.
- Previous nephrectomy.
- Good performance status (0–1) (📖 Performance status).

Combined biological and chemotherapy

Phase III trials are currently a combination of interleukin, interferon, and 5FU chemotherapy, against single agent interferon.

Management of transitional cell carcinoma (TCC)

Their biology, management, and prognosis are similar to that of TCC of the ureter, which is treated as if bladder TCC. See following pages.

Table 30.1 The Robson staging system

Stage	Description	% of cases	5-year Survival
I	Confined to the kidney	20–40%	50–60%
II	Extends into peri-renal fat but confined to Gerota's fascia	4–20%	30–60%
III	Involvement of renal vein or IVC or lymph node involvement	10–40%	20–50%
IV	Involvement of adjacent organs or metastatic disease	11–50%	0–20%

r of the bladder and ureter

miology

- his is the fourth commonest male cancer with a male: female ratio of 2:1.
- Two-thirds occur in people aged more than 70.
- More than 90% are transitional cell carcinomas.

Risk factors

- Cigarette smoking increases the risk by 2–6 times. 90% of bladder cancers are linked to smoking as a cause.
- Occupational exposure to aromatic amines and aniline dye e.g. tyre manufacture, printing, dyeing.
- Previous pelvic radiotherapy e.g. for gynaecological cancer.
- Chronic irritation of the bladder is associated with squamous cancer of the bladder.

Presentation

- 80–90% present with frank haematuria, usually painless.
- Frequency and dysuria.
- Recurrent UTI.
- Unexplained microscopic haematuria.
- Back, rectal, or suprapubic pain may suggest metastatic disease.

Pathology

- At least 70% of patients present with 'superficial' tumour, involving only the bladder epithelium.
- In 25% there is tumour invasion into the muscle of the bladder.
- 5% present with metastatic disease to the regional lymph nodes, lung, liver, or bone.
- 50% of carcinoma in situ can develop quickly into muscle invasive cancer.

Staging

Both the stage of disease and pathological grading are important. There is a strong association between well-differentiated tumours and early stage (☐ Diagnosis and classification).

- Low grade tumours rarely progress to advanced disease.
- There is a significant risk of metastatic disease with high-grade disease, and with increasing stage of muscle invasive disease.

Investigations

- FBC, biochemistry profile.
- IVU and US.
- Cystoscopy and transurethral resection of bladder tumour (TURBT).
- Staging with CXR and abdominal and pelvic CT/MRI if high risk of metastases. e.g. muscle invasive cancer or a suspicion of this.

Treatment options

Superficial tumours (70% newly diagnosed cases)

- Low-grade tumours are resected cystoscopically. A single post-resection dose of intravesical mitomycin reduces the risk of recurrence.
- Recurrent disease is managed by further surgical resection, intravesical chemotherapy or immunotherapy with BCG.
- Refractory disease is best managed by cystectomy.

Muscle invasive bladder cancer

Options are radical cystectomy or radiotherapy with surgical salvage, which offer equivalent results. Fit patients may be considered for chemotherapy prior to local treatment. This is contentious, with little difference between neo-adjuvant or adjuvant treatment.

Radical surgery

Cystectomy with urinary diversion, offers the best chance of cure if the cancer is localized to the bladder. The usual operation is either cystectomy and formation of ileal conduit or bladder reconstruction (neo-bladder). The conduit option is an incontinent diversion and reconstruction is a continent diversion. Patients may or may not have a choice depending on suitability for a diversion. If they do they should be counselled by both a stoma nurse and cancer CNS (☐ Care of the patient with a stoma).

Radical radiotherapy

- This is useful if the patient cannot tolerate surgery. It offers bladder conservation, although results are poor in multifocal disease.
- The side effects of radical radiotherapy include cystitis and diarrhoea (☐ Diarrhoea), plus a late effect of reduction in bladder capacity.
- Frail patients who are unfit for radical surgery or radiotherapy, may benefit from palliative radiotherapy to the bladder.

Neo-adjuvant chemotherapy

- Cisplatin-based chemotherapy given before cystectomy or radiotherapy affords a modest survival benefit of around 5% improvement at 5 years.
- For patients with good performance status, concomitant chemoradiotherapy may also offer improved response rates over radiotherapy alone.

Advanced disease

- Gemcitabine and cisplatin is becoming a common treatment due to reduced toxicity over older regimens, such as MVAC or MVC—about 50% of patients respond.
- Paclitaxel is also active in bladder cancer.
- Regimens can still be toxic, especially for patients with poor performance status and impaired renal function.

Treatment outcomes

The prognosis for superficial disease is good, with 5-year survival rates in excess of 80%. Survival from muscle invasive disease is 40–60%. For metastatic disease, median survival time is 1 year with around 10% living 2 years.

Prostate cancer

For many men with this diagnosis, the optimum management is uncertain, with a spectrum of treatment options ranging from no treatment at all to complex surgery or radiation therapy.

Epidemiology

- It is now the commonest male cancer in Europe and the US, with >30,000 new cases per annum in the UK.
- 85% of men are diagnosed at age 65 or older. It is rare in men under the age of 50 years though numbers are increasing due to screening.
- 70% of men >80 years have histological evidence of cancer in the prostate.
- African-Caribbean ancestry increases risk and these patients are more likely to have micro-metastatic disease at presentation.

Risk factors

- Age is the most important risk factor.
- Prostate cancer is androgen-dependent. Men who are castrated before 40 years rarely develop prostate cancer.
- 5–10% of cases appear to be linked to inheritance, i.e. those with a strong family history of prostate or breast cancer.

Pathology

- 95% are adenocarcinomas. Many are multifocal.
- Histological grade, assessed by Gleason score:
  - Low-grade cancers (Gleason 6 or less) are typically small and slow-growing, confined to the prostate gland.
  - High-grade cancers, Gleason > 7, grow faster and frequently reflect occult metastatic disease.

Investigations

- Digital rectal examination.
- PSA assessment (🕮 Cancer screening).
- High PSA (based on age-related PSA table) or palpable abnormality requires transrectal US scan and prostatic biopsy.
- Locally advanced disease, high-grade cancer, and high PSA level at presentation are all indications for more complete staging.
- MRI scan of the prostate and pelvis provides the most accurate estimate of locoregional tumour extent.
- Isotope bone scan.
- Lymph node biopsy if stage is unclear and radical treatment is a consideration.

Presentation

- Around 50% are asymptomatic, via PSA screening.
- Urinary symptoms e.g. frequency, nocturia, poor stream, retention, haematuria.
- Advanced disease may cause bone or back pain, lymphoedema in legs and genitals, or weight loss.
- Haemospermia, erectile dysfunction.

Staging and prognosis

- Staging is carried out using the TNM staging system below
  (◫ Diagnosis and classification).
- Risk categories are shown in the box.

Metastatic spread

- Direct through the prostate capsule, into adjacent organs
  (seminal vesicles, bladder, rectum).
- Regional lymph nodes.
- Distant typically to bone, and rarely to lung and liver.

Table 30.2 TNM staging of prostate cancer

T0	No evidence of tumour
T1a	Tumour, incidental finding at TURP (<5% chippings)
T1b	Tumour, incidental finding at TURP (>5% chippings)
T1c	Impalpable tumour identified by raised PSA
T2a	Tumour involves half of a lobe or less
T2b	Tumour involves more than a half of a lobe but not both lobes
T2c	Tumour involves both lobes
T3a	Unilateral extracapsular extension
T3b	Bilateral extracapsular extension
	Tumour involves seminal vesicles
T4	Tumour invades bladder neck, rectum, pelvic side-wall

Prostate cancer, prognostic risk categories
(Using TNM, PSA, and Gleason score)

Low risk:	T1-2a and PSA < 10µg/l and Gleason 6 or less
Intermediate risk:	T2b-c, or PSA 10–20µg/l, or Gleason 7
High risk:	T3-4, or PSA > 20µg/l, or Gleason > 7

Treatment

Organ-confined prostate cancer

There may be several treatment options based on the following:

- Patient's age and comorbidities.
- Disease stage, PSA, and Gleason score.
- The patient's concerns about likely toxicities.

For fit patients Local radical therapy can be considered, either:

Radical prostatectomy: gives excellent disease-free survival rates. Postoperative problems include impotence in approximately 50%, strictures, penile shortening, and urinary incontinence. For most, the incontinence is minimal and improves over the first 2 years. However, a few will have severe, long-term incontinence.

Radical radiotherapy

Options are:

- External beam (EBRT) or iodine (I^{125}) brachytherapy.
- Combined high dose rate (HDR) (Ir192) brachytherapy in combination with external-beam radiotherapy (EBRT).
- Rates of disease-free survival compare favourably with surgery and EBRT can also be offered if unfit for surgery.
- Intermediate and high risk patients are given adjuvant anti-androgens.
- EBRT is also given adjuvantly if indicated following prostatectomy.

Toxicities of radiotherapy include acute radiation cystitis/urethritis, proctitis with tenesmus, pain, and passage of mucus and blood. About 50% of those treated will become impotent.

Hormone therapy alone

- For patients with high-risk disease, for whom radical treatment is not appropriate or feasible, immediate treatment with androgen deprivation is preferred to 'active surveillance'.
- For metastatic disease the median benefit is 18 months. However some patients still have benefits at 10 years.

Active surveillance

- Particularly used for patients with low-risk cancers, or patients concerned with quality of life issues arising from treatment.
- Involves regular monitoring of PSA levels and physical examination.
- Patients who develop progressive disease on active surveillance should be considered for radical treatment or androgen deprivation.

Locally advanced disease

Optimum management is controversial. Options include:

- Radiotherapy, with or without androgen deprivation.
- Hormone therapy alone.
- Active surveillance.

Metastatic disease

Advanced prostate cancer is incurable, but most are sensitive to androgen hormones. Excellent palliation can be achieved with a survival time of 3–4 years with appropriate therapy.

Common hormone treatments include surgical castration (rarely used now), medical castration using gonadorelin analogues or anti-androgen therapy, e.g. bicalutamide or flutamide.

There is no clear evidence that *maximal androgen blockade* (combining therapies) produces superior outcomes compared with castration alone. The impact of medical/surgical castration or androgen blockade include:
• Impotence and loss of libido (📖 Sexual health and cancer).
• Fatigue (📖 Fatigue).
• Mood disturbance.
• Muscle weakness.
• Flushing and sweats (📖 Hormonal therapies).
• Weight gain.
• Gynaecomastia (enlargement or tenderness of male breasts).
• Osteoporosis in long-term survivors.

Hormone refractory metastatic disease
A rising PSA level may suggest local recurrence or advancing disease. This occurs after median of 2 years. Options are active surveillance, 2nd line antiandrogen therapy, androgen deprivation, or salvage local therapy e.g. prostate cryotherapy

There is controversy surrounding the benefits and timing of these interventions. The most common problem of advancing disease is painful bone metastases (📖 Metastatic bone disease).

Radiotherapy and chemotherapy for metastatic disease
Radiotherapy
• Local radiotherapy can effectively treat painful bone metastases, spinal cord or nerve root compression, or symptomatic soft tissue disease.
• Radioactive strontium as a single IV injection can be effective in treating multiple bone metastases, but it does cause significant myelosuppression.

Chemotherapy
• Mitoxantrone, usually in combination with low-dose prednisolone, offers symptom relief in about one third of patients. Docetaxel has recently been shown to cause more frequent PSA responses and the median survival time is two months greater than mitoxantrone.
• Bisphosphonate therapy, using monthly infusions of zoledronic acid, has recently been shown to delay symptomatic progression of bone metastases.

Treatment outcomes
• Median survival times >10 years for patients treated by either radical prostatectomy or radiotherapy.
• The natural history of recurrent disease may be very slow.
• For metastatic disease, the median duration of response to hormone therapy is 18–24 months.
• The median survival time after development of hormone refractory disease is 12 months.

Testicular cancer

This is one of the few solid tumours for which the majority of patients with metastatic disease can expect to be cured.

Epidemiology

- 95% of testicular tumours are of germ cell origin.
- It is the commonest cancer in men aged 20–40 years.
- Incidence has doubled over the last 30 years.
- 55% are seminomas—peak incidence age is 30–40 years.
- 45% are non-seminomatous germ cell tumours (NSGT)—peak incidence age 20–30 years.

Risk factors

- History of undescended testis (relative risk 8x).
- Previous testicular cancer (relative risk 25x).
- Testicular carcinoma in situ.
- Family history of testicular cancer.

Pathology (see Table 30.3)

Seminomas

Tumour growth can be very slow. 75% present with disease confined to the testis. The spread tends to be predictable, vertically via the lymph nodes, and then to other metastatic sites. Tumour markers are not very reliable. Only 30% of seminomas present with raised human chorionic gondotrophin (HCG). Lactic acid dehydrogenase (LDH) may be raised in advanced cancer. Tumours that appear to be seminoma histologically should be treated as NSGCTs if they have elevated alpha fetoprotein (AFP) levels.

Non-seminomatous germ cell tumours (NSGCT)

Lymphatic spread occurs earlier. NSGCT produce markers: human chorionic gondotrophin (HCG) and/or alpha feta protein (AFP) in 75% of cases. (📖 Diagnosis and staging: tumour markers).

Presentation

- Testicular lump, either painless or painful (slightly less common).
  - May be mistaken for infection.
  - If symptoms persist despite one course of antibiotics, patients should be referred to a urology clinic for assessment.
- Gynaecomastia (swollen breasts in men)—due to HCG.
- Metastatic disease may present with:
  - Lumbar back pain with bulky paraaortic lymphadenopathy.
  - Cough and dyspnoea with multiple lung metastases.
  - SVCO with mediastinal lymphadenopathy (📖 Superior vena cava obstruction).
  - CNS symptoms/signs with brain metastasis.
- Asymptomatic relapsed spread, often picked up on routine monitoring of serum markers, chest X-ray, or CT scan.

Investigation of testicular germ cell tumours

- US of both testicles.
- Chest X-ray.
- Tumour markers (AFP, HCG, LDH).
- Inguinal orchidectomy ± biopsy of other testis.
- Further staging investigations postoperatively:
  - CT scan of the thorax, abdomen, and pelvis.
  - Brain or bone scan if clinically indicated.
  - Post-operative tumour markers (falling AFP and HCG).

Sperm storage

- Sperm count and storage should be considered at an early stage where patients are likely to require further therapy, though up to 50% of patients with testicular germ cell tumour may be sub-fertile at presentation.

Table 30.3 Pathological classification of testicular cancers

British	WHO
Seminoma	*Seminoma*
Spermatocytic seminona	Spermatocytic serinoma
Teratoma	*Non-seminomatous germ cell tumour*
Teratoma differentiated (TD)	Mature teratoma
Malignant teratoma intermediate (MTI)	Embryonal carcinoma with teratoma (teratocarcinoma)
Malignant teratoma undifferentiated (MTU)	Yolk sac tumour, embryonal carcinoma
Malignant teratoma trophoblastic (MTT)	Yolk sac tumour; choriocarcinoma

Treatment of testicular cancer

Stage 1 seminoma treatment

Primary treatment is inguinal orchidectomy. Approximately 20% of patients develop recurrent seminoma, mainly in paraaortic nodes.

There are three options post-orchidectomy:
• Surveillance, including an annual CT scan.
• Adjuvant radiotherapy to the paraaortic nodes.
• One cycle of carboplatin chemotherapy.

Note: almost all patients with relapsed disease are cured by salvage therapy.

Stage 1 NSGCT

Primary treatment for seminoma is as above. The relapse rate is around 30%, higher if there is vascular invasion in the tumour.

There are two options post orchidectomy:
• Surveillance—chest X-ray, tumour marker monitoring, and
  regular CT scans.
• Adjuvant chemotherapy—particularly if vascular invasion. Two
  cycles of BEP chemotherapy offers 97% disease-free survival.
• Outcome even for relapsed stage I disease is excellent, with cure
  rates >95%.

All other stages of seminoma and NSGCT

BEP (bleomycin, etoposide, cisplatin) chemotherapy is the current gold standard treatment—three courses for good prognosis, and four for intermediate and poor prognosis. Poor prognostic factors are:
• Mediastinal primary.
• Non-pulmonary visceral metastases.
• High tumours markers, e.g. AFP, HCG.

BEP chemotherapy is potentially very toxic. Nausea and vomiting, neutropenic sepsis, neuropathy, nephropathy, and pulmonary fibrosis are all common (📖 Chemotherapy).
• Granulocyte colony stimulating factors are used to avoid dose
  delays and reductions if possible.
• Lung toxicity due to bleomycin can be fatal—four cycles of EP
  chemotherapy can be used in older patients with poor lung function.

Residual tumour masses post chemotherapy

• Seminomas generally regress on serial scans.
• Surgical resection should be performed for NSGCT.
• Most are in the retroperitoneum, and extensive and difficult surgery is
  often necessary. There is an anaesthetic risk due to patient exposure
  to bleomycin. If the residual mass contains a viable tumour, further
  chemotherapy is recommended.

Relapse

Patients who relapse or who do not have a complete response can have salvage therapy with further combination chemotherapy regimes. Regular follow-up is necessary as, in those patients who relapse, salvage therapy can be effective in approximately 25% of cases.

Penile cancer

Epidemiology

This is an uncommon cancer, with around 350 new cases per annum in the UK. The majority occur in people over 70, but up to 20% occur under the age of 40. The disease is relatively more common in Africa, India, and South America.

Risk factors

- Human papilloma virus (HPV 16 and 18) infection.
- Associated with poor hygiene and un-retractable foreskin.
- Increased risk with cigarette smoking and immuno-suppression including HIV infection.
- Neonatal circumcision gives lifelong protection.

Pathology

The vast majority are squamous carcinomas. Spread is initially via lymphatics to inguinal and then pelvic lymph nodes. Distant spread may include liver, lungs, bone, and skin.

Staging

The TNM system is commonly used (📖 Diagnosis and classification).

Investigations

- Inspection of the penis and biopsy of any lesion.
- Inguinal lymph node palpation—FNA of suspicious lymph nodes.
- Further staging if clinical suspicion of metastatic disease.

Presentation

- Erythema, warty tumour, or ulceration on the glans or foreskin.
- Advanced disease can cause considerable destruction of the penis.
- Metastatic disease e.g. inguinal and pelvic lymphadenopathy.

Treatment

Primary tumour

- Early stage disease may be successfully managed with organ conservation. For tumour in situ, topical 5FU, laser therapy, cryotherapy or local excision are all options. Excision or radiotherapy is used for stage I disease.
- More advanced disease or local recurrence often requires at least partial amputation of the penis. Reconstruction surgical techniques are now excellent. Patients with inoperable disease may be treated with chemotherapy and radiotherapy.

Regional lymph nodes
- With high grade and stage II tumours, regional lymphadenectomy may be considered. Patients who are unfit for surgery or have inoperable disease may benefit from chemotherapy and radiotherapy. Lymphoedema is a major side effect of radiotherapy and lymphadonectomy.
- The disease is moderately chemo-sensitive, and active regimens include methotrexate, bleomycin, and cisplatin (MBP). Chemotherapy is recommended both for advanced disease, and as adjuvant therapy for node positive disease.

Outcomes
Overall 50% of men with penile cancer survive disease-free beyond 5 years, with better results in node negative (60%) compared with node positive (30%). The majority of relapses occur in the first 2 years, and close follow-up is recommended at least during this time.

Nursing management issues

The nursing issues in these cancers will vary considerably depending on the disease site and on the extent of cancer spread. Common nursing management issues are briefly described below.

Sexuality

There are many potential assaults on an individual's sexuality due to genitourinary cancer and its treatment. Surgery can cause impotence, reduced ejaculate, and incontinence. It may involve formation of stomas for urinary diversion, removal of testis or the penis, or shortening of the vagina. Hormonal therapy can cause impotence and reduce libido. Chemotherapy and radiotherapy may impact on fertility, and multiple side effects may impact on an individual's body image and sexuality.

Nurses need to involve patients and their partners in open discussions about potential problems as a crucial part of care.

Pre-surgery

Patients may be extremely anxious about the impact of surgery. Their fears should be openly explored, along with straightforward explanations of likely impacts.

Post-surgery

It is important that nurses feel able to initiate discussions and proactively support patients with what might feel like embarrassing difficulties. Sexual issues may not be uppermost in a person's mind early on after diagnosis and during treatment. Post-treatment follow-up is needed to assess the psychosexual impact of treatment and the disease (📖 Sexual health and cancer).

Fertility

Many patients with testicular cancer are young, and will not have children at the time of their diagnosis. Sperm banking should be offered as a matter of course, though many patients will be sub-fertile at diagnosis. BEP chemotherapy causes infertility. Around half of patients will regain normal sperm counts two years post-chemotherapy, though others will have long term damage to their sperm.

Younger prostate cancer and penile cancer patients may also require sperm banking.

Urinary incontinence

After bladder surgery patients will require support in adjusting to and managing their stoma and possible incontinence. This includes skin care, using pouches, signs and symptoms of healthy stoma, and possible signs of infection. For those with continent pouches teaching of self-catheterization or rigorous bladder training may also be included. For those with a stoma, support and advice from a stoma therapist will be invaluable at this time (📖 Care of the patient with a stoma).

Radical prostate surgery and radiotherapy for prostate or bladder cancer can all cause long-term continence problems. Nursing management includes accurate assessment of the degree of the problem, teaching use of pelvic floor and biofeedback exercises, providing equipment such as pads and condom-like continence devices. Occasionally urinary catheterization is required. Long-term problems may require medical or surgical input. An incontinence expert is recommended to aid patients and nurses in providing effective support.

Lymphoedema
Advanced pelvic disease in both prostate and bladder cancer can lead to lower limb lymphoedema. This needs to be managed actively with advice from lymphoedema specialists to help prevent major complications (□ Lymphoedema).

Pain issues
Patients with advanced bladder and prostate cancer can get pelvic pain, with a neuropathic element, making it complex to manage. Bone pain is also common in advanced prostate cancer, due to bone metastases, and pathological fractures can occur. Pain can often be managed with bisphosphonates and radiotherapy. Physiotherapy and occupational therapy input may assist with mobility, and adaptation to bone metastases. Occasionally, orthopaedic surgery can be used to stabilize affected areas (□ Management of pain).

Financial issues
Many patients undergoing treatments struggle financially, especially those who are young and supporting a family, e.g. many testicular cancer patients. Advice and contact details should be offered of where to get help and advice (□ Social experience).

Further reading

Fillingham S, Douglas A (2003). *Urological Nursing*, 3rd edn. London: Bailliere Tindall.
Kirby R S and Brawer M K (2004). *Prostate Cancer*, 4th edn. Abingdon: Health Press.
National Institute for Clinical Excellence (2002). *Guidance on Cancer Services-Improving Outcomes in Urological Cancers: The Manual.* London: NICE.
Raghavan D and Bailey M (2006). *Bladder Cancer*, 2nd edn. Abingdon: Health Press.

Gynaecological cancers

Introduction

Gynaecological cancers are associated with the female reproductive organs. This includes the ovaries, fallopian tubes, uterus, cervix, vagina, and vulva. They account for about 15% of cancer in women and about 10% of cancer deaths.

Enhanced cervical screening in the UK has led to a dramatic decrease in the incidence of and deaths from cervical cancer. Abnormal development changes (dysplasia) in cervical cells are diagnosed when the disease is still curable. Unfortunately, ovarian cancer is usually diagnosed at an advanced stage, due to its asymptomatic early nature.

There are additional rare tumours called gestational trophoblastic tumours, which arise from pregnancy and include:
• Pre-malignant complete hydatidiform mole (CHM).
• Partial hydatidiform mole (PHM).
• Malignant invasive mole, gestational choriocarcinoma.
• Highly malignant placental-site trophoblastic tumour (PSTT).

This section will not look at gestational tumours. Further information on these can be found at: *Clinical Obstetric and Gynecology*, Vol 46(3), September 2003. The whole edition of this journal explores gestational trophoblastic disease.

Ovarian cancer

- It is the fourth commonest cancer in women in the UK, with a peak incidence in the 65–75 age group.
- Less than 5% of cases are clearly hereditary.
- Risk of ovarian cancer is related to an increasing number of ovulatory cycles, thus some protection from the oral contraceptive pill and pregnancy.

Presentation
80% of women present with disease that has spread beyond the ovary to involve the peritoneum and other abdominopelvic organs.

Common symptoms include:
- Bloating.
- Urinary urgency.
- Constantly swollen stomach.
- Indigestion.
- Ongoing fatigue.
- Back/abdominal pain.
- Weight loss.

Note: primary fallopian tube and peritoneal cancers are rare and behave similarly to ovarian cancer. They can be found on histology when suspicious of ovarian cancer and are treated in the same way.

Diagnosis and staging
The two main prognostic factors in ovarian cancer are the stage, and the amount of residual disease after surgery (see Table 31.1).
- Patients with more than a 2cm area of disease after surgery have a poor prognosis, with only 20% surviving 3 years.
- 80% of women with advanced ovarian cancer have elevated serum CA-125 (see below). A raised CA-125 with an abdominal mass or ascites on CT scan are highly suspicious of ovarian cancer.
- Full histological staging is carried out surgically via total abdominal hysterectomy, bilateral salpingo-oophorectomy, omentectomy, lymph node biopsies, and multiple peritoneal biopsies. Staging is carried out using the TNM staging system (📖 Diagnosis and classification).

CA-125 tumour testing
CA (cancer antigen)-125, is a protein produced on the surface of cells including ovarian uterine and cervical cells. It is measured via a blood test. It can be a useful tumour marker in ovarian cancer diagnosis in conjunction with other tests such as abdominal CT scan. It is also valuable in monitoring response to therapy and in the detection of early relapse. CA-125 can also be raised in some benign situations.

Table 31.1 Diagnosis and staging

Stage	Level of spread	5-year survival %
Stage I	Confined to ovaries	75
Stage II	Tumour spread within pelvis only	45
Stage III	Peritoneal spread outside the pelvis, e.g. omentum	20
Stage IV	Distant metastases	<5

Treatment

Radical surgery

Optimal tumour debulking (no tumour >1cm left). Other than stage 1a, combined surgery and chemotherapy is the best approach. There is uncertainty about the best order for treatment i.e. surgery pre- or post-chemotherapy. Both offer significant survival improvement.

First-line chemotherapy

Platinum/taxane combinations, normally 6 cycles, are generally regarded as the optimum treatment. Median survival rates are 2–3 years, with some patients cured of their disease.

Treatment at relapse

Patients with a treatment-free interval of greater than 12 months should be re-challenged with a platinum-containing regimen. The longer the treatment-free interval, the greater the likelihood of a worthwhile second response. For those relapsing sooner, a number of new agents, including liposomal doxorubicin, topotecan, and gemcitabine, can be used.

New approaches

Possible new approaches to improve management include:
• Intra-peritoneal chemotherapy.
• High-dose systemic chemotherapy.
• Biological response modifiers.
• Anti-angiogenic agents.

Cancer of the cervix

Introduction
Rates of cervical cancer vary enormously between countries. It is the commonest female cancer in South East Asia and Africa. Incidence drops rapidly where national screening programmes have been introduced.

Risk factors
- Early onset of sexual intercourse (before 17 years old).
- Non-barrier forms of contraception.
- HPV—particularly HPV types 16 and 18—is present in approaching 100% of cervical cancers seen in the UK. A vaccination programme is being developed for testing in trials.
- Cigarette smoking.

Presentation
- 80–90% are squamous cell cancer. Adenocarcinoma is less common but increasing in incidence.
- Normally asymptomatic until late presentation.
- Increased vaginal discharge.
- Post-coital bleeding.
- Inter-menstrual bleeding.

For management of screening detected abnormalities see (📖 Cervical screening).

Investigation
If patient is symptomatic, pelvic and abdomen CT or MRI scan can define tumour size and any lymph node involvement. Cystoscopy is used to assess evidence of bladder disease. Sigmoidoscopy may be used if there is evidence of bowel disease.

Staging
Staging is based predominantly on the extent of the primary tumour. The spread is usually from the cervix into the vagina and then into the pelvic wall. Metastatic spread is normally by the lymphatic system and can involve the bladder and rectum (see Table 31.2 opposite)

Treatment
Surgery
Radical hysterectomy is the main treatment option for early stage disease. Trachelectomy, where the cervix only is removed, may be offered to women who wish to conserve their fertility. Future pregnancies should be monitored by a consultant obstetrician and Caesarean section is required.

Combined chemotherapy and radiotherapy
Combined chemotherapy (cisplatin) and radical pelvic radiotherapy should be used if surgery is unlikely to remove the complete tumour. Both external beam radiotherapy and brachytherapy are used routinely within this setting. This can still be a curative treatment.

Pelvic radiotherapy can also be used in very advanced disease to palliate pelvic symptoms.

Chemotherapy

For advanced disease platinum based chemotherapy gives best results.

Prognosis

Survival at five years is typically—stage 1a, 100%; stage 1b, 70–90%; stage 2, 60–80%; stage 3, 35–45%; stage 4, 10–20%. These wide ranges reflect the large variation in disease volume seen within the present staging system; it is based on tissue involvement rather than volume of disease. Relapse after five years of remission is unusual.

Table 31.2 FIGO staging system for cervical cancer

Stage	Definition
Ia	Micro-invasive disease (max. depth 5mm, max. width 7mm)
Ib	Clinical disease confined to the cervix
IIa	Disease involves upper one-third of vagina but not parametrium
IIb	Disease involves parametrium but does not extend to pelvic wall
III	Disease involves lower two-thirds of vagina and/or pelvic wall
IV	Involvement of bladder, rectum, or distant organs

Endometrial cancer

Introduction

Endometrial cancer occurs principally in post-menopausal women, and the incidence rises with age. Its aetiology has not been fully determined, but risks include unopposed oestrogen HRT, endometrial hyperplasia, women with breast cancer taking tamoxifen, diabetes, nulliparity, and obesity.

Presenting features

- 80% present with vaginal bleeding, mainly post-menopausal.
- 10% present with purulent vaginal discharge.
- 5% present asymptomatic after a hysterectomy or follow up of abnormal pap smear.
- Pain and pelvic pressure are usually manifestations of advanced disease.

Diagnosis

- Pelvic examination.
- Endometrial biopsy.
- Further examinations depend on signs and symptoms.

Treatment

Surgery

The mainstay of treatment for stage I disease is total abdominal hysterectomy and bilateral salpingo-oophorectomy. Lymphadenectomny may enhance survival.

Radiotherapy

Radiotherapy can be used as a primary treatment for women unfit to undergo surgery or as adjuvant therapy following hysterectomy if high risk disease. It is also used to treat local recurrence and advanced disease.

Chemotherapy

Combination chemotherapy and progesterones can be used in advanced disease to shrink tumours and provide palliation.

Prognosis

It generally presents early and 5-year survival rates are around 75%.

Vulval and vaginal cancer

Vulval cancer

- Primary invasive vulval cancer occurs as commonly as cervical cancer in women over 60 years.
- One in four tumours occur in women under the age of 65 years.
- The majority (85%) are squamous carcinoma.
- Other types include basal carcinoma (10%) and malignant melanoma (4%).
- Associations with oncogenic HPV.

Symptoms

- Chronic vulval skin symptoms such as pruritus and irritation.
- Painful lump.
- Abnormal genital tract bleeding or haematuria may occur.

Treatment

Surgical excision with clear margins and removal of groin nodes. Extensive disease may require radical vulvectomy in combination with complex reconstruction. Chemo-irradiation can be used for advanced disease.

Prognosis

5-year survival of 85% if node negative. Poor prognosis if:

- >3 regional nodes involved.
- Stage III, IV disease.
- Large tumour bulk.
- Node metastases.
- Poor performance status (□ Performance status).

Vaginal cancer

Most vaginal cancers are metastatic spread from the cervix, endometrium, or vulva.

Presentation and diagnosis

- Presenting symptoms include abnormal vaginal bleeding, vaginal discharge, and bladder or rectal symptoms.
- It is diagnosed via a vaginal examination with an MRI scan being used to evaluate local spread.

Treatment

Radical pelvic radiotherapy—a combination of external-beam and utero-vaginal intra-cavity brachytherapy.

Prognosis

Overall 5-year survival is 40%, and salvage after first relapse is uncommon.

Nursing management issues

Treatment support

Many of the treatments available for managing gynaecological cancers are aggressive, and can have a profound physical, psychosocial, and sexual impact on women and their families.

Psychosexual concerns

Loss of fertility, onset of menopause, rectal and bladder dysfunction and vaginal dryness and tightness are all common difficulties that these women face. Changes in body image, sexuality and fertility may require referral for specialist psychological/psychosexual support.

It is important not to underestimate the significance of loss of fertility. Even if patients had not planned to have children, or to have more children, the knowledge that this is no longer possible can be devastating.

Concerns regarding sexuality may not emerge until well after major treatment, when women are back at home. Pre-treatment assessment, education and counselling, often by the clinical nurse specialist, is therefore essential in preparing individuals and their families.

Post-surgery patients need to be informed of what has been removed and the effect this treatment will have on them. It is helpful in planning their care to establish if they are sexually active, planning to have children or are menopausal.

Appropriate nurse follow-up and assessment is required to ensure any problems are not missed. Primary care involvement may be useful in this area. Early close liaison with the GP and District Nursing services is useful (📖 Sexual health and cancer).

Other common concerns problems include the following:

Ascites

This is particularly common in ovarian cancer and can be difficult to manage (📖 Malignant effusions).

Pain

Perineal and pelvic pain becomes more common in advanced disease. It often has a nerve-based element, making it difficult to completely resolve (📖 Pain management).

Hormonal symptoms

In most cases where the menopause has been induced early because of treatment (surgery to remove both ovaries or radical pelvic radiotherapy), Hormone replacement therapy may be given until the average age of the menopause, i.e. 51 years old. Exceptions to this are hormone dependant tumours such as some endometrial or some cervical tumours. (📖 Hormonal therapies: menopausal symptoms)

Lower limb oedema

When patients have extensive pelvic disease this is increasingly common. It needs active management including specialist compression bandaging and skin care (☐ Lymphoedema).

Vaginal discharge

This can be offensive and extremely embarrassing. Topical antibiotics, and deodorizing dressings can help.

Further reading

Hoskins, W J, Mitchell, W A, Randall, M E et al. (2004). *Principles and Practice of Gynecologic Oncology.* Philadelphia: Lippincott Williams and Wilkins.

Katz A (2003). Sexuality after hysterectomy: a review of the literature and discussion of nurses role. *J Adv Nurs,* **42**(3), 297–303.

Moore G J ed (2000). *Women and Cancer a gynaecologic oncology nursing perspective.* Boston: Jones and Bartlett.

NHS Executive (1999). *Guidance on commissioning cancer services: Improving outcomes in gynaecological cancers-the manual.* London: Department of Health.

White I (2005). The impact of Cancer and Cancer therapy on Sexual and reproductive Health. In Kearney N and Richardson A (2005). *Nursing Patients with Cancer: Principles and Practice* pp.675–700. Edinburgh: Churchill Livingstone.

Richard Smith J R and Barron B A (1999). *Gynaecological Oncology (Fast Facts Series).* Abingdon: Health Press.

Haematological cancers

Introduction

Haematological cancers are cancers of blood cells. All blood cells are made in the bone marrow from a haemopoietic (blood forming) stem cell. The stem cell divides and gradually turns into one of the mature blood cells, passing first through several immature stages (see Fig. 32.1).

Haematological cancers include acute and chronic leukaemias, high and low grade non-Hodgkin's lymphomas, Hodgkin's lymphoma and myeloma. These conditions can be divided according to the principal site of involvement, the cancerous cell type and the speed of progression (see Table 32.1).

Investigations

The following tests are useful in diagnosing a haematological cancer:
- Full blood count.
- Blood film.
- Bone marrow aspirate from posterior iliac crest (back of the pelvis)—particularly useful for diagnosing acute leukaemia.
- Bone marrow trephine—a piece of intact bone with the marrow, is removed from the posterior iliac crest. This is particularly useful in diagnosing lymphoma and myeloma.
- Immunophenotyping—can refine diagnosis. It detects surface molecules on a cell and can help define what type of cancer it is. It is useful for distinguishing between acute myeloid leukaemia (AML) and acute lymphoblastic leukaemia (ALL).
- Cytogenetics—are vital in diagnosing chronic myeloid leukaemia, which is nearly always associated with the presence of the Philadelphia chromosome (📖 CML). It can also determine how aggressive an acute leukaemia is likely to be.
- Lymph node biopsy—a full core or excision biopsy is required.
- CT scan—for staging lymphoma.

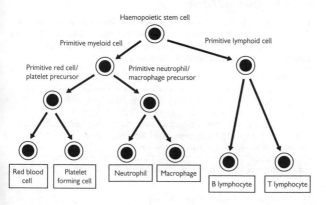

Fig. 32.1 Formation of the cellular components of the blood from a single haemopoetic stem cell.

Table 32.1 Outline of the main hematological cancers

Disease	Usual site of involvement	Cell type affected	Speed of progression
Acute myeloid leukaemia (AML)	Bone marrow	Immature myeloid forming blood cell	Rapid
Acute lymphoblastic leukaemia (ALL)	Bone marrow	Immature lymphocyte forming blood cell	Rapid
Chronic myeloid leukaemia (CML)	Bone marrow	Immature neutrophil forming blood cell	Initially slow
Chronic lymphocytic leukaemia (CLL)	Blood, lymph nodes, and bone marrow	Mature lymphocyte	Slow
High grade lymphoma	Lymph nodes and spleen (but can occur anywhere)	Mature lymphocyte	Rapid
Low grade lymphoma	Lymph nodes and spleen	Mature lymphocyte	Slow
Myeloma	Bone marrow	Plasma cell (antibody secreting cell)	Moderate

Acute leukaemia

Acute leukaemia is a rapidly progressive malignancy of an early blood-forming cell. It originates in the bone marrow and may or may not be seen in the blood itself. The two main types are acute myeloid leukaemia and acute lymphoblastic leukaemia.

Presentation

- Bone marrow failure—anaemia (fatigue, breathlessness, headaches) thrombocytopenia (bruising, bleeding, petechial rash, disseminated intravascular coagulation), leucopenia (infections, sepsis).
- Hyperviscosity of the blood due to a very high white cell count—can cause shortness of breath, headaches, alteration in neurological status, confusion, and visual disturbances.
- Infiltration of tissues—can cause skin lesions (chloromas), swelling of the gums, swelling of the testicles, enlarged liver and/or spleen, CNS.
- Bone pain.

Acute myeloid leukaemia (AML)

This is the commonest type of acute leukaemia in adults. Its incidence is 3 per 100,000. The risk increases with age.

Predisposing factors

- In most patients no cause is found.
- Myelodysplasia, myeloproliferative conditions, previous chemotherapy and radiotherapy, Down syndrome and other rare congenital abnormalities can all increase the risk.

Risk/prognosis

AML is divided into good risk, intermediate, and poor risk disease based on cytogenetic analysis.

Poor prognostic factors are:
- Older age at diagnosis.
- Failure to enter a remission after the first course of chemotherapy.
- A very high white cell count at presentation.
- Leukaemia secondary to previous chemotherapy or myelodysplasia.

Treatment

There are three broad approaches to the treatment of AML:

1. Intensive, potentially curative treatment involving high doses of combination chemotherapy:

- Induction: two courses which aim to get the patient into a remission.
- Consolidation: two further courses to prevent relapse.
- An allogeneic bone marrow transplant may be used instead of consolidation for poor risk disease, particularly if the patient has an HLA-matched sibling (🕮 Allogeneic haematopoietic stem cell transplant).
- Acute promyelocytic leukaemia, (a subset of AML with a specific cytogenetic abnormality) is also treated with all trans retinoic acid (ATRA). These patients are also at risk of disseminated intravascular coagulation (🕮 Oncological emergencies).

In the event of relapsed disease, a cure is very unlikely with more chemotherapy. An allogeneic stem cell transplant is an option depending on the age and physical status of the patient, and if a suitable donor can be found. Otherwise the outlook is very poor.

Side effects

These are often severe due to high doses of chemotherapy:

- General side effects include nausea, vomiting, diarrhoea, hair loss, reduced fertility, mucositis, infections, bruising, or bleeding due to profound bone marrow suppression.
- Specific side effects of the chemotherapy agents include conjunctivitis and neurological impairment (high dose cytarabine) and cardiac impairment (daunorubicin).

2. Palliative chemotherapy

In a patient not fit enough to receive combination chemotherapy, lower dose chemotherapy may be offered to treat the symptoms. This can induce a remission, but early relapse is highly likely.

3. Supportive care

No specific treatment is offered for AML if patients are elderly or have very poor performance status, because they are unable to tolerate treatment. In such cases, supportive care is important. This may include:

- Red cell or platelet transfusions.
- Antibiotics to treat infections.
- Analgesia and antiemetics.
- Psychological support.

Acute lymphoblastic leukaemia (ALL)

ALL accounts for *only* 20% of leukaemias in adults. It may also arise from chronic myeloid leukaemia. The outcome is poor, especially if the Philadelphia chromosome is positive (□ CML).

Risk stratification

The following factors suggest a poor prognosis:

- Increasing age.
- Initial white blood cell count of $>50 \times 10^9$/L.
- Adverse findings on cytogenetics, specifically:
  - The Philadelphia chromosome—which is more typically seen in CML (and in adult ALL).
  - Genetic abnormalities—involving chromosome 11.
  - Less than 45 chromosomes—termed hypodiploidy.
- Slow early response to treatment.
- Failure to achieve a complete remission by day 28 of treatment.

Treatment

Treatment of ALL is long and complex and often occurs as part of a clinical trial. The various phases of treatment are as follows

Induction
Combination chemotherapy is used to achieve a remission. Steroids are an important part of treatment, but frequently produce severe side effects.

Consolidation—intensification
The aim is to rapidly reduce the burden of leukaemia, which is known to be present, in spite of not being seen by routine testing. Further combination chemotherapy is used.

Central nervous system (CNS) prophylaxis
ALL commonly relapses in the CNS, so CNS prophylaxis is essential. Intrathecal chemotherapy (into the spinal fluid) is used, and in some cases, additional cranial radiotherapy.

Maintenance
This is used to reduce the risk of relapse. Typically, it involves a combination of oral chemotherapy tablets and intermittent injections, lasting for up to two years.

Treatment of relapsed disease
Early bone marrow relapse is particularly hard to treat, whereas late relapse outside of the bone marrow has an excellent cure rate.

Options for treatment include further chemotherapy or an allogeneic stem cell transplant. Stem cell transplantation is also used as first line treatment in poor prognostic disease, e.g. Philadelphia chromosome positive disease.

Nursing issues
Acute leukaemia patients can be challenging to nurse for a number of reasons.

Diagnosis
Within 1–2 days of attending the GP for a possible viral infection or other seemingly minor symptom, patients may have been diagnosed and started treatment. This frequently involves the insertion of a central venous catheter, being enrolled onto a clinical trial, commencing chemotherapy, with the prospect of many painful and life threatening side effects.

It can be a bewildering time, with patients facing a sudden loss of control over their lives, whilst trying to come to terms with a life threatening illness. Patients and their families will require intensive psychological and informational support to help them through diagnosis, and prepare them for the treatment phase.

Treatment

Patients often face a combination of side effects due to the high doses of chemotherapy and their already altered physical state. These include profound neutropaenia mucositis, hair loss, infertility, and nausea and vomiting. Patients are often already acutely unwell due to their disease, and can deteriorate very rapidly. Specific risks can include life-threatening infections leading to septic shock (📖 Bone marrow suppression), bleeding (📖 Bleeding), renal failure, and in ALL tumour lysis syndrome (📖 Tumour lysis syndrome). Patients require close regular observations, a strict fluid balance, daily weight, close electrolyte monitoring, multiple intravenous medications, and blood product support.

Patients who are profoundly neutropaenic may be nursed in strict isolation, and the visiting rights of family may be restricted, depending on local policies. Some patients can find isolation reassuring, but other patients will feel lonely and can become anxious and depressed. They may require additional psychological and emotional support.

Chronic leukaemia

There are two main types of chronic leukaemia: chronic myeloid leukaemia (CML) and chronic lymphocytic leukaemia (CLL). These are very different conditions, the only thing they have in common is the fact that they initially progress slowly.

Chronic myeloid leukaemia (CML)

CML is rare, affecting 1–2/100,000 per year. The median age at diagnosis is 50–60. Individuals exposed to radiation have an increased risk of developing CML. In the vast majority of patients the cause is unknown.

Philadelphia (Ph) chromosome

95% of people with CML have an abnormal chromosome 22, formed by an unequal exchange of genetic material between chromosomes 9 and 22 (Philadelphia (Ph) chromosome). This exchange creates a protein, which drives the abnormal cell growth.

Presentation

- Abdominal discomfort with nausea and feeling of fullness due to a massively enlarged spleen.
- Hyperviscosity due to a very high white cell count—headaches, breathlessness, visual disturbances.
- Tiredness, weight loss, drenching night sweats.

There are several distinct phases of the disease:

- *Chronic phase:* most patients first present during this relatively stable, slowly progressive period. It is easily controlled by medications and can last a few months to several years (typically 3–4 years).
- *Accelerated phase:* the disease becomes more rapidly progressive and difficult to control. It nearly always precedes a blast crisis.
- *Blast crisis:* this phase represents transformation to an acute leukaemia, either AML or ALL. It is rapidly fatal if untreated, and is often resistant to treatment.

Diagnosis

Blood film and bone marrow biopsy is taken. The diagnosis is confirmed by the demonstration of the Ph chromosome.

Treatment

There are two main modes of treatment in chronic phase CML.

Imatinib (Gleevec®) (📖 Chemotherapy)

This targets the abnormal protein produced by the Ph chromosome. It is a tablet taken daily, and is generally well tolerated.

- The vast majority of patients respond to imatinib. Nearly all have a haematological remission, and a majority become Ph chromosome negative. Fewer still have a complete molecular remission. Continued response is monitored by specialized blood tests.
- Due to the recent development of imatinib, it is currently unknown how long the drug will hold people in a remission, and if anyone will be cured.

Allogeneic stem cell transplantation (📖 Allogeneic haematopoietic stem cell transplant)

- This was the preferred treatment for a young, fit patient with CML, before the introduction of imatinib. It can lead to a cure in 60–80%.
- For selected individuals, preferably with an HLA-matched sibling, this approach is still valid.
- For older patients, and for those without an HLA-matched sibling, imatinib is the usual recommendation.

Other treatment approaches

These include subcutaneous interferon (which still has a role for women who plan to become pregnant), hydroxyurea (for initial control of the white cell count and spleen size), splenectomy or splenic irradiation (for uncontrolled, symptomatic splenomegaly), and autologous stem cell transplantation (although the role for this treatment remains controversial).

Future developments

Higher doses of imatinib are currently being trialed to see if more patients can have complete molecular response. Imatinib is also being trialed in combination with other agents such as interferon and also in combination with 'mini' allogeneic transplants (📖 Allogeneic haematopoietic stem cell transplant).

Key nursing issues

Patients with CML are often fairly well at diagnosis, and frequently respond well to treatment. However, certain problems are unique to these patients:

- Patients can feel that their disease is a 'time bomb'. They know that they are in the chronic phase, but may transform to a life-threatening acute leukaemia at any time. This can cause considerable anxiety and concern for the future and for dependent relatives.
- The introduction of imatinib is good news, but it leaves many questions unanswered. It is simply not known if it will cure some people, or if everyone on imatinib will eventually transform into acute leukaemia and die of this disease.

These 'unknowns' can leave a patient confused and with a feeling of being unable to make an informed choice. This is particularly the case for someone in their late 30s or early 40s, where the decision between imatinib or allogeneic stem cell transplant is a very difficult one to make. Though allogeneic stem cell transplants can offer a potential cure, there is a high mortality rate with the treatment. The patient generally needs as much information as possible, along with support for the decision he or she eventually makes (📖 Patient and family involvement in decision making).

Chronic lymphocytic leukaemia (CLL)

This is the commonest leukaemia in adults, but it can be very hard to treat. The incidence of CLL rises with age, reaching a peak in men of 40 per 100,000. It is commoner in men and in developed countries.

Presentation

- On a routine blood test in a healthy patient (increasingly common).
- Lumps in the neck, axillae, and groin (enlarged lymph nodes).
- Bone marrow failure (anaemia, low platelets, low white cell count).
- Autoimmune haemolytic anaemia (jaundice, dark urine, and symptoms of anaemia).
- Weight loss, loss of appetite, and night sweats.

Staging

- Bone marrow biopsy ± a CT scan.
- Cytogenetic analysis can also aid prognosis.
- Widespread lymph or organ involvement and bone marrow failure are poor prognostic factors.

CLL can be thought of as a type of lymphoma, and so staging is important.

Treatment options

'Watch and wait'

- Treatment is offered only if there is evidence of disease progression.
- Treatment is indicated if symptoms develop (see presentation above) or when there is rapidly rising white cell count.

Chemotherapy

Generally, this is single agent chlorambucil or fludarabine. It is often very well tolerated, although fludarabine can cause profound immunosuppression. Adding in cyclophosphamide or rituximab may increase effectiveness, although both the side effect profile and financial cost increase.

Other options include alemtuzumab (Campath-1H®), which is a monoclonal antibody used mainly in cases of refractory CLL. Autologous or allogeneic stem cell transplantation is an option for a fit, younger patient.

Supportive care

In the palliative care setting, radiotherapy may be used for specific sites of disease that are causing symptoms. Blood product support may be required for more intensive chemotherapy regimens and prompt treatment of infections is required. In the terminal stages of CLL, patients most commonly succumb to an infection such as pneumonia.

Nursing issues

With CLL, there is often no initial indication to treat, and patients may remain well for many years on no treatment. However, once diagnosed, patients often latch onto the word leukaemia with its associations of intensive therapy, major side effects, and immediate threat to life. It can be very difficult to accept if individuals are then not offered a specific treatment.

Patients need specially tailored and accurate information regarding their own condition, and in particular the stage of their disease. General leukaemia information leaflets may be too broad, and may lead to confusion or increased anxiety.

Hodgkin's lymphoma (Hodgkin's disease)

This is a cancer of B lymphocytes. It affects one in 100,000 people per year. In the majority of cases the cause is unknown although in a proportion, the Epstein–Barr virus is thought to be involved.

The peak age at diagnosis is 20–29, with another smaller peak in older age (over 60s). Men and people over age 45 have a poorer prognosis.

Presentation
- One or more visible lumps, representing enlarged lymph nodes.
- Breathlessness and cough due to enlarged lymph nodes in the chest (called mediastinal lymphadenopathy).
- Weight loss, fever, and drenching night sweats (called 'B symptoms').

Diagnosis
A biopsy of the affected region is taken. The hallmark of the disease is the Reed–Sternberg cell. The biopsy should distinguish between the two main types of Hodgkin's lymphoma. Treatment and prognosis is very different for each type.

The two types of HL are:
- Nodular lymphocyte predominant Hodgkin's lymphoma (NLPHL).
- Classical Hodgkin's lymphoma (the most common variety).

Staging
- CT scan of the chest, abdomen, and pelvis.
- Bone marrow trephine biopsy.
- The Ann-Arbor classification is used (see Table 32.2).

Treatment
NLPHL
The vast majority of patients present early, and are treated with radiotherapy alone. It is generally an indolent condition and the prognosis is excellent.

Classical Hodgkin's lymphoma
This is a more aggressive condition and requires aggressive treatment. Treatment varies according to staging:
- *Early stage (IA or IIA):* in very early disease, radiotherapy alone is an option. However, most centres recommend 2–4 cycles of chemotherapy (usually the ABVD regimen), with radiotherapy to the affected regions.
- *Advanced stage (III, IV or early stage with B symptoms):* the standard of care is 6–8 cycles of ABVD (doxorubicin, bleomycin, vinblastine, dacarbazine) combination chemotherapy + radiotherapy to residual disease post-chemotherapy.

Table 32.2 The Ann-Arbor staging system for Hodgkin's lymphoma

Stage	Regions affected
I	Single lymph node group
II	More than one lymph node group restricted to either above or below the diaphragm
III	Lymph node groups both above and below the diaphragm. III-S indicates additional involvement of the spleen
IV	Extra-nodal regions such as the liver or bone marrow

In addition, each stage is termed either 'A' or 'B' depending on the absence or presence of the following symptoms: fever, drenching night sweats or weight loss of >10% body weight over 6 months. B symptoms indicate a worse outlook.

Other poor risk factors include anaemia white cell count >16 x 10^9/L, low lymphocyte cell count, and Low albumen (<40g/L)

Side effects
ABVD is an intensive regimen. Common side effects include bone marrow suppression, nausea, lung toxicity, peripheral nerve damage, fatigue, and hair loss. G-CSF is often administered to stimulate neutrophil production (📖 Biological therapy).

Note: ABVD is often not tolerated well in elderly patients. Alternative regimens may then be considered.

Prognosis
With combination chemotherapy, long-term survival rates are around 75–80% overall. In early stage, good risk disease this rises to >90%. Even in advanced stage disease this can be as high as 80%. In patients with poor risk disease long-term survival falls to around 50%.

Relapsed HL
It is still possible to offer curative treatment. This normally involves two phases:
- *Salvage chemotherapy:* normally 2–3 courses of a platinum-based chemotherapy regimen, often with stem cell collection planned for after the 2nd or 3rd course.
- *High-dose therapy with autologous stem cell support:* BEAM (carmustine, etoposide, cytarabine, and melphalan) is the usual conditioning therapy. It is thought that around 50% of those who relapse after chemotherapy can be cured (📖 High dose therapy).

Long-term toxicity
Due to the excellent cure rates, many patients live long enough to experience long-term toxicity from the treatment. Two major problems are:
- *Secondary cancers*—breast cancer and lung cancer for those who received chest radiotherapy. Acute leukaemia for patients treated with very aggressive chemotherapy regimens.
- *Heart disease*—particularly for older patients treated with radiotherapy to the chest and those treated with anthracycline chemotherapy.

At around 15 years after treatment, the risk of dying from a complication of the treatment becomes greater than the risk of dying from relapse of the Hodgkin's lymphoma. Efforts are being made to reduce the treatment intensity whilst maintaining cure rates and ensuring close monitoring and long-term follow up.

Nursing issues

Hodgkin's lymphoma frequently affects young people. Particular concerns include:

Fertility

Standard ABVD chemotherapy does not generally render the patient infertile (male or female), although many men are offered sperm storage as a precaution.

Long-term toxicity

It should be emphasized that heart disease and secondary cancers are by no means inevitable later in life—although the risk is increased. The patient should be encouraged to participate in any screening programmes offered after therapy (such as for breast cancer), and to optimize a healthy style of living (giving up smoking, taking regular exercise, eating a balanced diet).

Transfusion-associated graft-versus-host disease

It is important to remember that **any** patient who has had Hodgkin's lymphoma in the past should receive only irradiated blood products, due to an increased risk of this very rare but fatal complication of blood product transfusion.

Age related issues

Because the peak incidence falls in late adolescence, when young people have left home and are independent, there may be family conflicts and issues centred around the parents need for control and to care for their child. This occurs whilst the patient still needs to maintain their newly developed sense of self, maintain control and independence. Families should be encouraged and supported to discuss the issues that are arising.

Non-Hodgkin's lymphoma (NHL)

NHL is a broad term, which covers a number of very different conditions all of which are cancers of lymphocytes.

The classification of NHL is a confusing and changing area. The most clinically relevant way of categorizing NHL is in terms of high grade or low-grade disease. (See Table 32.3)

Presentation
- Enlarged lymph node, commonly in the neck, axillae, and groin.
- Symptoms of NHL are due to extranodal disease, so presentation depends on the site of the disease. NHL can occur anywhere in the body e.g. brain, eye, bone, kidney, bowel, and can present with quite severe complications e.g. bowel obstruction, renal failure, seizures.
- Cough, breathlessness, tracheal deviation, superior vena cava obstruction due to mediastinal lymphadenopathy.
- 'B' symptoms—weight loss, fever, drenching night sweats.

Diagnosis and staging
- Core or excision biopsy of the lymph node or extra nodal disease.
- It is important to establish the exact subtype of lymphoma as the treatment depends on this.
- CT scan of the chest, abdomen and pelvis ± brain.
- Bone marrow trephine biopsy.
- The staging system is the same as for Hodgkin's disease (see Table 32.2).

Prognostic factors
Patients are categorised into risk groups depending on the number of poor prognostic factors they present with
- Poor prognostic factors include age >60, high serum LDH, poor performance status, stage III or IV disease and the existence of extranodal disease.

High grade lymphoma
- For low risk patients 5-year survival is around 73%.
- High-risk 5-year survival rates are nearer 25% (these statistics apply to diffuse large B cell lymphoma, the most common high-grade lymphoma).

Low grade lymphoma
- For low risk patients 5-year survival is around 90%.
- High-risk 5-year survival rates are nearer 50%.

Note: although low-grade disease is not curable the 5-year survival rates are better than for high-grade disease. However, survival rates continue to fall with time due to the disease continuing to relapse and/or transform into high-grade disease.

Treatment
Treatment depends on the exact subtype, stage and perceived aggressiveness of the disease, the age, and general fitness of the patients.

High grade lymphoma
Chemotherapy
Combination chemotherapy is standard therapy for high-grade lymphoma. For diffuse large B cell lymphoma, the standard treatment is CHOP-R (cyclophosphamide, doxorubicin, vincristine, and prednisolone in combination with the monoclonal antibody rituximab). (For further information on monoclonal antibodies, see biological therapy).

This treatment is generally well tolerated. It will cause a predictable neutropaenia, and rituximab can cause an infusional hypersensitivity reaction most common on the first dose (📖 Anaphylaxis). Other side effects include mucositis, cardiac and peripheral nerve toxicity.

Other forms of high-grade lymphoma may be treated differently.
For example:
- Burkitt's lymphoma regimens contain high doses of methotrexate and intrathecal chemotherapy, so as to prevent CNS relapses. Multiple doses of cyclophosphamide are also thought to be important.
- Lymphoblastic lymphoma is treated in the same way as acute lymphoblastic leukaemia (📖 Acute leukaemia).

Table 32.3 Classification of NHL into high or low grade disease.

High grade	Low grade
- Diffuse large B cell lymphoma	- Follicular lymphoma
- Burkitt's lymphoma	- Small lymphocytic lymphoma
- Lymphoblastic lymphoma	- Marginal zone lymphoma
	- Lymphoplasmacytoid lymphoma

Grade	High grade	Low grade
Speed of progression	Rapid	Indolent
Usual stage at presentation	More commonly early stage	More commonly late stage
Sensitivity to chemotherapy	Very sensitive	Less sensitive
Risk of tumour lysis syndrome	High	Low
Potential for cure	40–50% chance of cure	Usually incurable

Radiotherapy

Radiotherapy can be used in combination with a reduced number of chemotherapy courses or to target sites of bulky disease after chemotherapy has been given in order to prevent relapse.

Relapsed disease

For patients who relapse after treatment, the aim is normally to get the patient into another remission by using different forms of chemotherapy, and then a high dose therapy in order to consolidate the remission (📖 High dose therapy).

Low grade lymphoma

Low grade lymphoma is often not treated actively until it causes one of the following:

• Generalized symptoms such as weight loss, night sweats, and fevers.
• Falling blood counts due to bone marrow involvement.
• Progressive enlargement of the liver or spleen.
• Symptoms such as painfully enlarged lymph nodes, due to local disease.
• Evidence of high-grade transformation such as asymmetrically rapidly enlarging lymph nodes.

Once treatment is indicated, it can take a number of different forms:

• Oral chemotherapy: rarely curative, but is well tolerated and may induce a remission.
• Intravenous combination chemotherapy: several regimes are used in combination with the monoclonal antibody rituximab.
• Radiotherapy may be used to treat symptoms caused by local deposits of disease.
• High dose therapy with autologous stem cell support (📖 Chapter 20).
• Allogeneic stem cell transplantation for younger, fit patients (📖 Chapter 21).

Note: early trial results of radioimmunotherapy are encouraging. This involves attaching a radioactive compound to an antibody similar to rituximab, enabling the radioactivity to be targeted to the lymphoma cell.

Nursing issues

Patients with high grade lymphoma pose similar challenges to patients with acute leukaemia (📖 Acute leukaemia). It can be hard to adjust to a diagnosis of a rapidly progressive, life-threatening lymphoma, and bewildering when treatment is started within a few days of diagnosis. The intense treatment regimens bring a range of severe and potentially life-threatening side effects. For the very high grade lymphomas such as Burkitt's lymphoma, there is also a high risk of tumour lysis syndrome (📖 Tumour lysis syndrome).

Patients with low grade NHL on the other hand, face similar issues to CLL patients. They may find it confusing to be given a diagnosis of cancer, but not to be offered specific treatment straight away. If the patient is young, then to be told they have a life expectancy of 10 years is potentially devastating.

Myeloma

Myeloma is a cancer of plasma cells—the antibody producing cells which represent the final step in the development of a B-lymphocyte. In myeloma, the cancerous cells secrete a single type of antibody into the bloodstream called a paraprotein. As well as being a marker of myeloma, the paraprotein may lead to clinical problems. These include thinning bones, reduced immunity and obstruction of the renal tubules.

The incidence of myeloma increases with age. Presentation before the age of 50 is unusual. Incidence is around 5 per 100,000 in the UK. For unknown reasons, myeloma is more common in the African-Caribbean population.

Presentation
- Bone pain: predominantly due to bone thinning, causing fractures in any part of the body. This may also result in spinal cord compression.
- Hypercalcaemia: presenting with confusion or alteration in mental status, dehydration (📖 Hypercalcaemia).
- Anaemia due to bone marrow involvement or renal failure.
- Infections: the most common infection is pneumonia.
- Acute renal failure.

Diagnosing myeloma
The main tests required for a diagnosis of myeloma are:
- Blood tests to find the paraprotein.
- Urine tests to find the paraprotein—when present in the urine the antibody is called the 'Bence–Jones protein'.
- Skeletal survey: multiple X-rays to find any 'lytic lesions' where the myeloma is eroding away bone.
- Bone marrow aspirate and trephine.

Note: if a patient presents with any symptoms suggesting compression of the spinal cord, then an urgent MRI of the spine is indicated. (📖 Spinal cord compression).

Treatment
Myeloma is generally considered to be incurable; median survival is around 3 years. Symptom control is therefore an important part of treatment. Treatment options include:

Single agent oral chemotherapy
This offers around 50% response rate. Generally only used first-line in more elderly patients.

Combination chemotherapy
The main aim of this is to debulk the disease, making it more amenable to high-dose therapy.

High-dose therapy with autologous stem cell support
Available evidence suggests that this can prolong life expectancy by about one year. That extra year is often treatment-free and therefore of reasonable quality (📖 High dose therapy).

Thalidomide-based regimens
This is used frequently for relapsed myeloma. It is also being trialed as first line therapy in combination with other agents. It is not well tolerated, with sedation, constipation, nerve damage, and thrombosis being well recognized side effects.

Thalidomide and the risk of pregnancy

Women of child-bearing age must be counselled to use at least two forms of contraception (one being a barrier method), due to the well known toxic effects of thalidomide on a developing fetus. Men must also be told to wear a condom during sexual intercourse as thalidomide is excreted into semen.

Bortezomib-based regimens
Bortezomib is a new agent, which targets enzymes involved in controlling cell growth. It has shown good activity in relapsed patients who have been unresponsive to other forms of treatment. However, it is generally fairly poorly tolerated with diarrhoea, vomiting, and nerve damage all proving to be troublesome side effects.

Bisphosphonates
Adding bisphosphonates to myeloma treatment reduces pathological fractures and pain but does not improve overall survival.

Solitary plasmacytoma
- These are rare single-site plasma cell tumours. They account for less than 10% of all plasma cell tumours.
- Can occur in bone (SPB) or soft tissue (extramedullary plasmacytoma—EMP).

SPB
- Commonly presents in spine, pelvis, or femur. Pain is the most common presenting symptom.
- Diagnosis is through histological examination and ruling out other sites of disease.
- Treatment is with fractionated radiotherapy and curative in 50% of cases. If there is evidence of dissemination (the majority of patients will relapse with myeloma), treat with myeloma regimens.

EMP
- Commonly presents in upper airways but can occur at almost any site.
- Treatment is with radial radiotherapy possibly including regional lymph nodes.
- Progression to myeloma can occur but less commonly than SPB.

Nursing issues
Myeloma can be a very challenging condition to nurse; it can cause a variety of problems, which frequently require specialist input. An important role for a specialist myeloma nurse is to coordinate this care, and to help the patient assimilate all the information.

Key problems faced by patients include the following:

Bone pain: radiotherapy, opioids, and bisphosphonates all have a major role in managing this. In selected cases surgery or vertebroplasty can also be used to manage collapsed vertebral bodies (📖 Metastatic bone disease).

Spinal cord compression (📖 Spinal cord compression)

Immunosuppression: although myeloma patients may not be neutropaenic, they should be considered immunosuppressed, and prompt antibiotic treatment should be given for proven or likely episodes of infection.

Acute renal failure: dialysis may be required for patients who present with acute renal failure, and this may be needed long term if their kidneys fail to recover.

Further reading

National Institute for Clinical excellence (2003). *Guidance on Cancer Services-Improving Outcomes in Haematological Cancers: The Manual* London: NICE.

Hoffbrand A V, Pettit J E, Moss P A H, (2001). *Essential haematology 4th ed.* Oxford: Blackwell Science.

Grundy M (2006) *Nursing in haematological oncology* 2nd ed. Edinburgh: Elsevier, Baillière Tindall.

Souhami, R L, and Tobias J S (2005). *Cancer and Its Management.* 5th edn. Oxford: Blackwell.

Head and neck cancers

Introduction

- Head and neck (H&N) cancer is the sixth most common cancer worldwide. These cancers account for over 8000 cases per year in England and Wales, and 2700 deaths per year.
- H&N cancer describes a group of solid tumours of the upper aero-digestive tract, often arising from surface mucosa. The most common type of tumour is squamous cell carcinoma.
- There are over 30 specific sites in the H&N where cancer can occur, including the oral cavity (the most common site), the pharynx, hypo-pharynx and larynx. Rarer sites include the saliva glands, post-nasal space and sinuses, and the middle ear.
- Metastatic spread is not uncommon, and the lymph glands in the neck tend to be the first area where deposits occur.

Risk factors

Smoking and alcohol

- Around 75% of H&N cancers are associated with smoking and alcohol use.
- Combined cigarette and alcohol use has a potentiating effect.
- The risk of oral cancer in this group is over 35 times higher than for non-smokers and non-drinkers.
- For those who smoke but do not drink, the risk of developing H&N cancer is 10 times higher than for non-smokers.
- Nurses can help the patient to manage their alcohol and tobacco use in order to optimize treatment outcomes (📖 Alcohol withdrawal; Smoking cessation; Cancer prevention and screening).

Diet

- People who drink and smoke heavily may have a poor diet and be malnourished which exacerbates the risk of H&N cancer.
- Low risk associated with well-balanced diet rich in vegetables and fruit.
- Increased risk with a poor diet, particularly deficient in vitamins A and C.

Presentation

Depending on the site of tumour, H&N malignancies may present with:
- Hoarseness.
- Difficulty in swallowing.
- Local or referred pain.

Some tumours are detected during a dental examination.

Diagnosis and staging

- Clinical examination.
- Panendoscopy and biopsy.
- FNA for cytology is useful in patients presenting with neck lumps.
- CT or MRI scan.
- Staging is carried out using the TNM staging system (📖 Diagnosis and classification).
- Most tumours invade locally; bone involvement usually occurs in advanced disease.

Prognostic factors

Metastatic nodal involvement is more important prognostically than the size of primary tumour: i.e. smaller tumours and extensive nodal involvement have a worse prognosis than a large tumour and no nodal involvement. Other prognostic factors include age and the histopathology of the tumour.

Further reading

British Association of Head and Neck Oncology Nurses (BAHNON). Provides guidelines and protocols for health professionals: www.bahnon.org.uk

Clarke L M and Dropkin M J (2005). *Site-specific Cancer Series: Head & Neck Cancer.* Oncology Nursing Society.

Feber T (2000). *Head and Neck Oncology Nursing.* London: Whurr Publishers.

Russell C, Matta B, eds (2004) *Tracheostomy: a Multiprofessional handbook.* Cambridge: Cambridge University Press.

Websites

The following charitable organizations can play an important role in supporting the patient and their family:

- Changing Faces: www.changingfaces.org.uk
- National Association of Laryngectomy Clubs: www.nalc.ik.org
- British Red Cross Camouflage Service: www.redcross.org.uk

Treatment of head and neck cancer

The main treatment approaches for H&N cancer are radiotherapy and surgery. Chemotherapy is occasionally used in combination with radiotherapy, or as a palliative treatment.

Treatment of early stage disease (30–40% of presentations)

The main options are surgery, radiotherapy, or a combination of both. Postoperative chemoirradiation is also an option for specific high-risk, fit patients.

- Cure rates with primary radiotherapy, appear to be equivalent to surgery for early stage disease of many H & N tumours.
- The specific cancer site, patient health and their own preference will be major factors in which treatment option is chosen.

Surgery alone

Potential advantages of surgery alone include:

- It provides complete staging of the disease and quick local clearance.
- It avoids radiotherapy toxicities, including the risk of radiotherapy-induced second malignancies.

Radiotherapy alone

Options are external beam radiotherapy treatment (EBRT) ± a boost to the tumour site, either with further EBRT or interstitial therapy e.g. using iridium wires. EBRT is given in divided doses (20–30 fractions) of between 55–70 Gray (Gy) for solid tumours (commonly squamous cell carcinoma).

Potential advantages of primary radiotherapy include:

- Avoidance of operative mortality in patients who have significant co-morbidities.
- Organ conservation is more likely including preservation of the voice and swallowing.
- Radiotherapy treats clinically occult regional lymph node disease with relatively little extra morbidity.
- Surgery remains an option as treatment after radiotherapy if that is unsuccessful though this is associated with greater morbidity.
- It allows the treatment of multiple primary tumours.

Combined surgery and radiotherapy

- Bulky tumours are generally best treated by a combination of surgery and radiotherapy to minimize the risk of locally advanced disease recurrence.
- Risk factors for recurrence include large tumour size, positive resection margins, vascular invasion, and lymph node spreads

Post-operative chemo-radiotherapy

- Radiotherapy with concurrent cisplatin in oropharyngeal cancers shows fewer local and regional relapses and improvements in disease-free survival.
- An improvement in overall survival has not been consistently demonstrated.
- Toxicity is significantly increased in patients receiving both cisplatin and radiotherapy.
- May be considered for selected high risk, fit patients with resected squamous cell H&N cancers.

Management of involved neck nodes

Options include: therapeutic neck dissection, radiotherapy, or surgery for any relapsed disease after radiotherapy.

Neck dissection

Neck dissection involves removing the affected lymph glands, along with the other glands in the lymphovascular chain.

H&N surgery is complex, with associated complications and a potentially huge impact on a patient's long-term quality of life (see nursing management, next page).

Treatment of locally advanced unresectable disease

Chemoirradiation

- The majority of squamous cell H & N cancers have locally advanced unresectable disease at presentation.
- Surgery is often not technically possible or may produce unacceptable morbidity.
- Primary radiotherapy offers 5-year survival of only 10–30%.
- The addition of cisplatin offers a modest survival advantage over treatment with radiotherapy alone (4–8% increase in 5-year survival).
- This is associated with increased toxicity, in particular mucositis. It is most appropriate for patients with a good performance status and relatively few co-morbidities.

Biological therapies

Cetuximab (Erbitux®) (📖 Biological therapies)
Early trials suggest that in combination with radiotherapy (versus radiotherapy alone) cetuximab may offer improved 2 year survival in locally advanced squamous cell carcinoma of the head and neck.

Treatment of metastatic disease

Chemotherapy

Certain chemotherapy agents e.g. cisplatin, 5FU, methotrexate, and bleomycin have been shown to be effective in advanced squamous cell carcinoma. Highest response rates appear to be achieved by combination regimes. The risk vs. potential benefits have to be carefully considered for each patient.

Radiotherapy

Radiotherapy is used in metastatic disease to give short-term local con and to palliate symptoms such as bleeding and pain.

Laryngectomy and tracheostomy

Anatomy and physiology of the airway

The upper respiratory tract (URT) consists of the nasal airway, the naso-pharynx, oral cavity, oropharynx, hypopharynx, larynx, and trachea. The nose has an important role in humidifying, warming, and filtering the air. The whole URT is lined with mucous-secreting columnar ciliated epithelium. This prevents debris and microorganisms from entering the respiratory tract.

If the airway is altered due to tracheostomy or laryngectomy, it is exposed to cold air, large quantities of particulate matter and bacteria, pathogens and debris, and there is a rapid increase in the production of mucous.

Laryngectomy care

Stoma care is aimed at maintaining the patient's airway, preventing infection, including secondary chest infection and tracheitis, and promoting healing.

The main priority of post-operative support for laryngectomy patients is self-care and independence, through individualized teaching plans. Family members or carers should be included.

Basic information needs to be provided and individual coping strategies developed for dealing with the following: loss of normal speech, loss of smell, inability to sniff or blow one's nose, loss of sphincteric function of the larynx (affecting lifting and ability to 'push' during defecation), using bronchodilator inhalers, avoiding water entering the stoma when showering or swimming. A number of devices are available to help with this.

Tracheostomy

A surgeon will perform a tracheostomy when the airway is obstructed by tumour or postoperative oedema. A tube is inserted into the tracheostomy and a tract develops after 4 days—a tube change should not be attempted before this, unless in the case of emergency.

A tracheostomy can be temporary or permanent.
- Temporary: to protect the airway from oedema and swelling following surgery or radiotherapy.
- Permanent: following laryngectomy, airway obstruction caused by an inoperable tumour, or the effects of a tumour, for example, when there is a fixed vocal cord.

Nursing management of tracheostomy

Pre-operative counselling

Counselling should be given to the patient and their family if possible. A permanent tracheostomy can have life-long effects on speech, swallowing, and respiration. Input from a clinical nurse specialist (CNS), speech and language therapist (SALT), dietitian, and physiotherapist is essential if the patient is to achieve optimum rehabilitation.

For patients undergoing laryngectomy, a meeting with a patient who has already had a laryngectomy (a laryngectomee) can help the process of adjustment. Some areas operate a 'buddy' system of support.

Suction and humidification: patients with tracheostomy will produce increased pulmonary secretions. These are difficult to remove with coughing and can block breathing. Patients will need suction to help to clear them. Heated humidified oxygen is administered at prescribed rate immediately postoperatively. If oxygen support is not needed, consider using a heat-moisture exchanger (HME). The patient must take adequate fluids.

Neck tapes and keyhole dressing: these should be changed daily, or more frequently if required. This should only be undertaken by two practitioners, as there is a risk of the tracheostomy tube being coughed out when the neck tapes are removed. If the tube is stitched into the neck, the flange of the tube can cause pressure necrosis of the skin inferior to the stoma. The condition of the peri-stomal skin should be monitored, and any concerns raised with the surgical team.

Cuff pressure: this should be checked every 8 hours using a manometer. If cuff pressure is too high, tracheal stenosis may be caused. If it is too low, the patient may be at risk of aspiration. Inner tubes should be cleaned replaced every 8 hours, or more frequently if required.

A fenestrated tracheostomy tube: this may be used in combination with a speaking valve to facilitate speech. Where a tube is cuffed with fenestration, the cuff MUST be deflated before attempting to use a speaking valve, or the patient will not be able to breathe.

When the patient is capable, the nurse should support the patient in becoming independent with care of the stoma and change of tube. Give the patient a pen and paper or a magnetic writing board to facilitate patient communication.

Complications of tracheostomy
Obstruction of the tube: a blocked tube can be fatal. Warning signs of tube occlusion include increased respiratory rate and decreased oxygen saturation. If a tube without an inner cannula becomes blocked, then the tube must be changed immediately to prevent cardio-pulmonary arrest.

Haemorrhage: erosion of the tracheal wall is possible by excessive tube or cuff pressure causing a haemorrhage from the inominate or right common carotid arteries—this can be fatal. Surgical repair of the damaged vessel is undertaken if the patient survives long enough.

Infection: as tracheostomies bypass the immune system provided by the upper airways, chest infections can be a problem. Tracheitis can be due to infection or irritation. Fungal infection is not common, but can be seen by signs of fungal growth on the tracheostomy tube.

Other complications include tracheo-oesophageal fistula, tube displacement, excessive granulation tissue, and pressure sore formation inferior to the stoma.

Nursing management issues

H&N cancers can have a profound effect on a person's quality of life, as they affect the most visible parts of the body, and the critical functions of eating, drinking, breathing, and speaking. A large multidisciplinary team is needed to manage the complex nature of the disease and the side effects of treatment.

The patient's journey through the health care system can be complex, so continuity of care is important. The H&N cancer nurse specialist has an important role in providing continuity; other professionals may take a key-worker role at different points. Developing effective links with community services, i.e. GP, district nurse and/or community palliative care teams is essential in providing long-term support of these patients.

Effective nursing care involves supporting the patient through a complex series of treatments, helping them manage the side effects and complications of treatment, and changes to their self-image.

Impact of radiotherapy

Side effects

The upper aero-digestive tract is extremely sensitive to radiotherapy It can have a profound, long-term impact on the quality of life of the H&N cancer patient. Common side effects include:

- Mucositis; causing severe pain, taste loss, dysphagia, sleep disturbance.
- Xerostomia: mouth pain, loss of appetite, chewing difficulties, taste changes, halitosis.
- Fatigue.
- Skin damage.
- Loss of hair.

For management of each of these side effects, see the appropriate section under (📖 Symptom management).

Impact of surgery

Pre-operative management

Counselling is essential to prepare patients for the possible long-term side effects of neck dissection, e.g. body image, swallowing, nutrition, communication (see speech and language therapy below). In addition, the nurse should discuss post-operative pain and how to deal with numb skin on the neck. A physiotherapy referral enables a baseline assessment to be undertaken, and post-operative management to be discussed. A nutritional assessment is also required (see Nutritional support below)

Post-operative management

For standard post-operative care (📖 Surgery). Specific issues in H&N surgery include management of skin flaps and grafts, meticulous oral hygiene, pain, swallowing, and speech therapy. Laryngectomy and tracheostomy have been explored earlier in this chapter.

Potential emergencies
Carotid haemorrhage
Bleeding from the neck is uncommon, but it can occur following neck dissection, particularly if the tumour has involved a main artery or vein. This is an emergency situation. Very firm pressure should be applied to the bleeding point, the resuscitation team and the surgeon should be alerted for immediate return to theatre if possible, and the patient resuscitated with fluids (📖 Bleeding).

Chylous fistula
Any leak into a surgical drain which appears milky, may be a chylous fistula. The patient should have a pressure dressing applied, and be commenced on a totally fat-free diet for up to 6 weeks to allow the fistula to heal. Surgical repair of the thoracic duct may be required.

Later complications include lymphoedema and subcutaneous fibrosis. This is more frequent with combined surgery and radiotherapy.

Nutritional support
Many patients with H&N cancer are nutritionally compromised prior to treatment. A full dietitian assessment is essential prior to their treatment to plan appropriate nutritional support (📖 Nutritional support).

Enteral support
H&N cancer and its treatment may compromise or obstruct the GI tract. In these situations short- or long-term enteral support is required, such as a naso-gastric feeding tube or a gastrostomy tube (📖 Nutritional support).

Psychological support
Over time, the cumulative effects of disease and multiple treatments can result in 'patient burnout'. This is a severe state of mental and physical exhaustion and demoralization. A referral to a psycho-oncology team may be required (📖 Psychological support).

Speech and language therapy
Patients should be referred to a speech and language therapist as early as possible, so that baseline assessments can be made. Potential problems include.

Difficulty in swallowing
This may be caused by anatomical changes in any part of the oral cavity, pharynx or oesophagus. New swallowing techniques may need to be mastered in the post-operative period.

Speech
Most centres use tracheoesophageal puncture and prosthetic valves to facilitate speech following laryngectomy. Many patients are taught how to change their own speech valve following the surgery. Some patients are not eligible for prosthetic valves and will need an alternative method of communication e.g. an electrolarynx (a vibration device that is placed on the neck).

HIV related cancer

HIV related malignancies

Epidemiology

Human immunodeficiency virus (HIV) represents the worst epidemic of the twentieth and twenty-first centuries. There are approximately 38 million cases worldwide. The highest prevalence is in sub-Saharan Africa with around 7.5% of the adult population infected. In Western Europe there were 20,000 new cases of HIV infection in 2003.

Aetiology

Transmission is through direct contact with blood or body fluid of infected individual. Usually spread through:
- Unprotected sex or sharing needles for drug use.
- Infants can get HIV from their mother if she is infected.

Highly active antiretroviral therapy (HAART) has increased survival for many people with HIV infection. However, the rate of malignant disease in HIV-infected patients has increased to over 25% due to:
- A reduction in competing causes of deaths.
- The effects of chronic immuno-suppression.
- The influence of other oncogenic viruses in these individuals, e.g. *Epstein–Barr* (EBV) and HPV.

25–30% of deaths in patients with HIV are due to malignancy. Cancers associated with HIV infection include:
- Kaposi's sarcoma (KS).
- Intermediate and high-grade NHL.
- Primary CNS lymphoma.
- Invasive cervical cancer in HIV-positive females.
- Hodgkins disease.

Management

Management of HIV is complex, involving management of the cancer, of the underlying immune deficiency, and of the complex psychological and social issues which usually co-exist.

AIDS

AIDS stands for acquired immuno-deficiency syndrome. When HIV infection becomes advanced it often is referred to as AIDS. It is characterized by the appearance of opportunistic infections such as *Pneumocystis carinii* pneumonia and malignancies such as Kaposi's Sarcoma.

HIV disease is a more current name for the condition. It is more accurate because it refers to the pathogen that causes AIDS and encompasses all the condition's stages, from infection to immunodeficiency and the onset of opportunistic diseases.

Specific cancers

Kaposi's sarcoma (KS): this incurable multi-focal soft tissue sarcoma is the most common HIV or AIDS related malignancy. Cutaneous involvement of multiple red-purple lesions affecting the upper body, face, and legs is characteristic. Disease progression is generally slow, although it can behave aggressively causing significant morbidity. Death is usually from opportunistic infections.

Treatment
- Is usually palliative in intent.
- Local therapy options (for local control and cosmesis) include cryotherapy and laser therapy.
- Intralesional chemotherapy or radiotherapy can produce short-term regression in ~75% of cases.
- Systemic therapy—with HAART ± chemotherapy *(Liposomal doxorubicin)* are front line treatment for systemic disease.
- Immunotherapy using *Interferon–α (IFN– α)* is most effective if the disease is non-visceral.

Supportive care
- Camouflage with cosmetics.
- Psychosocial support.
- Palliation of symptoms.

Systemic non-Hodgkin's lymphoma
NHL is the second most common malignancy to affect those with AIDS. The risk is 60–160 times greater than in the HIV negative population, with increasing incidence with worsening immuno-suppression. Most people present with widespread disease.

Treatment
- The optimal approach is to be in a centre with specialist expertise in AIDS-associated lymphomas.
- Systemic chemotherapy with concomant HAART is the normal approach (☐ Haematological malignancies for NHL treatment).
- Response rates to treatment are less good than in patients with non-AIDS related lymphoma, with only a small percentage of long-term survivors.
- Use of the monoclonal antibody *rituximab* in AIDS-associated NHL is controversial, with no data yet supporting its use.

Primary CNS lymphoma (PCNSL) is usually a late manifestation of AIDS, and patients often have other serious opportunistic infections. It presents with a range of CNS symptoms, and also lymphoma 'B' symptoms (☐ Haematological cancers). It needs to be distinguished from cerebral toxoplasmosis.

Treatment
- Whole-brain radiotherapy in combination with corticosteroids, combined with appropriate HAART.
- Median survival from diagnosis remains just 2–4 months due to severe immunocompromisation. Death is usually due to opportunistic infections.

Cervical cancer in HIV-positive females
The prevalence of cervical intraepithelial neoplasia (CIN) is up to 40% in HIV-infected women. It is advisable to screen patients frequently e.g. every 6–12 months. Effective antiretroviral therapy is associated with regression of CIN (☐ Cervical Screening).

Nursing management issues

People with HIV disease can face social isolation for a number of reasons including homophobia, prejudice against drug users, lack of family acceptance, or discrimination. It is a slow, progressive disease causing chronic wasting and an increasing risk of death as it progresses. Having to deal with a diagnosis of cancer on top of this may reassert the feeling of living with a death sentence.

Nurses are in an important position to support patients with their symptoms, the side effects of treatment and the social and psychological impact of both illnesses.

Patient education

After a diagnosis of HIV, it is extremely important to prevent further infection, to prevent the spread of HIV infection, and because further exposure to infections may increase the individuals risk of progressive disease[1].

Topics for patient education include:
- Safer sex techniques.
- Use of clean drug equipment.
- Perinatal transmission risks.
- Advice about rest, nutrition and stress reduction, to reduce the risk of opportunistic infections.
- Education about the signs and symptoms of specific cancers such as KS or NHL, and the importance of early treatment.

Support can come from specialist HIV counsellors. Contact your local Sexually transmitted Infections (STI) unit for a list of appropriate services that may be helpful. Useful information may also be obtained from support organizations such as the Terrence Higgins Trust[2].

Treatment decisions

Many patients are very immuno-suppressed, and may not tolerate full dose chemotherapy or radiotherapy regimens. Dose reductions and delays are common. Patients need advice and explanations about the reasons for these difficult decisions.

The risk of life-threatening infections can be high with immuno-suppression, due to both HIV and systemic chemotherapy. Good patient education is required on both the early signs of these infections, e.g. *Pneumocystis carinii*, or cytomegaly virus and the need to contact their treatment unit immediately with any suspected signs.

Body image disturbance

This is common due to KS lesions and severe weight loss. In addition, hair loss or steroid effects can add to body image disturbance (📖 Altered body image).

---

1 Health Development Agency (2001). HIV *prevention and sexual health promotion with people with HIV.* London: HDA.
2 Terrence Higgins Trust. Website: www.tht.org.uk/home/

Palliative care

Early access to hospice and palliative care services will be important for many people. The outlook for AIDS patients with NHL or PCNSL is often bleak. Specialist hospices for those with AIDs do exist in a few areas of the country, though most care in the UK is now integrated into general hospices.

Further reading

National Institute for Clinical Excellence (2003). *Guidance on Cancer Services- Improving Outcomes in Haematological Cancers: The Manual*, London: NICE.

Pattman R, Snow M, Handy P et al (2005). *Oxford Handbook of Genitourinary Medicine, HIV and AIDS*. Oxford: Oxford University Press.

Watson M, Lucas, C, Hoy A and Back I (2005). *Oxford Handbook of Palliative Care* pp.555–70. Oxford: Oxford University Press.

Websites

▣ Medscape- website of educational articles. http://www.medscape.com/hiv

▣ National AIDS Manual (NAM) excellent website with up-to date treatment news http://www.aidsmap.com/

Lung cancer

Introduction

Lung cancer is a mainly preventable disease, the main cause being cigarette smoking. It was relatively rare until the 20th century, but is now the leading cause of cancer death in the UK, Europe, and the USA. This is despite changes in treatment modalities, diagnostic procedures, and recent falling smoking rates amongst many sectors of society.

Much criticism has been leveled at the lack of attention and research funding given to lung cancer relative to other cancers. Recent government policy in the UK has emphasized the importance of smoking cessation clinics. There are moves to ban smoking in all public places in the UK as in some other European countries, though this policy remains controversial. The key to reducing deaths from lung cancer remains smoking prevention and cessation work (□ Smoking cessation).

The impact of a diagnosis of any lung cancer is devastating, with a poor overall prognosis for most individuals. Coupled with complex symptom management issues, nursing these patients is particularly challenging. The following section covers the key treatment approaches for the two main types of lung cancer and mesothelioma. Key nursing issues are highlighted at the end of the section.

Epidemiology
- Second most common cancer in UK, comprising 14% of all cancers.
- It is the most frequent cause of cancer death in UK men and women.
- Incidence and mortality rate is falling in UK men but rising in UK women.
- The worldwide incidence is continuing to rise, particularly in developing countries, as cigarette smoking becomes more prevalent.
- Survival rates remain dismal with 5 year survival at 6–7% in the UK.

Risk factors
- 80–90% of lung cancers are due to smoking.
- Risk relates to the number of cigarettes smoked and the number of years of smoking.
- Passive smoking.
- Exposure to asbestos (mesothelioma).

Common presenting symptoms and signs
Presentation is often late, as symptoms such as persistent cough and dyspnoea are attributed to smoking.
- Persistent cough, haemoptysis, dyspnoea.
- Recurrent chest infections.
- Chest or shoulder pain (constant, progressive).
- Hoarse voice (vocal cord palsy).
- Anorexia, weight loss.
- Superior vena cava obstruction.
- Finger clubbing.
- Symptoms from metastatic disease.
- Fatigue.

Investigations

After a physical examination and a chest x-ray, patients with suspected lung cancer require further imaging with a CT scan of their chest and abdomen, and a tissue diagnosis, obtained by the least invasive route e.g.

- Sputum cytology.
- Bronchial brushings and washings.
- Bronchoscopy with biopsy.
- CT guided biopsy.

Other important assessments include performance status, pulmonary function tests, FBC, and a biochemical profile. Patients with symptoms suggestive of metastatic disease may require a bone scan or CT of the brain.

Table 35.1 TNM staging of lung cancer

T1	Tumour 3cm or less in diameter, surrounded by lung or visceral pleura, distal to the main bronchus
T2	Tumour >3cm diameter; or involving main bronchus 2cm or more distal to carina; or invading visceral pleura; or associated with atelectasis which extends to the hilum but does not involve the whole lung
T3	Tumour invading chest wall, diaphragm, mediastinal pleura, or pericardium; or tumour in main bronchus <2cm distal to carina; or atelectasis of the whole lung
T4	Tumour invading mediastinum, heart, great vessels, trachea, oesophagus, vertebra, or carina; or intralobar tumour nodules; or malignant pleural effusion
N0	No regional node metastases
N1	Ipsilateral peribronchial or hilar node involvement
N2	Ipsilateral mediastinal or subcarinal nodes
N3	Contra-lateral mediastinal nodes; scalene; or supraclavicular nodes
Stage grouping	
I	T1–2 N0
II	T1–2 N1; or T3 N0
IIIa	T1–2 N2; or T3 N1–2
IIIb	T4 any N M0; or any N3 M0
IV	Any M1

Pathology

For the purposes of management, lung cancers are grouped as NSCLC and SCLC. Staging is via the TNM system.

Common sites of metastatic spread

- Regional lymph nodes.
- Bone.
- Liver.
- Adrenal glands.
- Lung.
- Central nervous system.
- Skin.

In SCLC it is estimated that >90% of patients have either overt or occult metastases at presentation.

Mesothelioma arises from the serosal lining of the chest. Metastatic spread is normally to the peritoneum (▢ Mesothelioma, p.460).

Management of non-small cell lung cancer (NSCLC)

Surgery

Complete surgical removal of NSCLC offers the best possibility of a cure. This is appropriate for patients with stage I–II disease who are fit for surgery with adequate lung function. Advanced stage of the disease and significant co-morbidity reduce the number of people who are offered surgical resection.

Major lung resection carries significant risks of morbidity and mortality. Post-operative mortality rate should be less than 3% following lobectomy and less than 5% following pneumonectomy (see Table 35.2).

Surgical resection

The aim is to resect the primary tumour with clear margins and regional draining nodes. This may require lobectomy, bi-lobectomy, or pneumonectomy. Partial lobectomy is not recommended because of the risk of incomplete resection, but may be appropriate occasionally in patients with small tumours and poor lung function. The operation should include regional lymph node sampling.

Post-operative management

Patients should be nursed in an intensive care or high-dependency unit. Excellent pain control, oxygen therapy and regular chest physiotherapy is essential.

Results of lung resection

Overall 5-year survival for patients undergoing resection may be as high as 40%, approaching 70% in cases without nodal involvement (N0). When mediastinal nodes are involved (N2) only 15% of patients will survive five years.

Multidisciplinary team meetings (MDT)

The MDT discussion of each case is key to the optimal management of lung cancer, with input from radiologists and pathologists, as well as the chest physician, thoracic surgeon, clinical and medical oncologists, clinical nurse specialists, and specialist palliative care team.

Non-surgical treatment for NSLC

Chemotherapy

NSCLC is not as sensitive to chemotherapy as SCLC. However regimens with a platinum agent in combination with newer chemotherapy agents have shown improved success in recent years. Chemotherapy has a developing role prior to surgery to downstage tumours and also as adjuvant therapy for stage I–II.

In advanced disease, chemotherapy offers modest survival benefit, but improved symptom relief and quality of life in more than 50% of people:
• Cough, haemoptysis, and pain are relieved in 70%.
• Anorexia in 40%.
• Dyspnoea in 30%.

Table 35.2 5-year survival after surgery for NSCLC by stage

Stage	5-year survival
I	60–80%
II	25–40%
IIIa	10–30%
IIIb and IV	<5%

There is little evidence to justify more than 4 cycles of chemotherapy. Patients with poor performance status 2 or worse, (📖 Performance status) may be treated with single agent chemotherapy such as gemcitabine or vinorelbine. New therapies e.g. monoclonal antibodies are currently showing some promise in this setting.

Radiotherapy

External beam radiotherapy is used as the local treatment for thoracic disease in the majority of NSCLC patients. Radical radiotherapy can be offered to selected stage I–II patients who are unfit for surgery and can produce a cure in some of this group.

- The UK recommended approach is continuous hyper fractionated radiotherapy (CHART): 54 Gy in 36 fractions over 12 days (this is not yet offered in all centres).
- Difficulties of this treatment include inconvenience for patients and staff and increased acute toxicity.

For many patients with advanced NSCLC, palliative radiotherapy is a key component in alleviating symptoms from thoracic disease, in particular:

- Haemoptysis.
- Chest pain.
- Cough.
- Large airway obstruction or stridor.
- Superior vena cava obstruction (📖 SVCO).
- It also produces useful palliation for many metastatic sites including lymph nodes, bone, brain, and soft tissue (📖 Radiotherapy).

Chemo irradiation

There is preliminary evidence that concurrent radiotherapy and chemotherapy may be more effective than sequential radiotherapy, but toxicity, in particular oesophagitis remains a major problem. Should be offered to those with Stage III NSCLC.

Management of small cell lung cancer (SCLC)

SCLC accounts for 15–20% of all lung cancers. The staging and management of SCLC is quite distinct from NSCLC because:
- SCLC demonstrates rapid growth and early dissemination with more than 90% having systemic disease at presentation.
- Chemotherapy is the key primary treatment and has an important impact on survival.

Staging and prognostic factors
A two-stage system applies:

Limited-stage disease
The tumour is confined to one hemithorax and regional lymph node, and can be covered by tolerable radiotherapy fields.

Extensive-stage disease
The disease is beyond the bounds stated for limited disease.

Treatment
Surgery
In general, surgical resection is not recommended for SCLC. If SCLC is treated by primary surgery, the systemic relapse rate is high, and adjuvant chemotherapy is recommended.

Chemotherapy for SCLC
Without treatment, median survival is:
- 6 weeks for patients with extensive disease.
- 3 months for those with limited disease.

Combination chemotherapy leads to a response in the majority, with improved survival times, and is now the standard primary treatment for both stages of the disease (see Table 35.3).

Principles of treatment
4–6 courses of etoposide plus cisplatin or carboplatin has been established as the best first-line treatment.

The response rate is around 80% of all patients. Complete responses in:
- 30–40% patients with limited stage disease.
- 10–20% with extensive disease.

Almost all patients relapse after chemotherapy only. There is a high risk of CNS relapse after chemotherapy, and this can be reduced by prophylactic cranial irradiation. This is given at the end of chemotherapy in an effort to minimize CNS toxicity.

Note: chemotherapy can be considered for elderly patients and those with poor performance status (2–3) (📖 Performance status). Careful selection is required and mortality rates may be high during chemotherapy treatment.

Second-line chemotherapy
SCLC can remain chemo-sensitive at relapse after primary chemotherapy. If the patient is fit enough 2nd-line regimens can be considered.

Radiotherapy
SCLC is a highly radiosensitive disease
- For those with limited stage disease, thoracic irradiation in addition to chemotherapy can improve survival. Dose: 40–50gy in 15–25 fractions.
- Concurrent radiotherapy appears to be most effective, but toxicity, especially severe oesophagitis, may prevent its use.
- Prophylactic cranial radiation reduces the risk of brain metastases.
- Palliative radiotherapy is an effective treatment in patients relapsing after, resistant to, unfit for, or refusing chemotherapy.

Table 35.3 Outcome of chemotherapy for SCLC

Stage of disease	Median survival (months)	1-year survival	3-year survival
Limited	18–24	50–70%	10–20%
Extensive	8–10	20%	
Relapsed[*]	6		

[*]Limited to patients who remain fit to receive chemotherapy for relapsed disease

Mesothelioma

Malignant pleural mesothelioma (MPM) is an aggressive tumour arising from the serosal lining of the chest. It often leads to encasement of the lung by a solid tumour and has a poor survival rate.

Epidemiology

- Rare, around 2200 cases each year in the UK.
- The peak age is 60–70 years.
- Male: female ratio is 5:1.

Aetiology

- Most mesothelioma is caused by asbestos exposure. All types of asbestos fibre are implicated.
- 90% have an occupational history of exposure e.g. builders and shipyard workers have a high risk.
- Clinical presentation is often 30–40 years later.

Clinical presentation

Late presentation is common. Classic symptoms are:
- Non-pleuritic chest pain.
- Dyspnoea.
- Systemic symptoms of fatigue, weight loss, sweating, and fever.

Spread

- Peritoneal involvement, through direct spread.
- Advanced spread to other organs such as the liver.

Investigations

- CXR: pleural effusion/thickening.
- CT/MRI scan: extent of pleural mass and effusion, and encasement of lung.
- Histological diagnosis should be obtained in the majority of cases, using the least invasive technique.
  - Aspiration cytology (30% positive).
  - Thoracoscopy and biopsy (80% positive).

Note: there is a high incidence of false negative biopsies, leading to the need to repeat it. There is a risk of seeding the tumour along biopsy tracts.

Staging

The TNM classification is not commonly used. Staging is vital if patients are considered for surgery. The Brigham staging system provides an alternative straightforward method, based on key disease characteristics, that stratifies survival.

Treatment

Without treatment, the average patient with MPM survives less than one year from the time of diagnosis.

Surgery
For the vast majority of patients radical surgical resection is not an option, with high mortality reported. Palliative pleurectomy/decortication (removal of the pleura without removing the whole lung) can provide excellent relief from effusions and pain from the tumour.

Radiotherapy
Prophylactic irradiation of chest drain, biopsy and wound sites prevents the development of chest wall tumours. Short course palliative radiotherapy can be used for painful chest disease/masses.

Chemotherapy
The role of chemotherapy is uncertain. Platinum regimens have shown some objective response, with palliative benefit. Recent promising results are reported with the anti-folate pemetrexed.

Palliative care
Symptom control is often difficult, in particular pain and dyspnoea; the early involvement of specialist palliative care services may be beneficial.

Compensation and notification

Patients may be entitled to claim compensation in two ways:
- A claim for Industrial Injuries Disablement Benefit from the Department of Social Security (via the Benefits Agency)
- A Common Law claim for damages from the firm/firms where exposure to asbestos occurred

All deaths of patients with mesothelioma must be notified to the coroner (procurator fiscal in Scotland) unless it is clearly not industry related. It is important that patients and their family are aware of their right to pursue a compensation claim.

Nursing management issues

The poor prognosis of all types of lung cancer can make nursing these patients extremely challenging. The approach is often for palliative support from diagnosis. Co-morbidity due to smoking may prevent access to effective surgical or pharmacological treatments. Patients and their families often have little time to come to terms with the diagnosis before facing the reality of dying from their disease. Multidisciplinary team involvement, including surgeons, oncologists, site-specific CNS, palliative care specialists, and social workers is crucial to the effective management of these patients.

Treatment issues

Lung cancer treatment raises a number of important nursing support issues. Patients will require high levels of support in making decisions about different treatment options. The success rates of many of these treatments are low. The balance between toxicity and potential benefit means that choices are not straightforward. The lung cancer CNS is a very useful support at this time.

Particular treatment issues include:

Surgery
- Fear due to high surgical mortality and morbidity rates.
- Respiratory problems: breathlessness, pneumonia, acute respiratory distress syndrome (ARDS).
- Cardiac arrhythmias and MI.
- Chronic post-thoracotomy pain can last for many months.
- Longer-term patients may need to make lifestyle changes and cope with reduced activity.

Thoracic radiotherapy: fatigue, oesophagitis, pneumonitis.

Chemotherapy: has a wide range of side effects including fatigue, risk of infection, mucositis, nausea, and vomiting (for management of each individual side effect ☐ Symptom management).

Psychosocial issues

- The poor prognosis of lung cancer means that patients and families often have little time to come to terms with the diagnosis. Because of its link with smoking, patients and their families can also have feelings of guilt and anger. These require skilled and sensitive nursing support.
- The highest incidence of lung cancer is in people from lower social classes, and there can be difficult social and financial support issues to be resolved. A specialist cancer or palliative care social worker can be an invaluable support in these circumstances.
- Pain and breathlessness often cause panic and anxiety. Patients may need to use anxiolytics. Nurses can support patients to develop effective relaxation techniques (☐ Anxiety management).
- Cerebral metastases can lead to altered behaviour and personality, as well as difficulties with communication. This can be extremely distressing for patients and relatives (☐ Acute confusional states).

Breathlessness

This is common in all lung cancers. It can be particularly severe in meso-thelioma due to pleural involvement limiting lung capacity. Treatments such as chemotherapy and radiotherapy may be effective in SCLC but are less likely to work for mesothelioma or NSCLC (☐ Breathlessness).

Pain

Many lung cancer patients present with chest pain. This can be a major problem. Specific pain issues include:
* Pleuritic pain: which often responds well to NSAIDS.
* Bone pain: from bone metastases.
* Nerve pains: caused by mesothelioma and also Pancoast's tumour—a tumour high in the lung apex causing classic shoulder pain radiating down ulnar nerve distribution (☐ Pain management).

Cough

This often exacerbates pain and breathlessness and causes sleeplessness, which can be extremely debilitating. Codeine linctus or morphine may be helpful (☐ Breathlessness).

Superior vena cava obstruction (SVCO)

Due to regional tumour spread can be extremely frightening, with severe breathlessness and a feeling of drowning. It is also potentially life-threatening (☐ SVCO).

Haemoptysis

This can be distressing, and is often a symptom that makes patients see their GP prior to diagnosis. Palliative radiotherapy and tranexamic acid can both be helpful. There is also a real, though rare, potential risk of catastrophic bleed (☐ Bleeding).

Further reading

Souhami R L and Tobias J S (2005). Tumours of the lung and mediastinum. In *Cancer and Its Management*. 5th edn. pp.195–215 Oxford: Blackwell.

Knop C S (2005). Lung Cancer. In Yarbro C.H., Frogge M.H., Goodman M. (eds) *Cancer Nursing, Principles and practice*. 6th edn. Massachusetts: Jones and Bartlett.

Muers M, Macbeth F, Wells F, and Miles A, (eds), (2001). *The effective management of lung cancer*. London: Aesculpapius Press.

National Institute for Clinical Excellence (2005) *Lung cancer: The diagnosis and treatment of lung cancer*. Clinical Guideline 24. London: NICE.

Chest, **123**(1), Supplement January 2003. *Diagnosis and Management of Lung Cancer. ACCP Evidence-based Guidelines*. Complete volume of articles focusing on lung cancer management.

Useful website

☐ Oncology Nursing Society: Lung Cancer Clinical resource Area: www.ons.org/clinical/lung/index.shtml Excellent resource with access to evidence based guidelines on treatment and care.

Skin cancer

Malignant melanoma

Epidemiology

- Malignant melanomas arise from melanocytes, mainly found in the basal layer of skin. These cells produce melanin and are responsible for the tanning response after exposure to ultraviolet (UV) radiation.
- A few melanocytes exist elsewhere in the body—this explains the rare melanomas that can occur elsewhere, e.g. intracocular, oesophageal.
- Incidence rates are rising faster than for any other cancer worldwide.

Risk factors

- Sunlight is the highest risk factor, in particular excess exposure in early life.
- Caucasians have the highest risk (>1:80).
- There is a genetic risk. Approximately 10% of people affected will have a strong family history of melanoma.
- Benign pigmented moles.

Screening and prevention

(📖 Cancer screening and prevention)

Clinical presentation

- Alteration in a pre-existing pigmented mole on the skin: irregular pigmentation, irregular border or new asymmetry of a lesion ± oozing, crusting, itching, or bleeding.
- A new pigmented lesion—particularly relevant if ≥40 years.
- Less commonly, signs of metastatic disease.

Diagnosis

- Excision biopsy—complete excision with normal skin margins is optimal.
- CXR and serum biochemistry.
- Further imaging e.g. CT or MRI scan of the chest or abdomen guided by symptoms of metastatic spread, or thickness of melanoma.

Prognostic indicators

- Tumour thickness (Breslow depth), any invasion of dermal blood vessels, lymphatics, and the rate of cell division are key factors.
- Other factors:
  - Women seem to have better survival rates due to hormonal factors.
  - Head, neck, and trunk melanomas tend to fare worse than those on the extremities.

Surgical treatment

Surgery at the primary site

Complete excision of the lesion—the margin of excision varies according to the thickness of the tumour

- From in-situ disease only, 0.5cm to ≥4mm = 3cm margin.
- Excision must be adequate laterally and in depth.
- Sites such as foot sole, require tailored surgical techniques.
- A minority may require either a flap or a graft to achieve closure.

Surgery for the regional lymph nodes
This is indicated when there is clinical evidence of lymph node involvement, increasing cure and reducing risk of fungation. Complications include infection and seroma formation plus lymphoedema longer-term.

Lymph node dissection: when the spread is unknown this is controversial. The main benefit is for accurate staging, provided this will affect options for subsequent adjuvant therapy.

Sentinel lymph node biopsy: is being trialled in an attempt to reduce associated morbidity of lymph node dissection.

Prognosis and risk of relapse
In the early stage of the disease surgery is curative in 70–90% of cases. Relapse rates rapidly increase as the disease progresses. Median survival with metastatic disease is typically <9 months.

Chemotherapy, immunotherapy, and radiotherapy
Adjuvant therapy
Clinical trials with a high dose of intravenous interferon–α (HDI) are ongoing. The effect on overall survival is unknown.

Loco-regionally advanced disease
- If there is no evidence of disseminated disease, further resection should be considered.
- Alternative approaches include 'regional' chemotherapy treatment via hyperthermic isolated limb perfusion. This is only offered in specialist centres and provides regional effect with limited systemic side effects:

Treatment of metastatic disease
There is no curative treatment for stage IV disease. The aim is to palliate symptoms and maximize quality of life.

Surgery
Tumour debulking may occasionally be appropriate.

Chemotherapy and biotherapy
These offer limited benefit. Response rates of around 20% with median duration of 4 months are typical. Options include:
- Dacarbazine (DTIC), temozolomide.
- Self administerd interferon– α (IFN–α).
- High dose interleukin-2 (IL-2) is also being trialled.
- The lack of effective treatments means that entry into a phase I trial remains a reasonable option for some patients in this group.

Radiotherapy
- Can be used for pain from bone metastases.
- Cerebral metastases are relatively common. Cranial irradiation can be considered if symptomatic.

Non-melanoma skin cancer

The two main forms are squamous cell carcinoma (SCC) and basal cell carcinoma (BCC). Malignant skin lesions may also represent metastases e.g. from breast, lung, or GI primaries.

Epidemiology and aetiology

- These are the commonest malignancies in western populations.
- Main risk factors for development include:
  - Excess UV radiation exposure—main environmental cause.
  - Easily burned, fair-skinned individuals.
  - Outdoor work, outdoor recreational activities.
  - Psoralen ultraviolet A treatment (PUVA).
  - Immuno-suppression e.g. post organ-transplant.

Presentation

BCC—75% of non-melanoma skin cancers:

- Lesions arise on sun-exposed areas, normally hair-bearing skin.
- Slow-growing, pink papule with telangiectasia.
- Typically indolent, can be locally invasive, metastases are rare (0.1%).

SCC—20% of non-melanoma skin cancers:

- Arise on sun-exposed sites or at sites of chronic inflammation.
- Rapidly growing, red papule, or non-healing skin lesion.
- Ulceration and bleeding may occur.
- 5–10% metastasize, initially to regional lymph nodes—poor prognosis for the disseminated disease.

Management

- **Surgical excision**: allows assessment of histological features and adequacy of resection margin. ≥90% cure for primary disease.
- **Cryotherapy** (using cold) or **electro surgery** (using heat). Can be used for in-situ disease or small, low-risk lesions. The disadvantage of these techniques is that they prevent confirmation of clear margins.
- **Radiotherapy:** may be useful for poor surgical candidates, such as frail or elderly people, or where surgical excision is difficult e.g. eyelids, nose, and lips, and the cosmetic result is likely to be superior to surgery.
- **Chemotherapy:** imiquimod (immunotherapy) or topical 5-FU can be used for low-risk BCCs. Otherwise not as successful as other therapies.
- **Ongoing surveillance:** most recurrences will occur within the first 5 years.
  - Patients are also at risk of developing other non-melanoma skin malignancies.
  - Advise patients with a non-melanoma skin cancer about the importance of sun avoidance to minimize future risk.

Further reading

ional Institute for Clinical Excellence (2006). *Guidance on Cancer Services-Improving utcomes for People with Skin Tumours including Melanoma: The Manual.* London: NICE.
mi R L, and Tobias J S (2005). *Cancer and Its Management.* 5th edn. Skin Cancer, pp.369–85.
rd: Blackwell.

Section 7

Symptom management

Assessment

Introduction

Assessment is one of the most complex nursing activities. It involves interpersonal and communication skills, and decision-making skills.

Assessment has a number of purposes. It aims to:
- Establish a working relationship with the patient.
- Understand the patient's preferences and priorities.
- Identify their needs and match them with the services available.
- Record the patient's needs for the benefit of teamwork.
- Enable effective care planning and symptom management to take place.
- Assess risk.

Assessment tools can be used, but assessment is also a matter of clinical judgement. Although it is one of the most common activities in nursing, assessment is not always undertaken in a systematic or effective way.

The purpose of assessment can be related to *diagnosis* of specific conditions, in order to ensure that the necessary treatment is given. However, assessment is often focused on the assessment of *needs*, or health-related goals (📖 Quality of life). This enables needs to be matched with the appropriate care and services.

It is important to be aware that the patient and the nurse may view their needs differently. The subjective experience of a problem is not the same as the assessment of a need for care. For example, a patient may experience pain, but not want to accept the pain relief that is being offered.

The following factors will influence an assessment:
- The purpose of assessment.
- The skills of the nurse.
- The time and facilities available.
- The condition of the patient and their preferences.

Context of assessment

An assessment is influenced by the context in which it takes place:

The patient's context

It is very important to understand the patient's context—their current life circumstances, concerns, and priorities. Without this, key elements of the patient's experience may be missed or misunderstood by the nurse. For example, a nurse may assess the patient's main need as symptom relief, when their most pressing concern may be their relationship with their family. It is important to always identify the patient's key concerns, as part of the assessment process. There are assessment tools that can be used to structure the process of identifying concerns (📖 Assessment tools).

The family

Involving the family in the assessment process ensures a common understanding about problems, and information and decision-making can be shared. At times, however, a patient may feel more comfortable being seen on their own, so that they can be open about how they feel, without worrying about the reaction of family members. It is good practice to ask the patient if they give their permission for family members or significant others to be present.

Purpose of assessment

Assessment is undertaken at the start of a process of care, but it is an ongoing activity. Assessment should be interactive, a negotiation and information exchange between the nurse and patient, an opportunity for both to get to know each other and identify personal and health care priorities. It is important that assessment is a deliberate process. Information gathered incidentally may not be complete. It is important to share information and focus on concerns that are raised by patients in this way.

Amount of time available

Detailed assessment cannot always be undertaken at busy times. If time is limited, focus on the key information that you need to know. Be clear with the patient what you need to know and how much time you have, and gain their consent for this.

Space and privacy

The ideal context for assessment is one where the patient is comfortable and privacy is assured, for example in a room that is separate from other people. If it is not possible to find a room, make the context as private as possible, ensuring the patient's confidentiality is respected. In hospital, this could involve drawing curtains around a bed and talking quietly.

Timing of assessment

Assessment is an ongoing process, and should take place regularly across the patient's journey. Key points for assessment have been identified in the NICE Guidance on Supportive and Palliative Care for Adults with Cancer[1].

- Diagnosis.
- Prior to and during treatment.
- End of treatment—often a very difficult time when support is less available.
- Recurrence.
- Entering the terminal phase of illness.

Whilst it is important to bear in mind that key stages on the patient's journey may be significant, it is also essential to be aware of the wider personal context of the patient's life when undertaking an assessment. (📖 The personal experience of cancer—calendars).

---

1 National Institute for Clinical Evidence (2004) *Supportive and Palliative Care for Adults with Cancer.* London: NICE. http://www.nice.org.uk/

Process of assessment

The most important aspect of the assessment process for the nurse is to listen. Each patient (and carer) will have their own understanding of events (their story), their own priorities, and expectations. Assessment is an opportunity for them to tell the nurse what these are. This must be balanced with the clinical imperatives that drive care and treatment. The process of each assessment will vary according to circumstances, but the following are offered as guidelines:

• Be clear about why the assessment is being done.
• Establish mutual expectations of the purpose of the assessment, i.e. what is the patient's understanding of the purpose and likely outcome of the assessment?
• Introduce yourself and explain the reason for the assessment, how long it will take and what it will involve.
• Ask specific questions about the things you need to know.
• Give the patient the opportunity to respond to your questions in their own terms.
• Check that your questions are understood.
• Discuss the available care and treatment options, and what actions you or your team will take to deal with any problems.
• Care planning should be done collaboratively with the patient and their family as far as this is possible.
• Does the patient (or their family) have any questions?
• Combine data from different sources—clinical notes, other informants, colleagues.
• Ensure that the assessment and its outcome are documented in a way that is accessible to colleagues.

Self-awareness and assessment

Assessment can be influenced by the perceptions or the attitudes of the nurse. For this reason, it is important to develop self-awareness:
• Note your own responses to the patient.
• Do not make assumptions about the patient on the basis of their age, gender, diagnosis, or other personal characteristics.
• Develop sensitivity to your reaction to the needs of individuals from minority groups (e.g. ethnic minority, sexual orientation, socio-economic status).

Reflection points

• Can you recall an occasion on which you felt your attitudes or feelings towards a patient made the assessment more difficult for you or the patient?
• Is there anything that you would do differently if this happened again?

Dimensions of assessment and key questions to ask

Many wards or units have a proforma for assessment, which guides the questions asked. A holistic assessment will cover the different dimensions of a patient's experience of illness, treatment, and life.

Key questions are offered here to act as prompts, to be followed up with more specific questions. These are given in no specific order; in practice the way questions are asked will depend the context.

- Start with an open question:
    - *Can you tell me how you are feeling?*
- Psychological well-being.
    - *How are you feeling in yourself?*
    - *How would you describe your mood during the last few days?*
- Social.
    - *How are you getting on with family and friends?*
    - *Do you feel you are getting enough support?*
- Spiritual well-being.
    - *How do you feel about life at the moment?*
    - *How do you feel about your future?*
- Disease and symptoms.
    - *Do you have any physical problems that are bothering you?*
    - *Are you having any problems as a result of the illness or treatment?*
- Physical functioning.
    - *Are you concerned about any limitations to your activities?*
- Cognitive function.
    - *Are you having any problems with your concentration or memory?*
- Occupational and financial.
    - *Are you able to work?*
    - *Do you have any financial problems or concerns?*

The assessment of pain and sexual problems are dealt with in other sections of the book (☐ Pain management; Sexual health and cancer).

Assessment tools

Assessment tools are a means of ensuring consistency across assessments, or across different team members. They also serve as a guide or checklist, so that the nurse enquires about specific problems or symptoms. These tools will only be used if they are seen to have value within clinical practice, and their use varies considerably. Some assessment tools rely on patient self-assessment.

Examples of assessment tools used in cancer care

Cancer Care Monitor (CCM)[1]
Screening and assessment tool for symptoms and QOL in cancer patients.

Cancer Rehabilitation Evaluation System (CARES)[2]
Measure of rehabilitation needs and QOL.

Concerns checklist[3]
Aid to eliciting primary concerns of people with cancer.

Problems checklist[4]
Measure of the frequency and severity of psychosocial problems in cancer.

For a detailed review of these and other cancer-related assessment tools see Richardson et al[5].

1 Fortner B, Okon T, Schwartzberg L, Tauer K, Houts A C (2003). The Cancer Care Monitor: psychometric content evaluation and pilot testing of a computer administered system for symptom screening and quality of life in adult cancer patients. *Journal of Pain and Symptom Management*, **26**(6), 1077–92.
2 Ganz P A, Schag C A, Lee J J, Sim M S (1992). The CARES: a generic measure of health-related quality of life for patients with cancer. *Quality of Life Research*, **1**, 19–29.
3 Harrison J, Maguire P, Ibbotson T, Macleod R (1994). Concerns, confiding and psychiatric disorder in newly diagnosed cancer patients: a descriptive study. *Psycho-oncology*, **3**, 173–9
4 Bonevski B, Sanson-Fisher R, Girgis A, Burton L, Cook P, Boyes A (2000). Evaluation of an instrument to assess the needs of patients with cancer. *Cancer*, **88**, 217–25.
5 Richardson A, Sitzia J, Brown V, Medina J, Richardson A. (2005). *Patient's Needs Assessment Tools in Cancer Care: Principles and Practice*, London: King's College London.

Quality of life (QoL)

- Quality of life (QoL) is a key element of assessment. It is a complex, multifactoral concept in the context of cancer, and involves the individual's appraisal of their position in life, relative to their expectations.
- QoL can involve both positive and negative appraisals: there can be good features of life, like a sense of well-being, and bad effects of the illness, like symptoms, and these can occur together.
- QoL is subjective: only an individual can judge what their QoL is, but objective measures can also be used, for example, to assess levels of physical functioning.
- QoL is dynamic, and ideas about what it means have changed over time, for example, from treatment outcome to subjective feeling of well-being.

Concepts related to QoL

The following are terms you will come across in the literature on QoL:

Need: a need is a complex concept that can be viewed differently from the patient's or the professional's point of view, for example, a patient may perceive a need to be well, whilst a nurse may perceive a patient's need for care. It can have the following meanings:
- A health-related goal, e.g. to be free of a distressing symptom
- A measurable deficiency from a health-related goal
- A means of achieving a health-related goal, e.g. a treatment

Outcome: the achievement or failure to achieve defined health-related goals.

Health-related quality of life: quality of life conceptualized as involving a complex range of factors, including, for example, subjective feelings of social and psychological well-being.

Disease-related quality of life: quality of life relating primarily to the effects of illness and treatment.

Health status: can mean either:
- Absence of illness.
- Presence of physical, psychological, social, and spiritual well-being.

Functional status: ability to perform usual activities or roles within limitations imposed by illness.

Symptom distress: the degree of physical or mental distress or suffering experienced from a symptom.

Dimensions of QoL

QoL is multidimensional, it affects different aspects of the person's life. Dimensions of QoL include:

- *Physical well-being:* this includes features such as fatigue, pain, other symptoms and side effects of treatment.
- *Functional well-being:* this refers to the activities of living, including basic functions of eating, sleeping, washing, and also activities that support occupation and relationships.
- *Emotional well-being:* emotional reactions to cancer can be both positive and negative. Emotional well-being can be enhanced by the support of family and friends, or patients may experience distress or low mood.
- *Social well-being:* this is complex, and can include social support, family relationships, intimacy and sexuality.
- *Spiritual well-being:* this includes religion and cultural aspects of life, as well as the personal sense of meaning and purpose in life, and attitudes to death and dying.

There is considerable overlap between these dimensions, and improvement or decline in one area may or may not affect the others. For example, fatigue may not stop a person going out with friends, but it may be bad enough to reduce their enjoyment.

QoL measurement has a number of uses in health care, and this can lead to confusion. Within the context of cancer nursing, its meaning is primarily concerned with the assessment of needs and care planning, but it can also be used for:

- Research and clinical trials.
- Audit.
- Treatment planning and evaluation of treatment outcomes.

QoL measurement tools should be approached with caution for this reason. Measures designed for research purposes may not be suitable for care planning[1].

1 Bowling A (2005) *Measuring Health. A Review of Quality of Life Measurement Scales.* (3rd ed) Maidenhead: Open University Press.

QoL in practice

In day-to-day cancer nursing practice, QoL provides a means of focusing on the priorities of the patient and their family. QoL can be viewed as a global measure of how the patient feels about their life at that point. This can provide the patient with a means of monitoring their progress, in their own terms, and act as a balance to care or treatment outcomes. The simplest way to establish this is to ask the patient to rate their QoL today on a scale of 1–10.

Other strategies that you can use to monitor and enhance QoL are:
- Help patients and their family to identify what makes their QoL better or worse by reflecting on their progress.
- Encourage patients to participate in activities that improve their QoL.
- Monitor the effects of cancer treatments on the patient and their families' QoL.
- Address the negative impact of cancer treatments on QoL.
- Evaluate symptoms within the framework of QoL.
- Intervene to provide adequate symptom management.

Further reading

Cella, D F (1994). Quality of Life: concepts and definition, *Journal of Pain and Symptom Management*, **9**(3), 186–192.

Costain Schou, K Hewison J (1999). *Experiencing Cancer*, Buckingham: Open University Press.

King C R, Haberman M, Berry D L, *et al.* (1997). Quality of life and the cancer experience: the state-of-the-knowledge. *Oncology Nursing Forum* **24**(1), 27–41.

Bone marrow suppression

Bone marrow function

The bone marrow makes all of the cellular elements of the blood. These are:

- Red blood cells—carry oxygen around the body.
- White blood cells—fight infection.
- Platelets—assist in blood clotting.

The bone marrow is an extremely active organ, producing over a million red blood cells per second. It is also very adaptive, being able to selectively increase production of cells in response to depletion in the peripheral blood.

Active blood-forming (haemopoietic) bone marrow is not found in every bone in an adult. It is concentrated in the axial skeleton—the pelvis, vertebrae, ribs, shoulder girdle, and skull.

Bone marrow suppression results in a reduced number of blood cells in the circulation. This can produce a number of different problems depending on which cell type is mainly affected (see Table 38.1 below). Frequently, patients display features caused by a reduction in more than one type of blood cell; when all three cell types are low, they are said to have pancytopenia.

Table 38.1 Impact of bone marrow suppression

Condition	Definition	Symptoms	Other complications
Anaemia	Low red blood cell count. (Hb level <13.5g/dl for men, <11.5g/dl for women)	Fatigue, breathlessness, headache, palpitations, angina. (Cancer patients rarely symptomatic below 10g/dL).	Dependence on blood transfusions to correct anaemia–results in iron overload, which can be difficult to treat. Exacerbation of cardiac conditions, e.g. CHF
Neutropaenia	Low neutrophil count (<1 x 10^9/L)	Bacterial or fungal infections: fever, rigors, local signs (cough, chest pain, diarrhoea, pain on micturition, pain around central venous line). May be no specific signs	Overwhelming sepsis Mouth ulceration. Note: pus and normal inflammatory processes may not be present
Thrombocy topaenia	Low platelet count (high risk of bleeding when count below 10 x 10^9/L)	Petechial rash, nose bleeds, gum bleeds, haematuria, heavy menstruation, GI bleeds, retinal bleed, intracranial bleed (rare)	Dependence on platelet transfusions to correct thrombocytopaenia may result in formation of antibodies which makes further transfusions less effective

Anaemia

Anaemia is defined as a reduction in the oxygen carrying capacity of the blood. It occurs when the haemoglobin (Hb) concentration falls <13.5 g/L in a man and <11.5g/L in a woman.

Causes

Anaemia in cancer patients has a number of causes:
• Bone marrow suppression due to chemotherapy, radiotherapy, or infiltration by malignancy.
• Chronic blood loss.
• Iron deficiency.
• Anaemia of chronic disease—caused by persistent inflammation.
• Haemolysis—premature destruction of red blood cells.

Consequences

Common symptoms include:
• Fatigue (📖 Fatigue).
• Shortness of breath on exertion.
• Headache.
• Palpitations.
• Angina.

Severe anaemia can cause heart failure, resulting in peripheral oedema and breathlessness on lying flat.

Treatment

Assessment

It is useful to carry out a pre cancer-treatment risk assessment for anaemia
• Full blood count, anaemia-related symptoms, e.g. cardiac, pulmonary.
• Risk factors; advanced age, low starting Hb, lung, gynaecological, haematological malignancy, prior myelo-suppressive therapy.

Treatment of underlying cause

• Correct underlying cause if possible; e.g. iron, folate, vitamin B12 supplementation.
• Treatment of haemolytic causes.
• Prevention or stopping chronic/acute blood loss.

Blood product support

For correction of anaemia via blood transfusions and use of erythropoiesis stimulating proteins, see the section: Blood product support.

Neutropaenia

A normal neutrophil count for an adult is 2.5–7.5 x 10^9/L. Neutropaenia can be defined as any neutrophil count less than the lower limit. In practice it generally does not cause great concern until it has fallen to <1.0 x 10^9/L, and infections remain uncommon until the count is <0.5 x 10^9/L.

Causes

There are many causes of neutropaenia; in a cancer patient the main ones are related to bone marrow suppression. These include:

- Chemotherapy.
- Radiotherapy.
- Infiltration of bone marrow by cancer cells, most commonly:
  - Haematological cancers—leukaemia, myeloma, lymphoma.
  - Prostate cancer.
  - Breast cancer.
  - Lung cancer.
  - Thyroid cancer.
  - Renal cell carcinoma.

Infection risks

Neutropaenia is expected and reversible when caused by chemotherapy or radiotherapy. Most infections come from the patient themselves, rather than from relatives or friends with whom they come into contact whilst neutropaenic. Infections are common in neutropaenic patients, largely because mucosal barriers such as those lining the GI tract are broken down. This allows bacteria, which are normally resident there, to enter the bloodstream (bacterial translocation). Damage to skin integrity through treatment, or siting of a central venous line is another major source of bacterial translocation.

Those most vulnerable to serious infection are patients with haematological malignancy, neutropaenia >7 days, age >60, central venous catheters and mucositis.

Bone marrow infiltration

- Neutropaenia caused by bone marrow infiltration is often progressive, and is only reversible if the underlying cancer is effectively treated.
- Death often occurs from an overwhelming infection such as pneumonia or a line infection.

Prevention of infection in the neutropaenic patient

A number of measures are taken to reduce infection in the neutropaenic patient, although evidence for the effectiveness of many of them is limited.

Essential practices are:

- Scrupulous hand washing by the patient and those with whom they come into contact, e.g. health professionals, family, and friends (see box).
- Meticulous care of indwelling venous catheters, with scrupulous aseptic/non-touch technique when accessing these.

Hand hygiene

- The only sure way to reduce infection is scrupulous hand hygiene. Studies conclusively support reduced infection rates in many hospital settings due to the high level of hand hygiene.
- Use of alcohol gel rubs has been effective in reducing hand microbial colonization and infection rates.
- Easy access to hand cleansing equipment is an essential part of ensuring a high level of adherence to hygiene. Many hospitals have alcohol gel rubs available at the entry to wards and patient rooms, and staff may carry small bottles clipped onto their uniform.
- Alcohol gels strip away the outer layer of oil on the skin, destroying any transient microorganisms present. They combine a high level of immediate antimicrobial effect with ease of use. However, on visibly soiled hands frictional rubbing with soap and water is still the recommended approach.

Hand hygiene guidelines

- When hands are visibly dirty or contaminated they should be washed with soap and water.
- Decontaminate hands with an alcohol rub:
  - Before and after having **any** direct contact with a patient.
  - After contact with inanimate objects in the immediate vicinity of the patient.
  - Before and after manipulating any invasive devices.
  - After removing gloves.

If an alcohol rub is not available, wash hands with an antimicrobial soap and water.

Note: alcohol is less effective than soap and water against *Clostridium difficile* toxin.

Other commonly used practices include:
- Isolation: many neutropaenic patients are put in a side room when on a ward. Some units restrict the number of visitors. In some bone marrow transplant settings, protective laminar airflow, and/or high efficiency particulate air (HEPA) filter environments are used to nurse patients.

Note: there is limited evidence to suggest that different isolation procedures impact on patient long-term survival.
- Avoidance of crowded places and individuals who obviously have an infection, such as a cold.
- Neutropaenic diet—the rationale is to minimize the intake of bacteria in food. This includes avoiding unpasteurized milk products, blue cheeses, uncooked vegetables, salads, uncooked herbs and spices, raw nuts, raw or undercooked meat and fish.

- Good dental hygiene—including brushing with a soft toothbrush (📖 Mucositis).
- Prophylactic antibiotics e.g. oral ciprofloxacin: recent evidence suggests that this reduces the incidence of infections, but many units do not routinely prescribe antibiotics due to concerns that regular use may lead to the emergence of resistant organisms.
- G-CSF injections: these have been shown to reduce the neutropaenic period in patients treated with high-dose chemotherapy regimens, to reduce the incidence of infections in these patients and to allow full dose and schedule of drugs to be given in a number of standard chemotherapy regimens[1] (📖 Biological therapy).

Patient education

Many patients will spend a period of time at home when they may be neutropaenic and at risk of infection. It is essential to educate the patient and their family about why they are at risk of infection, how they might get an infection, and measures to try and prevent infection (see above).

- Patients should know about potential signs and symptoms of an infection, the potential dangers, and the need to respond quickly to any such signs, regardless of the time of day or night.
- Although a temperature is the most common and important sign of infection in the neutropaenic patient, other symptoms or feeling unwell, even without a temperature, should be reported.
- The patient and their family should be supplied with clear instructions on what to do and who to contact if they develop new or worsening symptoms, cough, sweats, feeling cold, diarrhoea, fever, or feel unwell.
- Give patients clear instructions on how to take their temperature and guidance on how frequently they should do this. The most important time to take their temperature is when they feel unwell.

Why patient education is crucial

Every year patients die because they do not seek advice quickly enough. Contact telephone numbers should be included in any written information, and on a card that can be carried easily.

Note: it must always be remembered that some patients may be septic without having a temperature. Ensure that patients know the temperature masking effects of paracetamol and aspirin, which can give false reassurance and potentially delay seeking advice or admission to hospital.

1 Dolan S, Crombez P, Munoz M (2005). Neutropenia management with granulocyte colony stimulating factors: From guidelines to nursing practice protocols. *European Journal of Oncology Nursing*, **9**, s14–23.

Treatment of febrile neutropaenia and sepsis/septic shock

Fever of >38°C in a neutropaenic patient is a medical emergency

The cut-off of 38°C is rather arbitrary and **any symptoms** in a neutropaenic patient should be taken seriously, regardless of the temperature.

- Patients with neutropaenic sepsis may become very ill rapidly with a risk of developing septic shock and multi-organ failure leading to death. The mortality rate of septic shock is high (over 40%).
- Such patients may require cardiovascular support with inotropic medications such as dobutamine and support by the ICU.

The ITU should be informed if any neutropaenic patient with an infection has hypotension that is resistant to initial fluid resuscitation.

Physiology

Sepsis and the resulting endotoxin release from the bacteria stimulates a systemic inflammatory/immune response causing:

- Damaged pulmonary and systemic vasculature, vasodilation and increased permeability of vessels.
- Systemic activation of clotting cascades and coagulation abnormalities. These lead to:
  - Hypovolaemia.
  - Pulmonary oedema.
  - Thrombocytopaenia, bleeding, and low clotting factors.
  - Disseminated intravascular coagulation.
  - Cardiac and renal dysfunction.
  - Multi-organ failure.

Management

- Identify and treat sources of infection.
- Support the patient symptomatically.
- Detect any onset of organ/multi-organ failure.

Nursing management includes

- Ensuring the patient's safety regarding line management and administration of drugs and blood products.
- Close constant observation and monitoring.
- Maintaining comfort.
- Hydrating and maintaining nutritional needs.
- Supporting the patients symptomatically.
- Supporting the patient and family psychologically (see box for specific nursing measures).

Nursing management of neutropaenic sepsis

- Take routine observations: temperature, pulse, blood pressure, oxygen saturations, respiratory rate and reassess at frequent intervals,
- Ensure that an urgent chest X-ray is taken
- Take the following blood tests: blood cultures (from any indwelling lines and from the peripheral blood), full blood count, clotting screen, blood chemistries, C-reactive protein (CRP).
- If symptoms are present send urine cultures, sputum cultures, and a specimen of diarrhoea (requesting microscopy, culture and sensitivity and *Clostridium difficile* toxin).
- The patient should be assessed by medical staff for any obvious source of infection.
- Administer prescribed antibiotics **urgently**—usually with two broad spectrum intravenous antibiotics.
- Perform regular observations: temperature, pulse, blood pressure, oxygen saturations, urine output. If the patient is clinically dehydrated, tachycardiac, hypotensive or oliguric then:
  - Administer any prescribed IV fluids or oxygen as required.
  - Increase frequency of observations, up to every 15 minutes.
- These patients are at high risk of pulmonary oedema (see physiology above). Maintain accurate fluid balance and central venous pressure (CVP) readings. Observe breathing sounds and lungs for signs of fluid overload.
- Any deterioration should prompt an urgent medical review.
- Assess skin, mucosal membranes, orifices, body fluids for signs of bleeding—patients with sepsis are at risk of clotting abnormalities and DIC (📖 Disseminated intravascular coagulation). If there is bleeding, administer prescribed blood products and drugs, e.g. vitamin K.
- Maintain the patient's comfort throughout. Assist with personal hygiene, including regular mouth and skin care. Assist with all activities to help the patient reserve energy.
- Keep the patient and their family fully informed. They may be extremely frightened by the situation, particularly in cases of rapid deterioration, or if the patient requires intensive care admission.
- Ensure that you offer calm and reassuring nursing management, despite the emergency nature of treatment.

Bleeding

Bleeding occurs in many patients with cancer, ranging from minor bleeds, which may be part of initial diagnosis to potentially life-threatening haemorrhage, e.g. haemoptysis or carotid artery rupture.

Bleeding can be obvious, e.g. nose bleeds, oral mucosa, haemoptysis, haematemesis. It can also be hidden:
- Gastrointestinal: malaena, anaemia.
- Pulmonary: breathlessness, pleural effusion.
- Genitourinary: haematuria.
- Cerebral: headaches visual disturbances, other neurological disturbance.

Causes

Altered platelet count/function
- Tumour: mainly haematological cancers but also secondary spread into the bone marrow, e.g. lung, breast, prostate cancer.
- Treatment:
  - Many chemotherapy agents.
  - Radiotherapy: dependent on volume of bone marrow in the treatment field.
- Enlarged spleen.
- Immune mediated damage, e.g. idiopathic thrombocytopaenia purpura.
- Altered coagulation mechanisms e.g. acute pro-myelocytic leukaemia causing DIC (📖 Disseminatetd intravascular coagulation).
- Liver primary or secondary cancer.

Direct tumour impact
- Invasion into bone marrow causing altered platelet count, as above.
- Tumour extension into blood vessels:
  - Can be minor and part of initial presentation, e.g. gynaecological, lung, bowel, genitourinary.
  - Can be extreme: e.g. Lung cancer-haemoptysis, head and neck cancer—carotid artery erosion.

Cancer treatment
- Chemotherapy/radiotherapy: causing thrombocytopaenia.
- Surgery: carotid artery rupture.

Other drugs: heparin, aspirin, NSAIDs

Infections: septic shock, causing DIC

Assessment
- Risk factors e.g. the tumour, cancer treatment, other drugs e.g. NSAIDs.
- Past medical history.
- Signs and symptoms of anaemia (📖 Anaemia).
- Physical examination: being aware of both obvious and less obvious signs of bleeding (see above).
- Screening tests: platelet count, clotting screen, bone marrow aspirate, INR.

Thrombocytopaenia (low platelets)

The normal adult platelet count is $150–400 \times 10^9$/L. Thrombocytopaenia can be defined as any count less than this. However, patients rarely bleed spontaneously unless the count falls to $<20 \times 10^9$/L and most invasive procedures can be performed with a count of $>50 \times 10^9$/L.

Causes of thrombocytopaenia

As with neutropaenia, there are many potential causes of thrombocytopaenia. The most common causes in a cancer patient are:
- Bone marrow suppression (see above).
- Drugs e.g. antifungals such as amphotericin.
- Enlarged spleen (splenomegaly) which results in pooling and destruction of platelets.

Consequences of thrombocytopaenia

The major types of bleeding associated with thrombocytopenia are:
- Nose bleeds.
- Gum bleeds.
- GI bleeds, rectal bleeding, blood in stool, or black coloured stool.
- GU bleeds, dark coloured, or blood in urine.
- Petechial rash (small, purple spots which do not blanch on pressure, often prominently seen around the ankle).

Bleeding into the brain is the most severe complication, but this is uncommon.

The bleeding risk is increased in the following situations:
- Concurrent infections.
- Concurrent coagulation abnormalities e.g. if the patient is on warfarin.
- Administration of antiplatelet medications such as aspirin.
- Recent history of a bleeding episode.
- Invasive procedure.

Prevention of bleeding

- Avoid antiplatelet medication e.g. aspirin, NSAIDs (ibuprofen, diclofenac).
- Avoid intramuscular injections—these can result in a very painful intramuscular haematoma.
- Administer a pool of platelets if the count falls to $<10 \times 10^9$/L (or $<20 \times 10^9$/L in the presence of another risk factor for bleeding).
- Ensure the platelet count is adequate to cover any planned invasive procedure.

Treatment of bleeding due to thrombocytopaenia

- Administer a pool of platelets.
- Correct any reversible factors contributing to the bleeding risk e.g. treat underlying infection, stop antiplatelet medication.
- In the case of nose bleeds, pressure and ice packs may help.

Nursing management

Patients require accurate advice if they are thrombocytopaenic. They may also be anxious about the risk of a serious bleed. Ensure that they are aware of potential risks, preventative measures and action to take if they are bleeding. Reassure them that most bleeds are short lived and can be effectively managed with platelet transfusions (📖 Blood product support).

Patient education

Educate patients about:
- The reason that they are at risk of bleeding.
- The first signs of a low platelet count (see consequences above).
- Give advice about bleeding risk with drugs such as aspirin or NSAIDs-use paracetamol for headache.

Preventative measures
- Do not use dental floss.
- Use a soft toothbrush or sponge.
- Maintain moist mouth and lips.
- Do not use tampons if menstruating.
- Avoid straining at stool. Use a stool softener or laxative if prone to constipation.
- Do not perform PR examination or use rectal thermometers, suppositories, or enemas.
- Use an electric razor for shaving.
- Use a water-based lubricant and avoid vigorous thrusting during sexual intercourse.

What to do if any signs of bleeding
- Patients should contact their cancer unit or centre immediately. They will normally require an immediate full blood count to assess their platelet count. They may need to be admitted for a platelet transfusion.
- If there is a major bleed or injury, the patient should immediately go to their local hospital emergency unit and inform them that they are at risk of thrombocytopaenia.

Bleeding in advanced cancer

Localized bleeding caused by cancer may be treated by radiotherapy. Examples of its use include, ulcerating skin tumours, haemoptysis caused by lung cancer, vaginal bleeding, caused by gynaecological cancers, and haematuria caused by bladder/prostate cancer.

Massive terminal haemorrhage

Occurs as a result of a major arterial bleed and causes death, usually in minutes. The most common cause is tumour erosion into either the

- Aorta or pulmonary artery: leads to haematemesis or haemoptysis.
- Carotid artery: external bleeding.
- Femoral artery: external bleeding.

May be preceded by smaller minor bleeds, allowing some warning or awareness of the risk.

Management

- The aim of management is to rapidly sedate the patient in order to relieve any distress. If the bleed is anticipated then it may be appropriate to discuss this with the patient and family members.
- For anticipated bleeds it is useful have the drugs available at the bedside, already drawn up—many wards have patient medication lockers, which can enable this to be done safely.
- Red, blue, or green towels mask the colour of blood and should be available to control the spread of blood.

Pharmcological

IV is the preferable route due to the quicker rate of action of the drugs.

- *Midazolam:* 10mg SC/IV or bucally.
- *Ketamine:* 150–250mg IV. Provides rapid sedation. For IM route the dose needs to be increased to 500mg.
- *Opioids:* these are less recommended, as they cannot be left at the patient bedside, take time to draw up and titration of the appropriate dose is more difficult[1].

1 Watson M S, Lucas C F, Hoy A M, Black I N (2005). *Oxford Handbook of Palliative Care.* Oxford: Oxford University Press.

Further reading

Hart S (2006). Prevention of infection. In Grundy M (ed). *Nursing in Haematological Oncology*, 2nd edn, pp. 32–338. Edinburgh: Bailliere Tindall.

Larson E, Nirenberg A (2004). Evidence-based nursing practice to prevent infection in hospitalized neutropenic patients with cancer. *Oncology Nursing Forum*. **31**, 717–25.

Todd J, Schmidt M, Christian J, Williams R (1999) Controversies in cancer care. The low bacteria diet for immunocompromised patients: reasonable prudence or clinical superstition. *Cancer Practice*, **7**, 205–7.

West F and Mitchell S A (2004). Evidence-based guidelines for the management of neutropenia following outpatient haematopoietic stem cell transplantation. *Clinical Journal of Oncology Nursing*, **8**(6), 601–13.

Blood product support

Blood products

The introduction of safe, reliable blood products has enabled the development of intensive chemotherapy programmes for a variety of malignancies. This has led to significantly improved remission rates.

It must be remembered however that blood product use is not without risks, and that these are a very expensive resource. The pool of acceptable donors is also diminishing because of more stringent screening. Blood products should only be used in appropriate situations in consultation with national and local guidelines. (See British Committee for Standards in Haematology, BCSH[1]). The advent of erythropoiesis stimulating proteins (EPS) such as erythropoietin (EPO) has started to change management of cancer-related anaemia.

Erythropoietin

Recombinant human erythropoietin (EPO) has been shown to reduce transfusion requirements, and potentially can improve quality of life by reducing fatigue and other anaemia-related symptoms in some cancer patients receiving chemotherapy or radiotherapy. However, only around 50% of patients respond and it is expensive. EPO is administered as a regular subcutaneous injection, which is not always popular with patients. There is an increased risk of thrombosis using EPO, though this is rare.

Guidelines on the use of EPO

The European EORTC guidelines[2] suggest that patients receiving chemotherapy and/or radiotherapy should have EPO commenced when:
- Their haemoglobin (Hb) is in the range of 9–11g/dl.
- This should take account of their anaemia-related symptoms.
The aim is to maintain a Hb range of 12–13g/dl. EPO should not be used prophylactically with patients with a normal Hb level.

Blood transfusion

Whole blood is almost never currently used in the UK. When a unit of blood is donated it is separated into the following fractions:
- Red cells.
- Platelets.
- Plasma.

Plasma is frozen and is subsequently used as fresh frozen plasma (FFP). It is most frequently used to correct problems with blood clotting in patients with coagulation disorders, such as those on warfarin or with liver disease.

Standards in Haematology (BCSH) website: www.bcshguidelines.com/
S, Courdi A et al. (2004). EORTC-guidelines for the use of erythropoiↄts with cancer, *European Journal of Cancer* **40**, 2301–6,

Red cells

Packed red cells are frequently administered to cancer patients who are anaemic. Most oncology and haematology units have a protocol whereby red cells are administered if the Hb concentration falls below a particular cut off e.g. 8 or 9g/L. The threshold may be higher with patients receiving radiotherapy. The disadvantage with this policy is that it leads to a high use of blood products, with attendant cost and risks. Some patients cannot tolerate such a low level of Hb e.g. those with symptomatic ischaemic heart disease. The Hb threshold for transfusion may be raised accordingly based on their symptoms.

Complications of red cell transfusions

Acute haemolytic transfusion reaction (AHTR)

This is the most severe complication of a red cell transfusion and is due to ABO mismatched blood being administered. This can cause:

- Fever.
- Hypotension.
- Oliguria.
- Abdominal or flank pain.
- Jaundice.
- A general feeling of 'impending doom'.
- Renal failure.
- DIC (📖 Disseminated Intravascular coagulation).
- Death.

The most common cause for this is clerical error e.g. blood samples being mislabelled, or patient checks being incorrectly carried out. It is therefore vital that local protocols for blood transfusion are strictly adhered to.

If AHTR is suspected, urgent medical attention should be sought. Treatment is supportive, involving careful fluid balance, IV fluids, treatment of DIC and renal support.

Febrile non-haemolytic reaction

This is less common since the introduction of universal white cell depletion during processing of blood donations. Management includes:

- Assessment of the patient, including pulse, blood pressure, oxygen saturations.
- Considering slowing or stopping the transfusion for a short period if the patient is well and continue to monitor vital signs.
- Administering paracetamol 1g orally, chlorphenamine 10mg IV/4mg orally, and/or hydrocortisone 100–200mg IV.
- Stopping the transfusion and seeking medical advice if the patient feels unwell or their observations are unstable. They should be investigated for an AHTR (see above).

Delayed haemolytic transfusion reaction

The patient becomes anaemic and jaundiced a few days after a transfusion.

- Management is largely supportive. Blood tests should be sent to the transfusion laboratory to determine the type of antibody causing the reaction.
- If the patient requires further transfusions any blood that they receive should be negative for the molecule that the antibody recognizes.

Note: any patient with an antibody that reacts against certain types of red blood cells, and has caused a reaction in the past, should carry a card stating the antibody type.

> **Transfusion reaction notification**
>
> Any complication of transfusion from any blood product should be notified to the blood transfusion department, so that the product can be screened and further complications for other patients prevented.

Other complications

These include:

- Bacterial contamination of the blood.
- Transmission of viral infection—this is rare. The risk is in the order of 1/250,000 for hepatitis B, 1 in 8 million for HIV, and 1 in 30 million for hepatitis C.
- Variant Creutzfeldt–Jakob disease (vCJD). Though the risk is very low, screening for this is likely to be instigated.
- Transfusion associated graft-versus-host disease: this is extremely rare but nearly always fatal (📖 Irradiated blood products).
- Iron overload: this commonly occurs after 25–30 units of blood and results in iron deposition within the liver, heart, and endocrine glands. It is potentially very serious, and is treated by an arduous regime of desferrioxamine treatment.
- Cardiac overload due to fluid overload/rapid transfusion.

Compatibility of red cell transfusions

Red cells of one ABO blood group should preferably be given to a patient of the same blood group. The main exceptions to this rule are:

- Group O (so called 'universal blood') can be given to any patient in an emergency, but it is still preferable to match the ABO group if at all possible.
- A patient who has had an allogeneic stem cell transplant may change their blood group, receiving different blood from their original type (📖 Allogeneic haemopoietic stem cell transplantation).

Rhesus D (RhD) group is also important. A woman of childbearing ho is RhD negative and does not have any RhD antibodies should iven RhD positive red cells if at all possible. This is to avoid the of antibodies that can subsequently cause haemolytic disease r newborn. RhD negative men and women who are beyond e can receive RhD positive red cells, as the formation of t have deleterious effects. Once RhD antibodies have nly RhD negative products should be given, to avoid a delayed haemolytic transfusion reaction. Certain patients should receive irradiated and/or CMV negative products only (see next topic).

Platelets

The most common indication for a transfusion of platelets is the prevention of bleeding for patients receiving chemotherapy and/or radiotherapy affecting the haemopoietic system. Most units have a 'cut off' point below which prophylactic platelets are administered. This is commonly 10×10^9/L but may be higher if the patient has other risk factors for bleeding, such as severe sepsis.

Note: in 2006 research was ongoing into comparing a platelet transfusion policy with no prophylactic transfusion vs. the current UK prophylactic transfusion policy.

Unlike blood, a platelet transfusion is given rapidly to avoid aggregates forming in the bag and IV line. There are two main sources of platelets:
- Those obtained by pooling together the platelets from four individual blood donors (most common source).
- Those obtained from a process called apheresis where a single donor can give enough platelets for a transfusion. If platelets of a particular type are required—e.g. HLA matched—they must be collected by apheresis (📖 Allogeneic haemopoietic stem cell transplantation). The blood service wants more platelet donations to come from apheresis donors, as it reduces the exposure of patients to numerous donors.

Complications of platelet transfusions
- Febrile reaction: this is less common since the widespread introduction of white cell depletion during donation processing. It may be accompanied by rigors and urticaria (hives). Management includes:
  - Stopping transfusion (if not already completed).
  - Administering hydrocortisone 100–200mg IV and chlorphenamine 10mg IV (or 4mg orally).
  - Considering pethidine 25mg IV for persistent rigors.
  - Pre-medicating the patient with hydrocortisone and chlorphenamine (doses as above) for further platelet transfusions.
  - Occasionally, patients who react badly to platelet transfusions may require HLA-matched platelets.
- Bacterial contamination: this is more common than with red cells because platelets must be stored at room temperature. Every bag of platelets should be visually checked for discolouration or cloudiness prior to administration.
- Viral transmission: as with red blood cells (see above).
- Development of anti-HLA antibodies: this can lead to platelet refractoriness whereby further platelet transfusions are ineffective and specially HLA-matched platelets are required.
- Transfusion related acute lung injury (TRALI): this is a serious co resulting in respiratory failure and possibly death. It is usually antibodies in the donor plasma. Treatment is supportive, mechanical ventilation.

Compatibility of platelets

Where possible, ABO matched platelets are given. It is perfectly acceptable to administer ABO mismatched platelets, but the patient's platelet count may not rise as much as expected. RhD negative platelets should be administered to RhD negative women of childbearing age who do not have RhD antibodies already. As with red cells, certain patients should receive irradiated and/or CMV negative platelets (see below).

Irradiated blood products

Packed red cells and platelets contain a small number of contaminating white blood cells. Normally, if these cells are transfused with the blood product, the host's immune system would rapidly clear them. In immuno-suppressed patients however, these white cells can grow, divide, and attack the recipient's tissues. This can lead to a very serious condition called transfusion associated graft-versus-host disease (TAGvHD).

This condition is characterized by bone marrow failure, severe rash, diarrhoea, and liver failure. It is nearly always fatal, but is extremely rare. TAGvHD can be prevented by exposing the blood product to gamma-radiation. The product is then said to be irradiated. Irradiated products should be used in the following situations:

- From the start of conditioning therapy in all patients receiving a stem cell transplant. For autologous transplants, this should continue for at least 3 months after the transplant; for allogeneic transplants, at least 6 months (📖 Allogeneic haemopoietic stem cell transplantation). Indefinitely for patients who have received a purine analogue in the past e.g. fludarabine, cladribine.
- Patients with Hodgkin's lymphoma.
- All HLA-matched platelet transfusions.

CMV negative blood products

Cytomegalovirus (CMV) is a common virus that can be transmitted by a blood transfusion. It is harmless in most cases, but it can lead to serious disease in patients who are immuno-suppressed. A number of blood products are assessed for the presence of CMV and many haematology units will administer only CMV negative products to the following groups of patients:

- Any patient who may be given a stem cell transplant in the near future, e.g. a fit patient with acute leukaemia and who is either CMV seronegative or who has not yet been tested.
- Any CMV seronegative patient who is undergoing an autologous or allogeneic transplant from a sero-negative donor.

If a patient is CMV sero-positive they will harbour the virus already and so there is no need to only give CMV negative products.

TAGvHD guidelines card system

To ensure adherence to these guidelines, the blood bank should be informed of any patient fulfilling one of the above criteria, and a note should be made on the computer system. The patient should be informed and given a card stating their need to have blood products irradiated. A card should also be attached to their medical notes. The patient should be assured that even if they were to receive non-irradiated blood products the risk of TAGvHD is still low.

The nurse's role in blood product transfusions

Educating the patient

Patients should be informed of the reasons for their blood product transfusion and consented for the transfusion. They should also be made aware of any risks and benefits and any potential alternatives, including autologous transfusion. Some patients may be anxious about receiving blood products, for fear of contracting infections such as hepatitis or for fear of transfusion reactions. Misconceptions need to be corrected and any particular fears dealt with sensitively.

Administration errors

Errors at the time of administration of blood or blood components are the most common cause of transfusing the wrong blood. It is essential to follow hospital blood administration policies when administering any blood product.

Checking blood products

- The bedside check is a vital step in preventing transfusion error. The nurse must be vigilant in ensuring that the patient is positively identified and that the patient's identification details on their wristband match those on the blood transfusion report form, and the compatibility label attached to the blood pack.
- Further checks must include the blood unit number, blood group, and special requirements such as CMV –ve or irradiated.
- Checks should be made between the following:
  - Patient's identification wristband and blood transfusion compatibility report form.
  - Compatibility label attached to the blood pack.
  - Prescription chart.
  - Medical notes.

Full national guidelines are available on the BCSH website (see Further reading)

Administration

- Blood should be transfused through a sterile blood administration set.
- Platelet concentrates should be transfused through a sterile blood or platelet administration set.
- Electronic infusion pumps should not be used for the administration of red cells, unless they are verified safe according to the manufacturer's instructions.
- ing sets should be changed every 12h to prevent bacterial growth.

Monitoring patients

- Visual observation is probably the most effective check. Patients having transfusions should be in areas where they are easily visible and accessible. There should also be quick and easy access to emergency resuscitation equipment if appropriate. Patients should be advised to report a rash, temperature, shivering, feeling unwell, feeling cold or pain at the site of the infusion.
- Patients should be monitored for signs of potential complications of transfusion. They should be most closely observed during the first 15 minutes of the start of each unit, when severe reactions are most likely to occur.
- Temperature, pulse, and blood pressure should be measured and recorded before the start, and at the end of each transfusion episode.
- Temperature and pulse should be measured 15 minutes after the start of each unit.
- Vital signs should be clearly dated and recorded separately from routine observations.

The use of further observations is at the discretion of each clinical area.

Further reading

Contreras M (2002). *ABC of Transfusion*, 4th ed. London: BMJ Books.

Dolan S, Crombez P, Munoz M (2005). Neutropenia management with granulocyte colony stimulating factors: From guidelines to nursing practice protocols. *European Journal of Oncology Nursing*, **9**, s14–23.

National Institute for Clinical Excellence (2005) Appraisal consultation document-erythropoietin for anaemia induced by cancer treatment. Available at http://www.nice.org/page.aspx?o=296882

Smyth D, Zumbrink S (2005). Optimising the management of anaemia in patients with cancer with practice guidelines using erythropoiesis stimulating proteins. *Europ*   *9*, s3–13.

BCSH http://www.bcshguidelines.com

Thrombosis

Venous thrombosis

Venous thromboembolic disease (VTE) includes thrombosis of superficial and deep veins (DVT), usually of the leg, thigh, and pelvis, pulmonary embolus (PE) and thrombosis associated with central venous catheters (CVCs).

Venous thrombosis can have a profound impact on a cancer patient's quality of life. It is a well recognized, major complication of cancer and the second leading cause of death in hospitalized patients with cancer. It remains an under-diagnosed and under-treated condition.

Aetiology
- Tumoural production of a range of procoagulant factors.
- Cancer treatments including surgery and chemotherapy.
- Use of CVCs.
- Venous thrombosis maybe the first sign of malignancy and the development of VTE in patients with cancer is often associated with a poor prognosis.

Signs and symptoms
- DVT: unilateral swelling of an extremity with oedema, erythema, and pain.
- PE: tachypnoea, tachycardia, dyspneoa, chest pain aggravated by inspiration, and unexplained haemoptysis.

Diagnosis
- Thorough patient history.
- Assessment of risk factors.
- Physical examination.
- Contrast venography or venous ultrasonography, for diagnosing DVT.
- Ventilation perfusion scan or pulmonary angiography, used for diagnosing PE.

Management
Prophylaxis
Primary prophylaxis should be considered for patients with cancer in the presence of additional risk factors such as immobilization, surgery, chemotherapy, hormonal therapy, or central venous catheters.

Surgery
Surgery in cancer patients is associated with twice the risk of thrombosis than in those without cancer. The use of graduated compression stockings in combination with unfractionated heparin (UFH) or low molecular weight heparin (LMWH) provides better protection than the use of other method alone. LMWH is more efficacious than low dose UFH in patients undergoing elective abdominal surgery, and extending prophylaxis weeks of treatment has demonstrated more benefit.

Central venous catheters for administration of chemotherapy

Long-term indwelling CVCs increase the risk of thromboembolic complications leading to significant morbidity, catheter malfunction, and treatment delays.

Pulmonary embolism has also been reported to occur in 5–12% of these patients[1]. However, overall rates of CVC-associated VTE have been decreasing over the last ten years due to improvements in catheters and catheter care. Results of recent large trials have shown low dose warfarin and LMWHs to be of no apparent benefit.

However, dose-adjusted warfarin to maintain the international normalized ratio (INR) between 1.5 and 2.0 seemed superior to 1mg warfarin in reducing VTEs but was associated with more major bleeding events.

VTE prophylaxis with low-dose warfarin or LMWHs is therefore currently not recommended for thromboprophylaxis.

Treatment of VTE

The management of DVT and PE are similar, with the initial administration of weight-adjusted LMWH by SC injection or UFH given intravenously to maintain the activated partial thromboplastin time at 1.5–2.0 times normal. Treatment with warfarin is generally started on day 1 during initial LMWH/UFH therapy, adjusted to maintain an INR of 2.0–3.0 and continued for 3–6 months. In cancer patients with acute VTE, even with the use of LMWH and an oral anticoagulant, there is a significant risk of recurrent thrombosis. Guidelines now recommend the use of LMWH instead of warfarin for the long-term treatment of acute VTE for 3–6 months.

Overview of nursing care

For those patients who survive a VTE, there is often reduced limb function (with DVT) or low respiratory function (with PE), resulting in immobilization, hospitalization, interruption of life-saving treatments (with CVC-related DVT), and heightened anxiety. The treatment puts patients at high risk of injury from bleeding. Identification of patients at high risk of thrombosis is crucial. Nurses firstly have to raise awareness of thrombosis with patients through counselling about the risk of VTE, followed by risk assessment. Active or passive exercise should be encouraged to support venous circulation and pharmacologic and non-pharmacologic measures to reduce anxiety, pain, or dyspnoea. Managing the complications of anticoagulant therapies and overall coordination of the patient pathway are crucial to optimal support for patient and carer.

Further reading

Haire W D (2000). Thombotic Complications. In M D Abeloff, J O Armitage, A S Lichter J E Niederhiber (eds) Clinical Oncology 2nd edn. pp.657–89. Philadelphia: Churchill Livingst
Van Gerpen R (2004). Thrombolic Disorders in Cancer Clinical Journal of Oncology Nursi
289–99.

1 Verso M and Agnelli G (2003). Venous thromboembolism associated w'
central venous catheters in cancer patients. Journal of Clinical Oncology, **21**('

Altered bowel function

Diarrhoea

Diarrhoea is an unpleasant and potentially embarrassing symptom for patients. It is defined as the passage of loose stools with urgency, with three or more stools within 24 hours.

It can have a major impact on an individual's quality of life potentially causing:
• Faecal incontinence.
• Social isolation.
• Malnutrition and dehydration.
• Stopping or reducing dose of anti-cancer therapy.
• Fatigue, exhaustion.

Diarrhoea may also be associated with abdominal pain, cramps, urgency, and tenesmus. Nausea and vomiting may be present if the upper gut is involved.

Causes
• Diet e.g. high-fibre diet, spicy food, alcohol.
• Drugs: chemotherapy, laxatives, antibiotics, antacids, non-steroidal anti-inflammatory drugs, and iron preparations.
• Surgery e.g. bowel resection, gastrectomy.
• Radiotherapy to pelvic area or gut.
• Bowel obstruction: faecal overflow.
• Malabsorption: particularly in pancreatic cancer and bowel cancer.
• Infection e.g. *Clostridium difficile*.
• Disease e.g. colorectal, pancreatic cancer.
• GvHD (Complications of allogeneic transplant).
• Non cancer-related, e.g. inflammatory bowel disease, coeliac disease.
• Anxiety.

Assessment
• Assessment needs to be carried out sensitively. Patients may be embarrassed and reluctant to talk about their bowel habits and diarrhoea may be seen as dirty.
• It is important to clarify both the range of potential causes and the patient's individual perception and interpretation of the term diarrhoea.
• Without a detailed assessment it can be difficult to plan appropriate treatment and support. Early management can prevent related consequences such as dehydration and exhaustion (see Table 41.1).

Management of diarrhoea

Accurate assessment

Where the cause of diarrhoea is not explicit further investigations may be required e.g. physical observation, abdominal palpation, stool specimens to rule out infection, and barium studies or endoscopy.

- Fluid and electrolyte replacement.
- Identification and treatment or removal of the cause.
- Symptomatic relief.
- A proactive approach to skin care and hygiene is essential to prevent burning and breakdown of skin. Consider using a barrier cream when diarrhoea persists for longer than 24 hours.

Table 41.1 Assessment of diarrhoea

Question	Rationale
• What is the patient's normal bowel habit?	• Provides a baseline, and determines when the problem started.
• When was the last normal bowel action?	• It may help in establishing a new 'norm' for the patient particularly if the cancer or its treatment has affected the bowel.
• What is the patient's perception of normal?	
• What is the patient's perception of the cause and the impact on their quality of life?	• It is important to establish the extent of the problem and impact on the patient's quality of life.
• How frequently does it occur? What does it smell like?	• This provides a benchmark to monitor and record improvement or worsening of the symptom.
• What does it look like (colour, consistency, and amount)?	• Dark stool may suggest need for FOB test.
• Is there obvious blood in the stool?	
• Is the diarrhoea a side effect of treatment?	• Consideration of the cause of the diarrhoea may affect how the diarrhoea is managed.
• Is the patient currently taking laxatives?	• Diarrhoea caused by increase in laxatives to treat constipation will normally resolve within 24–48hrs if laxatives are reduced or stopped.
	• Care should be taken not to reinduce constipation.

Note: stopping anti-cancer treatment may reduce persistent and unbearable diarrhoea but can have major consequences for the patient. The risk and benefit of stopping these treatments needs to be discussed with the patient and the health care team.

Further information on drug management of diarrhoea can be found in the *British National Formulary*: (www.bnf.org).

Management of cancer treatment-induced diarrhoea

Cytotoxic drugs

Cells within the GI tract have a high rate of reproduction. Effects of cytotoxic drugs on the mucosal stem cycle can be seen within days of treatment. Most chemotherapy-induced diarrhoea occurs during or immediately post-treatment until the gut settles. Immuno-suppression from treatment can increase risk of *Clostridium difficile* gut infection.

Note: diarrhoea from irinotecan (used to treat colorectal cancer) can be prolific and requires careful monitoring. It has the potential of causing severe dehydration if left untreated.

Management
• Most chemotherapy-induced diarrhoea can be managed with
  loperamide or codeine.

Radiotherapy

High dose radiotherapy to the abdomen or pelvis increases peristaltic activity by damaging the intestinal mucosa (acute radiation enteritis). Symptoms may be immediate but can occur several weeks into the course of treatment or after the radiotherapy has stopped.

Initial damage is due to immediate mucosal cell death. Progressive loss of cells, atrophy, and fibrosis of the bowel lining can occur in the following weeks. Patients suffering from acute enteritis may complain of nausea, vomiting, abdominal cramping, tenesmus, and watery diarrhoea.

Management
Generally as for cytotoxic drug induced diarrhoea, plus:
• Aspirin: can be helpful because of its effect in blocking prostaglandins.
• Cholestyramine: can also help in late chronic diarrhoea where there is
  evidence of bile salt malabsorption.
• If pain relief is required, opioids have the benefit of being constipating.

Stoma management

For bowel cancer patients who have a colostomy or ileostomy the management of diarrhoea follows the above guidance, however consideration should be given to:
• Is there adequate adherence, and comfort of stoma appliances?
• Does the patient have good skin protection?
• Is the stoma overactive?
• Could diet be used to manage over activity?
• Is fluid and electrolyte support required?

Table 41.2 Drug management for symptomatic relief

Drug	Action
Antimotility drugs 1. Loperamide Starting dose of 4mg, then 2mg 4hrly or after each bowel action. Maximum 16mg in 24hrs.	To reduce the motility of the gut in uncomplicated acute diarrhoea in adults e.g. diarrhoea of known cause and where there is a need to improve faecal consistency.
2. Codeine 10–60mg 4x daily. Maximum 240mg daily	
3. Octreotide Starting dose 250–500µg daily. Maximum 750µg.	Reduces motility, enhances fluid absorption, reduces secretions. Used in Graft versus Host Disease (📖 Allogeneic Haemopoietic stem cell transplantation) and chemotherapy-related diarrhoea.
Antispasmodic drugs Hyoscine butylbromide: 10–20mg 4x daily. Maximum 80mg daily.	Used to treat abdominal cramps but should not be used as a primary treatment of diarrhoea.
Antibacterial drugs Antibacterial drugs should be prescribed following the result of a stool sample and on the advice of the microbiologist.	Used to treat systemic bacterial infections e.g. campylobacter enteritis, shigellosis, and salmonellaosis.

For patients with an overactive ileostomy, loperamide (melts or tablets) could be considered 45 minutes prior to meals (📖 Stoma care).

Non-pharmacological management

There is a limited research evidence base to support one particular approach.
- Spend time with the patient assessing possible exacerbating factors, e.g. anxiety, diet, and alcohol and discuss behavioural modification.
- Diet: for many patients a high-fibre diet, alcohol, spicy food, milk products and caffeine all exacerbate diarrhoea. Getting patients to keep a diary of food intake and their pattern of diarrhoea can help to identify causal factors. Dietitian advice on dietary modification is a useful strategy.

Further reading

Doyle D, Hanks G, Chern N, Calman C (2004). *Oxford Textbook of Palliative Medicine*, 3rd edn. Oxford: Oxford University Press.

Websites

📖 Palliative Drugs.com: www.pallaitivedrugs.com
📖 British National Formulary: www.bnf.org

Constipation

Constipation is a commonly occurring symptom often exacerbated by cancer, its treatment and management.

It is defined as the infrequent passage of small hard faeces with difficulty, and less frequently than the individual's normal pattern. If untreated, constipation can lead to further symptoms: nausea, vomiting, poor appetite, weight loss, overflow diarrhoea, rectal bleeding, faecal incontinence, urinary incontinence, pain, tenesmus (an urgent and painful desire to defaecate), bowel obstruction, and confusion.

Nursing management should be proactive and anticipate the potential for constipation before it occurs as a problem. Potential causes of constipation in cancer patients are highlighted in Table 41.3.

Regular assessment for constipation is important and should include:

Accurate patient history
- Identification and possible removal of potential cause of constipation; identifying how long has the problem existed and establishing normal pattern. Patient diary is useful.
- Stool frequency, consistency, discomfort on passing stool, smell of faecal leakage. Stool chart may be helpful.
- Assessment of diet, including fluid intake.
- Use of laxatives.

Examination
- Physical observation including abdominal palpation.
- Plain X-ray of abdomen is helpful if an inconsistent clinical picture.
- Digital rectal examination can assess for presence of stool, haemorrhoids, and anal tone.

Record of potentially associated symptoms
Nausea; vomiting; abdominal pain; abdominal distension; malodorous breath.

Mobility
Access to toilet; lack of privacy; need for assistance/mobility aids.

Constipation can cause faecal leakage or watery faecal stained fluid to be passed. The fluid can contain small hard faeces and have a stale smell. This should not be confused with diarrhoea, which is more likely to have a soft consistency. If in doubt abdominal palpation or abdominal X-ray should be undertaken to determine the correct management.

Management of constipation
- Identify and remove the cause where possible.
- Set goals based on patient's normal bowel habits and established management regimen, taking into consideration the cancer treatment plan.
- Explore the potential for increasing fluid intake and adjusting diet.
- Consider measures to improve privacy.
- Appropriate encouragement to exercise.
- Consider prophylactic use of laxatives.

Table 41.3 Potential causes of constipation in cancer patients

Cancer related	Treatment related	Cancer impact
• Hypercalcaemia • Abdominal or pelvic disease • Cord compression • Cauda equina syndrome	• Chemotherapy (Vinca Alkaloids, particularly vincristine) • Radiotherapy (long term bowel fibrosis) • Opioids • Antiemetics (cyclizine & ondansetron) • Anticholinergics • Antispasmodics • Antidepressants • Neuroleptics • NSAIDs	• Weakness • Inactivity or bed rest • Poor nutrition • Dehydration/poor fluid intake • Confusion • Inability to reach toilet • Embarrassment due to lack of privacy

Note: multiple causes of constipation are common, particularly in advanced cancer.

Diet and other non-pharmacological measures
Diet
- Dietary advice is complementary to prescription of laxatives. Advice should be realistic and given with consideration to the patient's disease status, treatment plan and individual needs.
- Try to maintain a fluid intake of at least 2 litres a day.
- Where possible inclusion of fibre within the diet should be encouraged. This should not however be introduced too quickly or in excess to avoid flatulence and bloating. In dehydrated patients fibre may exacerbate constipation.
- Consider referral to dietician particularly for patients where constipation is an ongoing problem.

Other measures
- Assist with other symptom control e.g. patients with pain and/or nausea are unlikely to maintain adequate oral intake.
- Maintain good oral care and ensure that patients are comfortably positioned at meal times.
- Assist with maintaining mobility if appropriate.

Pharmacological management
Where the patient already has a management regime for their constipation it may be necessary to increase laxatives or intervene to achieve a bowel evacuation pattern which is normal for the patient. The evidence base supporting the management of constipation in cancer patients is limited. General guidelines on the use of laxatives based on best available evidence are covered in Table 41.4.

The use of oral laxatives should be considered for patients who may not be able to achieve a regular bowel evacuation by diet, increased fluid intake and exercise alone. Treatment should be preventative if possible, e.g. patients on opioids or vincristine should be on regular laxatives.

Enemas or suppositories can be undignified and painful and are generally not the first treatment option. They are useful in cases of faecal impaction and spinal cord compression.

Further information on laxatives and dosages can be found in the British National Formulary: www.bnf.org

Table 41.4 Guidance for use of laxatives

Classification	Action	Indication for use	Examples of drugs
Bulk-forming drugs	Increases faecal mass. **Note:** need high fluid intake	Of value in patients where fibre in diet can not be increased Useful in patients who have a colostomy, ileostomy to add bulk to stool Effect NOT immediate	Ispaghula husk (e.g. Fybogel Regular®) Methylcellulose Sterculia (e.g. Normacol®)
Osmotic laxatives	Draws water into the large bowel.	Discourages proliferation of ammonia-producing organisms Useful in the treatment of *hepatic encephalopathy* NB Cautious use in patients with low fluid intake or vomiting as can increase dehydration and volume of vomiting	Lactulose syrup MovicolMagnesium hydroxide suspension ('Milk of Magnesia') Phosphate enema Micro enema
Faecal softener/ lubricants	Lubricate and soften impacted faeces to promote a bowel action	Patients who have hard stools and difficulty in passing	Liquid paraffin/ mineral oil (**Note:** causes anal skin irritation) Docusate sodium Arachis oil enema Glycerol suppositories
Contact (stimulant) laxatives	Increase intestinal motility	For patients who may be taking opioids or other drugs which slow the action of the gut May cause abdominal cramp **Note:** should be avoided in bowel obstruction Prolonged use can cause diarrhoea and symptoms associated with diarrhoea	Bisacodyl Dantron (Danthron) Senna Sodium picosulphate (mild irritant to the bowel acting as a rectal stimulant)

Bowel obstruction

Obstruction occurs when digested food is unable to pass through the intestine due to tumour, impacted faeces, oedema, or motility disorders. It is commonly associated with intestinal and gynaecological cancers.

Causes

- Oedema caused by tumour.
- Faecal impaction.
- Intestinal muscle paralysis.
- Lumen occlusion; due to primary tumour enlargement, recurrence of abdominal mass, fibrosis, or adhesions.
- Carcinomatosis with concurrent infiltration of the mesentery or bowel muscles and nerves by the tumour.

Symptoms

The obstruction can be partial or complete. Presenting symptoms commonly include:

- Nausea.
- Vomiting, including occasionally faecal vomiting.
- Abdominal cramps and distension. (Can cause severe pain.)

Management

- The approach taken to manage bowel obstruction should be considered in collaboration with the patient and aim to promote the best quality of life. Treatment decisions should consider the: patient's prognosis and general health.
- Patient's expectations, wishes, and concerns.
- Clinical presentation.
- Potential impact of the chosen management approach on the patient's quality of life.

Partial bowel obstruction

In the case of partial obstruction, presenting symptoms may be inconsistent and resolve for short periods of time. If bowel obstruction is suspected an abdominal X-ray to determine air, fluid, and stool levels may be helpful. Proactive management of constipation can help to delay complete bowel obstruction.

It may be necessary to stop stimulant, osmotic, or bulk-forming laxatives as they could increase peristalsis. This causes abdominal pain and can lead to further complications such as perforation of the gut, if the bowel is obstructing.

It is preferable to use a faecal softener, e.g. docusate sodium 100–500mg in divided daily doses, to enable the faeces to soften sufficiently to pass through a narrowed bowel. For management of associated symptoms see Table 41.5.

Complete bowel obstruction

In advanced cancer bowel obstruction is unlikely to be a single acute event and more likely to become continuous. Management approaches include surgical intervention, stenting, or secondary symptom management.

Table 41.5 Management of symptoms associated with bowel obstruction

Management approach	Indications
Surgical intervention. Bypass procedures such as formation of a colostomy or ileostomy, dependant on the confinement of the tumour site	• Patient fit for surgery. • Tumour confined to a single site. • Low tumour grade.
Stenting under radiological guidance The stent enables the bowel to remain patent and allow passage of stool through area affected by tumour	• Less invasive than a surgical bypass. • Tumour not confined to one site. • Prognosis of weeks. • To facilitate symptom relief. • To improve quality of life.
Dexamethasone 8–16mg daily SC before midday	• To increase water and salt absorption. • To reduce oedema around tumour (limited evidence of its effectiveness). • Adverse effects: prolonged use may lead to problematic symptoms from steroid use, e.g. diabetes mellitus, agitation, depression, oedema, and Cushing's syndrome.
Naso-gastric tube	• Patient experiencing uncontrollable faecal vomiting. • Large volume vomits. • Adverse effects: impact on patients perception of body image, may reduce fluid absorption.
Octreotide Starting dose 250–500µg daily Maximum dose 750µg daily	• For reduction of, and to encourage re-absorption of gut secretions through: • Direct anti-cancer effect on solid tumours of gastrointestinal tract. • Decreases gut motility. • Increases water and electrolyte absorption. • Decreases carbohydrate absorption. • Decreases nausea and vomiting. • Adverse effects: insulinoma, dry mouth, flatulence, anorexia, nausea, vomiting, bloating, abdominal pain, diarrhoea, steatorrhoea.

Further information on drug management of bowel obstruction and contraindications can be found in the *British National Formulary*: www.bnf.org

For complete or partial bowel obstruction secondary symptom management is important to maintain patient's quality of life. Table 41.6 summarizes the management of secondary symptoms that may be experienced in complete or partial bowel obstruction.

Table 41.6 Management of secondary symptoms associated with bowel obstruction

Symptom	Management
Nausea and Vomiting (☐ Nausea and vomiting)	• First line: cyclizine 100–150mg SC in 24hrs. • Second line: haloperidol 3–5mg SC in 24hrs (this can be either with or without cyclizine). • Third line: methotrimeprozine 6.25–25mg in 24hrs. Low doses (6.25mg) are effective in the majority of individuals and should not cause sedation.
Abdominal cramp	• Hyoscine butylbromide 40–100mg SC in 24hrs. • It may also be necessary to consider centrally acting analgesic drugs if pain persists e.g. morphine.
Loss of appetite	• Control of associated symptoms that reduce appetite i.e. nausea and vomiting. • Small and frequent meals.
Constipation (partial obstruction only)	• Stop stimulant, osmotic, or bulk-forming laxatives to avoid pain from peristalsis. • Consider faecal softener e.g. Docusate Sodium 100–500mg in divided doses. • Consider rectal laxatives i.e. arachis oil enema to soften faeces in the rectum.
Diarrhoea	• Codeine 30–60mg orally 4xdaily. • Loperamide 2–4mg orally 4hrly. • This should be considered with caution if there is any chance of the obstruction being reversible, as it could make constipation and secondary symptoms of obstruction (i.e. pain) worse.

Further reading

Ripamonti C, Bruera E (2002). Palliative management of malignant bowel obstruction. *International Journal of Gynecological Cancer*, **12**, 135–43.

Ripamanti C, Mercante S (2004). Bowel Obstruction. In Doyle D, Hanks G, Chern N, and Calman C (2004). *Oxford Textbook of Palliative Medicine*, 3rd edn. pp.496–506. Oxford: Oxford University Press.

Scottish Intercollegiate Guidelines Network (2003). *Management of malignant bowel obstruction in relapsed disease*, Section 8. www.sign.ac.uk/guidelines

Seymour K, Johnson R, Marsh R, and Corson J (2002). Palliative stenting of malignant large bowel obstruction, *Colorectal Disease* **4**, 240–5.

Sykes N (2004). Constipation and diarrhoea. In Doyle D, Hanks G, Chern N, and Calman C (2004). *Oxford Textbook of Palliative Medicine*, 3rd edn. pp.483–95. Oxford: Oxford University Press.

Chapter 42

Cancer-related breathlessness

Causes, diagnosis, and assessment

Breathlessness is the experience of shortness of breath, of difficult or uncomfortable breathing. It is a very unpleasant and frightening experience, often associated with anxiety and distress, and a sensation of suffocating. It can cause profound disability, limiting the patient's function and drastically reducing quality of life, for the family as well as the patient. Breathlessness is a complex, multidimensional problem, with physiological and psychological components. It can be associated with a range of malignancies, but is most common in patients with primary lung cancer.

There is a role for specialist lung cancer nurses, social workers, and occupational and physiotherapists in the management of breathlessness. Patients being managed at home will need to have the full support of the primary care team to enable them to remain as independent as possible.

Causes

A central feature of the management of breathlessness is dealing with underlying processes, so it is important to establish the cause of the breathlessness.

Breathlessness as a direct consequence of malignancy

- Intrinsic or extrinsic airway constriction or obstruction with associated lung infection or collapse.
- Lymphangitis carcinomatosis or mediastinal lymphadenopathy.
- Involvement of the pleura.
- Pericardial involvement.
- Vessel involvement.
- Chest wall involvement.
- Phrenic nerve paralysis and diaphragmatic involvement.

Breathlessness as an indirect consequence of malignancy

- Embolism—e.g. pulmonary emboli.
- Pneumonia.
- Pneumothorax.
- Symptomatic anaemia.
- Chronic cancer folic acid and vitamin B12 deficiency.
- Respiratory muscle weakness (severe).
- Cachexia-anorexia syndrome.
- Drug induced (corticosteroids, benzodiazepines).
- Electrolyte imbalances/abnormalities.
- Paraneoplastic syndrome of malignancy.

Breathlessness as a consequence of treatment

- Surgery—e.g. pneumonectomy, lobectomy.
- Radiation-induced pneumonitis or fibrosis, pericarditis.
- Chemotherapy-induced pulmonary and cardiac toxicity, myelo-suppression.

Diagnosis

Physical signs such as nasal flaring, hyperpnoea (increased rate and depth of breathing), the use of accessory muscles, and tachypnoea (rapid breathing), are all associated with the subjective experience of shortness of breath.

Concurrent respiratory and general symptoms associated with breathlessness are important diagnostic features. For example; cough, sputum, haemoptysis, fatigue, insomnia, pain, loss of appetite, anxiety, and depression.

Accurate diagnosis is dependent on a thorough history, clinical assessment, examination, and targeted investigations. For patients with advanced disease, chest X-ray, routine blood tests, and pulse oximetry are the most useful investigations.

Assessment

Nurses have a considerable contribution to make to a comprehensive patient-centred approach to the assessment of breathlessness. To be effective, an assessment must be individualized. The essential areas an assessment should cover are:

- When did the breathlessness first become a problem?
- How did it start, was it acute or gradual?
- What does being breathless feel like? Ask the person to think about its emotional and physical characteristics.
- How frequently does breathlessness occur—is it continuous, occurring even at rest, or does it vary?
- Are there any precipitating or exacerbating factors—activity, wind, temperature, laughing, or eating for example?
- Has the person experienced any attacks of breathlessness, and if so, how long does it take to recover after an attack?
- Does the breathlessness—or the fear of it—stop the individual from doing things? What does the breathlessness mean to the individual and their family?

Management

Pharmacological approaches

Opioids, benzodiazepines, corticosteroids, bronchodilators, and oxygen (O_2) are the main pharmacological treatments used for relief of breathlessness. The primary aim in the management of breathlessness is to reverse any condition that may result in, or exacerbate existing shortness of breath. For example, if shortness of breath is caused by sepsis or fluid overload, antibiotics or diuretics may be prescribed. If breathlessness is caused by SVCO radiotherapy may treat the obstructive effects of the tumour, and corticosteroids reduce oedema (Superior vena cava obstruction).

Oxygen and air

O_2 therapy is commonly used as the first line intervention for symptomatic relief of an acute exacerbation of breathlessness. However, most breathless patients will not benefit from oxygen unless their oxygen saturations are below normal range (SaO_2 < 90%). Where O_2 is required, administration via nasal cannula rather than a face mask can reduce oral dryness and inhibition of social interaction.

If a patient's O_2 saturations are within the normal range (SaO_2 > 90%), the patient and family can be reassured that O_2 is not required, and that other interventions may be more beneficial. Strategies for aiding breathing without O_2 include a comfortable upright sitting position, and improving air flow by having a window open or using a small fan.

Opioids

Opioids are commonly used for breathlessness management within cancer palliation. In patients who have not taken opioids before (opioid naïve), doses should start at 2.5–5mg of oral morphine either 4-hourly or as needed to bring about therapeutic benefit. In patients already taking morphine, a dose increment may be indicated, although evidence to support this is equivocal. Morphine seems to alter the sensation of breathlessness for some patients by decreasing the ventilatory drive, and thus decreases the level of distress experienced from breathlessness. There is no evidence to support the use of nebulized morphine.

Benzodiazepines

Benzodiazepines, such as diazepam, can be used to ease the psychological aspects of breathlessness. Where this is associated with acute feelings of panic, lorazepam or midazolam may be used. Benzodiazepines with opioids may be used to provide a sedative effect for terminal breathlessness during the final hours or days of life.

Other pharmacological interventions

Commonly used methods to relieve breathlessness include: corticosteroids for inflammatory aetiology, bronchodilators for airway obstruction, antibiotics, anticholinergics, nebulised saline, anticoagulants, and diuretics.

Cancer-directed therapies and interventions

Chemotherapy, radiotherapy, and hormone therapy can provide some symptomatic relief for patients with treatment-sensitive primary and metastatic disease. Breathlessness associated with responsive anaemia, malignant pleural effusions, airway obstruction, ascites, and SVCO is often best managed by treating the underlying cause.

Non-pharmacological approaches

Relaxation techniques

Relaxation strategies can offer some simple steps to help 'undo' established reactions to breathlessness. This can increase a patient's sense of control in recovering their breath (🕮 Progressive muscle relaxation).

Positioning

Leaning forward from the hips, when sitting with forearms resting above the knees can increase abdominal pressure and promote improved respiratory muscle function. Directing a person to relax with a slow out-breath as they let their shoulders 'drop and flop' into a relaxed position, can help achieve greater relaxation of the shoulders, upper back, and neck. If accessory muscles are required for breathing, resting a hand on the upper back or moving it slowly in a downward movement can encourage slower breathing.

Controlled breathing techniques

Breathing retraining or controlled breathing techniques involve sitting upright, breathing in through the nose and out through the mouth, and focusing on using the diaphragm. Pursed lip breathing (PLB) helps slow breathing down by prolonging exhalation. These techniques help develop a slower, relaxed, and more efficient breathing pattern.

Activity pacing and planning

Helping the patient and family learn to plan and pace activities is central to promoting self-care and well-being. Finding ways of integrating controlled breathing techniques, relaxation, and new techniques for washing, dressing and climbing stairs into a person's daily life, requires sensitive, skilled, and knowledgeable caring.

Further reading

Bredin M, Corner J, Krishnasamy M, Plant H, Bailey C and A'hern R (1999). Multicentre random-ized controlled trial of nursing intervention for breathlessness in patients with lung cancer, *British Medical Journal*, **318**, 901–4.

Davis C (1997). Breathlessness, cough, and other respiratory problems: ABC of Palliative Care, *British Medical Journal*, **315**, 931–4.

Moore S, Plant H, and Bredin M (2006). Breathlessness. In Kearney N, Richardson A (eds). *Nursing Patients with Cancer. Principles and Practice*, pp.511–25. London: Elsevier Churchill Livingstone.

Website

🖥 Breathlessness Research Charitable Trust: www.breathlessness.org/

Cancer-related fatigue

Causes and assessment

Fatigue is one of the most common and distressing symptoms experienced by people with cancer. It is characterized by a lack of energy, being tired, weak, worn out, or exhausted, and is unrelieved by rest or sleep. This results in feeling less able to do mental or physical tasks. It can severely restrict activities, and this can lead to social isolation and impact on relationships. All patients should be informed of the likelihood of fatigue, and given self-care information, before it becomes a major impediment to their quality of life.

Multiple factors are associated with the onset of cancer-related fatigue, including psychological morbidity (particularly depression), serious viral infection, anaemia, and life events. Cancer-related fatigue is most commonly associated with treatment phases.

Treatment-related causes of cancer-related fatigue

Surgery
Post-operative fatigue may be linked to changes in muscle physiology, or they may occur as part of a general stress response to surgery.

Radiotherapy
Fatigue commonly occurs from the first day of treatment, and intensifies over a course of therapy, reaching a plateau between the second and fourth week.

Chemotherapy
Fatigue is one of the most frequent and distressing side effects of chemotherapy. It varies in intensity over the course of treatment, the length of cycle, within each cycle, and within each day.

Hormone therapy and biological response modifiers (BRMs)
Fatigue is recognized as an overwhelming side effect of biological therapy. However, our understanding of associations between BRM and fatigue is limited.

Assessment

Assessment should aim to identify:
- The nature and severity of the fatigue:
  - Onset and duration of the fatigue: at what point did the fatigue appear? How long has it been going on?
  - Nature and effects of the fatigue: what does it feel like and what effects does it have on the patient's lifestyle?
  - Treatable factors: pain, anaemia, depression, infection, cachexia, electrolyte imbalance and comorbidities.
- Behavioural factors that contribute to the continuation of the fatigue: sleep disturbance, inadequate balance of exercise and rest. Psychological factors: presence of distress, in response to the fatigue experienced.
  What helps to alleviate the fatigue? Does the patient already have strategies that help?

A number of instruments have been developed to measure fatigue. See Wu and McSweeney for a review[1]. However, in clinical practice, ask the following questions:
- Have you been experiencing fatigue?
- How has it been impacting on your life?

and then assess the above factors. This should enable an effective assessment to be carried out.

1 Wu H S and McSweeney M (2001). Measurement of fatigue in people with cancer. *O Nursing Forum* **28**(9), 1371–84.

Management

Many of the fatigue management strategies are behavioural. Therefore education and counselling are central to the effective management of fatigue. Patients on treatment may believe that fatigue is a sign of disease progression and may be cautious about discussing it. Reassuring them that fatigue is temporary in these situations can be reassuring.

The patient's clinical status, i.e. active treatment, comorbidities, stage of disease, will influence management and treatment strategies, e.g. the balance between exercise and rest.

Non-pharmacological approaches

A number of non-pharmacological interventions are available to help patients to live with fatigue. It is important to coordinate these interventions with other MDT members, including OTs and physiotherapists.

These include:

Exercise: evidence clearly supports the use of exercise to reduce the impact of fatigue. It promotes increased functional capacity and psychological well-being. Any programme of exercise needs to be individualized, taking into account the patient's age and gender, the type of cancer present, the treatment the patient is receiving for cancer, and the patient's physical fitness level.

It should be used cautiously if patients have comorbidities, such as bony metastasis, bone marrow immuno-suppression, or other treatment complications.

Rest: this complements exercise, but care should be taken not to detract from a restorative sleep pattern; naps should be reduced, and replaced by relaxation, e.g sitting quietly rather than lying down.

Energy conservation: patients can conserve energy through setting priorities, pacing themselves and delegating tasks. A structured daily routine, scheduling activities at times of peak energy can be helpful.

Attention-restoring interventions: promoting enjoyable pastimes increases the capacity to concentrate and direct attention.

Educational interventions: these help in promoting appropriate self-care activities to combat fatigue.

Psychosocial interventions: such as counselling, progressive muscle relaxation (☐ Progressive muscle relaxation), and group support, may result in higher energy levels and reduced feelings of tiredness.

Pharmacological approaches

The most commonly used pharmacological approaches include:

Treatment of anaemia: causes of anaemia need to be properly investigated. Iron or folic acid supplements may help. *Erythropoietin* has been demonstrated to increase energy levels after treatment in anaemic cancer patients receiving chemotherapy. Red cell transfusions may also be prescribed (📖 Blood product support).

Corticosteroids: such as prednisolone or dexamethasone, these are often prescribed for their effects on appetite, mood, and energy levels.

Progestogens: such as medroxyprogesterone acetate (MPA) or megestrol acetate (MA). These are prescribed to relieve anorexia and cachexia in patients whose fatigue may be related to cachexia.

Psychostimulants: limited evidence is available to support the use of psychostimulants, such as Ritalin®, to treat cancer-related fatigue, although there are clinically favourable reports of their use.

Treatment of depression: there is a clear association between cancer-related fatigue and depression, though whether the fatigue is a causative factor in the depression, or vice versa, has not been established. *Anti-depressants* may be particularly useful in managing fatigue that is accompanied by depressive symptoms.

Further reading

Ream E and Stone P (2004). Clinical Interventions for Fatigue, In J Armes, M Krishnasamy, and I Higginson (eds) *Fatigue in Cancer* pp.255–71. Oxford: Oxford University Press.

Richardson A (2004). Critical Appraisal of the Factors Associated with *Fatigue*. In J Armes, M Krishnasamy, and I Higginson (eds). *Fatigue in Cancer* pp.29–44. Oxford: Oxford University Press.

Ahlberg K, Ekman T, Gaston-Johansson F, *et al.* (2003). Assessment and management of cancer-related fatigue in adults. *Lancet* **362**, 640–50.

Nail L M (2002). Fatigue in patients with cancer. *Oncology Nursing Forum* 29, 537–544.

Website

National Comprehensive Cancer Network: www.nccn.org/default.asp

Malignant effusions

Introduction

Malignant effusions are abnormal collections of fluid. They most commonly occur in the peritoneal or pleural space. They are generally a sign of advanced metastatic disease. They can be managed but the fluid normally reaccumulates, often within a short space of time.

Malignant ascites (MA)

MA is accumulation of fluid in the peritoneal cavity. It occurs when the volume of naturally occurring fluid of the peritoneal lining (situated between the parietal and visceral peritoneal membranes) is too great to drain away through the diaphragmatic lymphatic vessels; or when the drainage pathways become blocked. It is most commonly associated with ovarian, colon, breast, and pancreatic cancers and adenocarcinoma of unknown origin[1].

Aetiology

MA may result from:
- Tumour compression of the hepatobiliary blood vessels.
- Increased permeability of the peritoneal lining and cavity (particularly the omentum); or the tumour itself may produce fluid.
- Obstruction of the diaphragmatic lymphatic vessels.

Presenting symptoms
- Abdominal discomfort (pain).
- Feeling bloated and uncomfortable.
- Nausea and vomiting.
- Inability to sit or bend easily.
- Loss of appetite, indigestion.
- Fatigue, breathlessness.
- Distress associated with altered body image.

Diagnosis
- Drainage and cytological examination of the fluid.
- Disease history.
- Detailed observation and assessment of patient problems.

Treatment

Treatment is suggested when the symptoms of MA are distressing, particularly abdominal pain and breathlessness.

Evidence is limited about which is the best treatment. The main approaches include:

Paracentesis: drainage of fluid from the peritoneal cavity using a catheter. The catheter may be placed by ultrasound guidance.
- Rate of drainage—practice varies. Some centres allow free drainage for the first 5 litres. There is little evidence of causing hypovolaemic shock. However, if the patient is hypotensive drainage can be stopped temporarily. Others guidelines are more cautious: 1 litre every 2 hours.

---

1 Dolan S and Preston N (2005). Malignant Effusions, In N Kearney and A Richardson (eds), *Nursing Patients with Cancer: Principles and Practice.* pp.619–31. London: Elsevier Churchill Living-stone.

- No evidence of benefit from albumin post drainage.
- Catheters are removed generally once drainage has slowed significantly or after 24 hours. Any longer increases risk of infection.
- Pain management. Insertion and removal of the catheters can be painful and patients may have abdominal pain/discomfort during the fluid removal. Adequate analgesia should be prescribed and administered throughout.

Indwelling catheter: a semi-permanent drainage catheter left in situ to enable drainage of fluid at home. This requires either stoma nurse or community nurse involvement. The rate of infection is higher than for paracentesis alone.

Diuretic therapy: although widely used to manage malignant ascites, there is uncertainty about its efficacy. It may cause dehydration with limited impact on peritoneal fluid volume.

Peritoneovenous shunt: a shunt is placed in the peritoneal cavity, under local anaesthetic. It tunnels under the skin and enters the vena cava. Fluid shifts along the shunt due to pressure changes during breathing. It can reduce the need for further paracentesis and can relieve symptoms. Limitations include shunts blocking or becoming infected.

Palliative chemotherapy: this may be given to try and shrink the tumour, therefore reducing obstruction and potentially relieving ascites.

Nursing management
Malignant ascites is a distressing and debilitating consequence of cancer. Abdominal discomfort, fatigue (📖 Cancer-related fatigue) and alterations in body image (📖 Altered body image) all require skilled nursing support. Comprehensive nursing assessment of this problem will allow nurses to support patients and their families to live with its demands, which often necessitate frequent hospital or hospice admission as the disease advances. Informational support about the different approaches to management is required, particularly as there is limited evidence about their effectiveness.

Malignant pleural effusion

Pleural effusion is the accumulation of fluid in the pleural space (between the parietal and visceral layers encasing the lungs). It can be caused by malignant and non-malignant triggers, such as infection, severe burns or congestive cardiac failure. Almost half of patients diagnosed with lung or breast cancer will develop an effusion during their illness, and malignant pleural effusions are present in approximately 50% of patients who die of cancer.

Aetiology
Malignant pleural effusions (MPE) may occur for several reasons:
- Infiltration of the pleura by the tumour.
- Alteration in the integrity of the pleural lymphatic system.
- Metastatic spread to the visceral pleural surface, or to the parietal pleura.
- Confounding co-morbid conditions such as renal failure, congestive cardiac failure, or pulmonary embolus.

Presenting symptoms
- Breathlessness, cough, chest pain.
- General flu-like malaise.
- Anorexia and weight loss may also be present.

Diagnosis
- Detailed observation and assessment of the patient's presenting problems.
- On auscultation, decreased breath sounds, dullness to percussion and decreased fremitus (vibration felt by hand placed on chest when patient speaks or coughs).
- Tracheal deviation—if the effusion is large.
- Chest X-ray.
- Ultrasound and CT may be helpful if the effusion is small or the fluid is loculated (in pockets).
- Thoracocentesis—if the effusion is confirmed in the absence of an enlarged heart or if cancer is strongly suspected.
- Other options include thoracoscopy, pleuroscopy, or surgical biopsy.

Treatment
- If a patient is asymptomatic, surveillance alone may be the treatment option of choice.
- If the primary tumour is amenable to treatment, the effusion may resolve once systematic treatment is established.

For symptomatic patients:

Thoracocentesis and tube drainage
- Small bore tube introduced after local anaesthetic under CT or ultrasound guidance.
- Position and absence of pneumothorax checked on X-ray.
- Tube aspirated and placed on low suction.
- Generally followed by sclerosis to prevent re-accumulation of the fluid.

Sclerosis (pleurodesis)
- Obliterates pleural space.
- Sclerotic agent introduced into the pleural space.
- Agents used include tetracycline or its derivatives, bleomycin, sterile talc.

Tunnelled long-term catheters and drainage
- Can be useful in community setting, reducing need for regular hospital admission.

Pleuroperitoneal shunting
- Can be used when pleurodesis is not possible or is unsuccessful.

Nursing management

Thoracocentesis
Patients should be premedicated with an opioid analgesic and have regular monitoring of pain post-procedure. Patients also need monitoring of temperature, signs of respiratory distress or bleeding, which could indicate infection, pneumothorax, or haemothorax.

Pleurodesis
Patients often get severe pleuritic pain with pleurodesis even with intrapleural local anaesthetic. Sedation and opioids may both be required. Patients need assistance with repositioning post procedure to enable the sclerosing agent to contact the entire pleural surface.

Effective nursing management of patients with MPE requires skill and expert knowledge. Presenting symptoms such as breathlessness (📖 Breathlessness) are frightening and patients normally have a poor prognosis with advanced disease. The choices of treatment are complex and involve procedures that are sometimes invasive, painful, and frightening.

Further reading
Antunes G, Neville E (2000). Management of malignant pleural effusions, *Thorax*, **55**, 981–3.
Smith E M, Jayson G C (2003). The current and future management of malignant ascites. *Clinical Oncology*, **15**(2), 59–72.

Nausea and vomiting

Treatment-related nausea and vomiting

Introduction

Nausea is an unpleasant feeling of the need to vomit, often accompanied by autonomic sensations. Vomiting is the forceful expulsion of gastric contents through the mouth. Nausea is generally the most distressing long-term symptom of the two, but it is often under-assessed.

Physiology

The physiology of nausea and vomiting is not yet fully understood. Evidence suggests that both are coordinated by the vomiting centre (VC) and the chemoreceptor trigger zone (CTZ) in the mid brain. Key chemoreceptors involved in the process of relaying messages from various organs to the VC include serotonin (5HT3), dopamine, substance P/neurokinin-1, histamine, and acetylcholine.

Common causes

- Chemotherapy or radiotherapy.
- Infection.
- Drugs, e.g. opioids, antibiotics, NSAIDs, digoxin.
- Gastrointestinal stasis, intestinal obstruction.
- Pain.
- Metabolic e.g. hypercalcaemia, renal failure.
- Brain metastases (raised intracranial pressure).
- Psychosomatic e.g. fear, anxiety.

Radiotherapy-induced nausea and vomiting (RINV)

The site of radiotherapy treatment will determine the risk of nausea and vomiting. Higher doses of radiation, longer duration of treatment and a larger treatment field will also increase the risk.

High risk	Intermediate risk
• Total body irradiation.	• Abdominal pelvic.
• Whole or upper abdominal.	• Cranium.
• Hemi body irradiation.	• Craniospinal.
• Lower thorax.	• Mantle.

For high-risk radiotherapy, administer a 5HT3 antagonist prior to each treatment. Add in dexamethasone if the nausea or vomiting is not controlled. If still unsuccessful, follow CINV guidelines.

For intermediate risk, use metoclopramide or domperidone. Swap to a 5HT3 antagonist if it is not controlled.

Chemotherapy-induced nausea and vomiting (CINV)

Nausea and vomiting are two of the most distressing symptoms of chemotherapy treatment. They impact on quality of life, cause a range of other side effects such as malnutrition and oesophageal injury, and can affect treatment compliance.

Up to 70% of patients receiving chemotherapy will experience some nausea and vomiting, although it is highly regimen-dependent.

High risk agents (>90%)	Moderate risk agents (30–90%)	Low risk agents
• Cisplatin >50mg/m^2 • Carmustine >250mg/m^2 • Cyclophosphamide >1g/m^2 • Lomustine >60mg/m^2 • Dacarbazine >500mg/m^2	• Cyclophosphamide <1g/m^2 • Carmustine <250mg/m^2 • Cisplatin <50mg/m^2 • Anthracyclines • Carboplatin • Irinotecan • Melphalan • Oxaliplatin • Methotrexate >1g/m^2 • Cytarabine >1g/m^2	• Methotrexate <250g/m^2 • Mitoxantrone • Asparaginase • Cytarabine • Docetaxel • Paclitaxel • Fluoruracil • Gemcitabine

CINV generally occurs in three distinct phases:

1. *Anticipatory nausea and vomiting*: this occurs prior to a new cycle of chemotherapy.
2. *Acute nausea and vomiting*: this occurs in the first 24 hour period after chemotherapy.
3. *Delayed nausea and vomiting*: this occurs more than 24 hours and up to 72 hours post-chemotherapy.

Management of CINV

Assessment

Prevention is the key, as once CINV occurs it can be difficult to control. Accurate assessment is a crucial part of management. The following must be considered:

• Emetogenic potential of the chemotherapy regimen—consider drugs, dose, and schedule.
• Other causes of nausea and vomiting (📖 Nausea and vomiting).
• Patient risk factors: those that increase the risk of CINV include age (being younger), female, history of motion sickness, previous uncontrolled nausea/vomiting after chemotherapy, severe pregnancy-related sickness, and high levels of anxiety.

A history of chronic alcohol ingestion actually reduces the risk of CINV.

Note: if a patient has two or more risk factors, consider starting them on a higher level of anti-emetic cover than normal for any specific chemotherapy regimen.

Nurses have a major role in both pre- and post-treatment assessment. A thorough initial assessment will establish any risk factors for nausea and vomiting, beyond the actual chemotherapy regimen.

Once treatment has started, nurses need to assess any nausea and vomiting, including:

• The number of episodes, their time, and duration. Ensure that you assess separately for nausea and vomiting.
• The effectiveness of any drug/non-drug measures.
• The behavioural, emotional, and physical impact of the symptoms.

Drug management

Anti-emetic drugs are the cornerstone of managing CINV. They usually act by competitively blocking receptors for serotonin, histamine, and dopamine at the CTZ and VC.

Table 45.1 highlights the main approaches for managing both acute and delayed symptoms. The anti-emetic course should be continued for 72 hours post-chemotherapy, if there is a risk of delayed symptoms. In the UK, each clinical area should have a protocol for management of CINV, which should be followed.

Side effects of anti-emetics

The side effects of the most common anti-emetics, plus their management are highlighted in Table 45.2.

Recent advances

Aprepitant (Emend®) is a substance P/neurokinin-1 antagonist. Substance P appears to have a key role in delayed nausea and vomiting. It interacts with dexamethasone, and doses of steroids may need reducing if aprepitant is added into regimens.

Palonosetron is a new 5HT3 antagonist, with a half-life of 37 hours—this increases its effectiveness in delayed nausea and vomiting.

Both drugs increase the potential cost of anti-emetic regimens; and further trials are required to establish their specific role within CINV.

Non-pharmacological management

There is some evidence that nausea and vomiting can be reduced by a number of non-pharmacological techniques, such as progressive muscle relaxation (📖 Progressive muscle relaxation), guided imagery, or acupressure (the use of 'sea bands').

These should not replace standard anti-emetic therapies, but they can be successfully added to care, to enable patients to increasingly take control and successfully manage treatment side effects (📖 Complementary therapy).

Other non-pharmacological management

- Reduce environmental triggers: a calm environment away from sight and smell of food, control of odours (colostomy, malignant wounds, distance from toileting facilities). A single room may be appropriate.
- If the person is nauseated at home, can someone else take over food preparation? Suggest ready prepared meals. Regular small snacks may be more effective than large meals.

Table 45.1 Pharmacological management of CINV[1]

Emetogenic risk	Acute symptoms		Delayed symptoms
High	5HT3 antagonist (e.g. tropesitron or granisetron) + dexamethasone		5HT3 antagonist + metoclopramide (or domperidone) + dexamethasone
Moderate	5HT3 antagonist + dexamethasone	Followed by:	Dexamethasone ± metoclopramide (or domperidone)
Low	Dexamethasone alone or either a dopamine agonist, prochlorperazine or haloperidol.		No prophylactic anti-emetics
Minimal	Nothing		No prophylactic anti-emetics

Notes

- There are no clinically meaningful differences between the currently available 5HT3 antagonists. Oral and IV regimens are equivalent when correctly dosed.
- If there is failure on one level, then move up to the next level, i.e. from *low to moderate or moderate to high*. If failure occurs at the top level, then a different 5HT3 antagonist can be used. Addition of lorazepam (given sublingually) can also be useful, but causes sedation.
- Levomepromazine antagonizes several receptors, so it can also be considered. Low doses (6.25mg) are effective in the majority of individuals and should not cause sedation. A small proportion of people will require 12.5–25mg od.
- Remember to reassess and consider other causes of nausea and vomiting in cases of resistant CINV, particularly in patients with advanced disease.

1 Miller M, Kearney N (2004). Chemotherapy-related nausea and vomiting—past reflections, present practice and future management. *European Journal of Cancer Care*, **13**, 71–81.
Antiemetic Unifying Consensus Meeting (2001). Use of Antiemetics prevent CINV. Meeting held at Columbia University, New York, 21–22 April.

Table 45.2 Side effects of anti-emetics

Drug classification	Side effects	Management
5HT3 antagonists	Headache, constipation, fatigue, dry mouth, dizziness	Analgesics for headache. Administration of laxatives as required or prophylactically for constipation
Phenothiazines, metoclopramide, and butyrophenones	Extrapyramidal reactions (EPRs) particularly for patients under 30 years of age. Phenothiazines can also cause sedation	Close observation for signs of EPRs, e.g. agitation, restlessness, tremor, muscular or facial twitching
Corticosteroids	Agitation, insomnia, increased appetite, dyspepsia, fluid retention. Perirectal burning when given IV	Give IV infusions slowly
Benzodiazapines	Sedation	Use cautiously if patients have poor respiratory status

Note: an antimuscarinic drug such as procyclidine can be used to stop any severe extrapyramidal reactions.

Anticipatory nausea and vomiting (ANV)

Anticipatory nausea and vomiting (ANV)

This is best described by the concept of 'Pavlovian' classical conditioning; the patient associates aspects of the treatment, such as the nurse or the hospital environment, with nausea or vomiting. On future occasions, these associations are enough to cause further nausea or vomiting, even before administration of the chemotherapy.

People who have had moderate to severe nausea or vomiting after their previous course of chemotherapy generally experience ANV more severely. Other risk factors include being under 50 years of age, susceptibility to motion sickness, being female and having a high level of anxiety. Screening for these risk factors could influence preventative management, e.g. increasing initial anti-emetic cover[1].

Prevention is the key, as once established, ANV can be hard to manage. Initial, effective anti-emetic management is crucial.

Due to the psychological aspects of the condition, the use of progressive muscle relaxation treatment (☐ Progressive muscle relaxation), the support of a psychological specialist (☐ Psychological support), or benzodiazepines such as sublingual lorazepam can be effective.

Further reading

Grunberg S M and Ireland A (2005). Epidemiology of chemotherapy induced nausea and vomiting. *Advanced Studies in Nursing*, **3**(1), 9–15.

1 Eckert R M (2001). Understanding anticipatory nausea. *Oncology Nursing Forum*, **28**(10), 1553–660.

Nausea and vomiting in advanced cancer

Nausea and vomiting are often multi-causal, with different chemoreceptors involved; and a combination of anti-emetics may be required to manage it successfully. Regular nursing assessment is crucial, as the causes of nausea and vomiting may change over time.

Management

Identify potential reversible causes, and ensure they are treated appropriately:
- Pain.
- Infection—give antibiotics.
- Cough—give an antitussive.
- Hypercalcaemia—give fluids and bisphosphonates (📖 Hypercalcaemia).
- Raised intracranial pressure—give corticosteroids.
- Emetogenic drugs—stop or reduce dose.
- Anxiety—give anxiolytics or psychological management (📖 Anxiety management).

Administer anti-emetic most likely to resolve nausea and vomiting
- Always give anti-emetics regularly, not prn.
- Oral medication can control nausea, but alternative routes will be required for vomiting, such as per rectum or SC.

If this is not successful or partially successful, the patient may require an increased dose or a different anti-emetic may be tried.
- If the cause is certain, then the first step is to increase the dose. Otherwise, combine anti-emetics that have different actions.
- Levomepromazine acts on several receptor sites and can be a useful broad spectrum antiemetic, though it can cause sedation at doses above 6.25mg bd.

Note: cyclizine may antagonize the prokinetic effect of metoclopramide, and they should not usually be given together.

The common causes of nausea and vomiting, and drug management options are highlighted in Table 45.3.

Table 45.3 Causes of nausea and vomiting and drug management

Cause of vomiting	Choice of antiemetics
Drug or endogenous toxins	Haloperidol 1.5mg twice a day
	Levomepromazine 6.25mg
Constipation	Metoclopramide
Gastric stasis	Domperidone
Intestinal obstruction	(📖 Bowel obstruction)
Raised intracranial pressure	Cyclizine 150mg/24 hrs po or SC
	Dexamethasone 4–16mg

Nursing management of nausea and vomiting

- Nurses have a key role in assessment. Separately assess nausea and vomiting. Identify potential causes and ensure treatment of any reversible causes.
- Ensuring regular, safe administration of anti-emetics, including frequent observations for common side effects such as extra pyramidal reactions, constipation, and sedation.
- Informing patients of the early signs of side effects, and the need to alert a health care professional about these. For example, contacting their GP or their cancer treatment centre if they are vomiting or nauseated at home.
- Assessing fluid balance and managing fluid replacement, including IV as required.
- Assessing weight gains or losses, and providing additional nutritional intake as required (📖 Nutritional support).
- Providing vomit bowls, privacy, and regular oral care to maintain comfort.
- Supporting and advising patients in using non-pharmacological measures as appropriate.

Further reading

Twycross R, Wilcock A (2001). *Symptom Management in Advanced Cancer*, 3rd edn, p.104. Oxford: Radcliffe Medical Press.

Warr D G (2005). Prevention and treatment of chemotherapy-induced nausea and vomiting after emetogenic chemotherapy. *Advanced Studies in Nursing*, **3**(1), 22–9.

Nutritional disorders

Nutritional issues

Malnutrition

Malnutrition is defined as a severe deficiency of protein and inadequate caloric intake. It occurs when there is an imbalance between dietary intake and nutritional requirements, resulting in wasting of muscle and multisystem dysfunction. There are usually clinical complications such as delayed wound healing, risk of infection, and increased mortality. Malnutrition is common in cancer patients and can adversely affect the patient's quality of life and survival.

Incidence

Ranges from 25–36% for tumours such as testicular and breast to much higher incidences for pancreatic, upper GI, and head and neck tumours (72–83%). Evidence has shown that 45% of all patients with cancer lose more than 20% of their pre-illness weight with 25% losing more than 20% pre-illness.

Causes of malnutrition

- Reduced oral intake—due to anorexia, nausea, and vomiting and altered taste and smell.
- Effects of tumour—due to odynophagia (pain on swallowing), dysphagia and catabolic effects of the tumour (see cancer cachexia, below).
- Psychosocial—due to depression, anxiety, and food aversions.
- Effects of cancer treatments—such as surgery, chemotherapy, and radiotherapy.

Cancer cachexia

This is a complex, multifactorial syndrome characterized by:
- Progressive involuntary weight loss.
- Anorexia and early satiety.
- Skeletal muscle atrophy.
- Generalized tissue wasting.
- Immune dysfunction.
- Metabolic alterations.
- Early satiety.

Cachexia is commonly associated with advanced cancer and the weight loss seen is due not only to the problems caused by the reduction in food intake but also by the metabolic abnormalities occurring. Metabolic abnormalities and immune system responses lead to:
- Increased resting energy expenditure.
- Competition between the tumour and the host for nutrients.
- Increased fat breakdown.
- Immune response: release of cytokines, e.g. interleukins, interferon, which increase metabolism and reduce appetite.

Clinical effects of cancer cachexia/malnutrition

- Poor tolerance of treatment and increased number of treatment breaks.
- Reduction in quality of life.
- Higher morbidity and mortality rates.
- Progressive weakness.
- Apathy and irritability.
- Skin breakdown.
- Impaired wound healing.
- Depressed immune system functioning.

See Van Cutsem and Arends[1] for in-depth discussion of metabolic disturbances leading to cachexia.

Table 46.1 Some common nutritional side effects of cancer treatment

Surgery	Chemotherapy	Radiotherapy (depends on site treated)
• Intestinal resection can cause malabsorption • Reduced capacity to take normal food portions • Problems associated with chewing and swallowing if surgery to head and neck region • Decreased intake due to preoperative starvation	• Nausea and vomiting • Mucositis • Diarrhoea • Anorexia • Stomatitis • Learned food aversions • Fatigue	**Head & neck:** • Mucositis • Dry mouth • Pain on swallowing **Chest:** • Oesophagitis • Dysphagia • Nausea and vomiting **Abdomen and pelvis:** • Diarrhoea • Nausea and vomiting • Radiation enteritis • Malabsorption

Note: effects may be exacerbated by combination therapies, e.g. surgery and radiotherapy or chemoirradiation.

1 Van Cutsem E, Arends J (2005). The causes and consequences of cancer-associated malnutrition. *European Journal of Oncology Nursing*, **9**, 51–63.

Nutritional support

The aim of nutritional support is to maintain or improve nutritional status and weight and to maintain strength and energy. This can lead to reduced side effects, improve toleration of treatment, enhance mobility and independence, and maintain or improve quality of life.

The main components of nutritional support are:
- Nutritional screening.
- Dietary advice.
- Oral nutritional supplements.
- Enteral nutrition.
- Parenteral nutrition.

Nutritional screening

Malnutrition can occur at any point during the course of the cancer journey, and screening must be performed at regular intervals. Screening should be carried out on admission to hospital or first attendance at outpatients to identify patients who are malnourished or at risk of malnutrition. A validated screening tool used nationally is the MUST tool (malnutrition universal screening tool) and there is also an American nutritional screening tool developed specifically for cancer patients known as the PG-SGA (patient generated—subjective global assessment). The screening tool is usually completed by nursing staff and is performed to identify those patients that need to be referred onto a qualified, registered dietitian for a full dietary assessment and individualized and specific dietary advice and support.

Dietary advice

Patients require advice and encouragement to modify their general healthy eating guidelines and regular meal patterns. For example they may currently be using a lot of low fat or low calorie food products, which may not be appropriate during cancer treatment. The dietitian can provide advice that is tailored to meet the individual patient's needs, whilst taking into account their personal food preferences. Regular follow-up from the dietitian or nursing staff can promote adherence to any nutritional regimens.

Oral nutrition support

Oral nutrition is the preferred source of support in patients who are able to consume food and fluid. It is important to keep the patient's diet as closely as possible to normal, as this reinforces the normality of their everyday life. This can be supplemented by commercially available supplements where necessary.

Dietary management
- Texture modification: such as adapting meals e.g. soft, mashed, or puree.
- Food fortification: including the addition of extra butter, cream, milk, and sugar to increase energy and calorie content.
- Adaptation of meal times: encouraging small frequent meals.

Oral nutrition supplements

Oral nutrition supplements are widely available, can be readily prescribed on the advice of a dietitian, and are useful when inadequate dietary intake is identified. Their use must be monitored and reviewed regularly (preferably by a registered dietitian) to ensure their effective use. However, if patients report taste fatigue, supplements can be incorporated directly within a meal without too much disruption. The benefits of oral nutrition supplements are to:

• Increase calorie and nitrogen intake.
• Stimulate appetite.

Types of oral nutrition supplements

Oral sip feeds
• Various types available e.g. milk, juice, yoghurt.
• High in calories and protein.
• Some nutritionally complete.
• Some contain eicosapentaenoic acid (EPAs which are n-3 fatty acids) and antioxidants which are thought to be of benefit to patients with cancer-related weight loss as they interfere with the mechanisms of cachexia at multiple levels.

Fortified puddings
• Useful in case of dysphagic patients who have a delayed swallow.
• Provide calories and protein in smaller volume.

Modular supplements
• Concentrated sources of calories/protein/fat either individually or in combination.
• Carbohydrate-based powders and drinks should only be given to diabetics under strict supervision.
• Can be incorporated into everyday foods.

Enteral nutrition

May also be referred to as 'tube feeding' where a tube is placed directly either into the stomach or small intestine via the nose or direct percutaneous route. Commonly used tubes are nasogastric, gastrostomy, and jejunostomy.

Enteral feeding can be used for patients who are not able to take sufficient nutrients orally due to a variety of reasons such as anorexia, dysphagia, or mucositis and when the patient has a functioning gut. It is *not* appropriate for the following patients:

• Patients with a bowel blockage.
• Patients suffering from severe nausea, vomiting and/or diarrhoea.
• Patients whose stomach or intestine are not working properly or have been removed.

The type of tube used will depend on the tumour site, anticipated duration of feeding, and patient's overall physical condition.

Benefits of enteral nutrition
- Nutrition can be delivered past obstructed areas, e.g. head and neck.
- Nutrition can be delivered at a slow, continuous rate permitting optimal use of a limited absorptive capacity over a long period of time.
- Prescribed feed may be tolerated better than oral nutrition products.

Enteral nutrition can be used as the sole source of nutrition or used in combination with oral or parenteral nutrition. The dietitian will calculate the patient's daily nutritional requirements and devise a feeding regimen that takes into account:
- Assessed nutrition needs.
- Patient's preference/wishes.
- Treatment regimen.
- Ability to administer the feed.
- Mobility.
- Prognosis.

The feed can be given continuously via a pump or intermittently as a bolus feed. Feeds are ready to use in a liquid form and contain energy, protein, fluid, and vitamins and minerals. Common complications of nasogastric feeding include tube displacement whereas for gastrostomy tubes complications include pneumoperitoneum, infections, leakage, hypergranulation, and erosion of the tube flange into the gastric mucosa (buried bumper syndrome).

Typical feeds are
- Standard feed: 1kcal/mL.
- High calorie: 1.2–2kcal/mL.
- Fibre feeds: combination of soluble and insoluble fibre added to the above.
- EPAs added.

Patients do not necessarily have to remain in the hospital whilst receiving enteral nutrition as it can be undertaken at home. To ensure a safe discharge, good communication between the hospital and community teams is required. There should be agreement on who will provide prescriptions for feed and equipment.

Parenteral nutrition

This is nutrition that bypasses the normal digestive system, instigated when the patient is unable to tolerate oral or enteral nutrition. Nutrients are administered by the IV route via a dedicated central or peripheral placed line.

The provision of parenteral feeding should be used only when all other forms of nutrition support have been tried or if the GI tract is not accessible. There are a number of complications including:
- Line infection.
- Thrombosis.
- Metabolic disturbances.

Indications
- Patients with a non-functioning gut.
- Patients suffering from severe nausea, diarrhoea, or vomiting.
- Patients suffering from severe sores in the mouth or GI tract.
- Patients with a fistula in the stomach or oesophagus.
- Patients who have received surgery to the head and neck.
- Patients with upper GI obstruction.

Commencing a patient on parenteral nutrition should be a carefully considered decision involving the patient and members of the multidisciplinary team, taking into account the potential benefits and risks. It is an invasive and relatively expensive form of nutrition support.

Complications
Though parenteral nutrition can be offered at home, this requires careful facilitation and planning and may delay discharge plans in some situations.

Further reading

Bozzetti F (2001). In Payne-James J, Grimble G & Silk D (eds) *Artificial Nutrition Support in Clinical Practice* pp.639–680. London: Greenwich Medical Media.

Brown J K (2002). A systematic review of the evidence on symptom management of cancer-related anorexia and cachexia. *Oncology Nursing Forum* **29**, 517–32.

Van Bokhorst-de van der Schueren M A E (2005). Nutritional support strategies for malnourished cancer patients. *European Journal of Oncology Nursing,* **9**, 74–83.

Elliott L (ed) (2006). *The Clinical Guide to Oncology Nutrition,* 2nd Edn. The American Dietetic Association.

Shaw C (ed) *Current Thinking: Nutrition and Cancer.* Norvatis.

Websites

British Association for Parenteral and Enteral Nutrition: www.bapen.org.uk/

NICE guideline: CG32 Nutrition support in adults February 2006: www.nice.org.uk/

Support of specific nutritional complications

Anorexia/weight Loss

The loss of appetite or desire to eat is a common symptom in patients. This leads to an energy deficit due to poor dietary intake, and results in weight loss.

Causes

Multifactoral and can include:
- Pain.
- Cancer treatment.
- Medication.
- Constipation.
- Depression.

Dietary management
- Serve smaller portions of food more frequently.
- Increase nutrient density of food, in particular energy, fat, and protein.
- Encourage participation in shopping and preparation at mealtimes.
- Advise methods for simplified meal preparation to reduce anxiety at mealtimes.
- Encourage a social atmosphere at mealtimes.
- Limit drinks at mealtimes to prevent early satiety, whilst ensuring adequate daily fluid intake.
- Drink liquids between meals such as milkshakes and oral sip feeds.
- Seek medical advice for appropriate appetite stimulants.
- Advise gentle exercise and/or small glass of alcohol pre-meal to stimulate appetite, if appropriate.

Anorexia can cause a great deal of anxiety and upset between the patient and the carer. The patient has no desire to eat and the carer is concerned and may prepare elaborate meals encouraging them to eat. Management needs to support both parties with advice and encouragement.

Xerostomia (📖 Oral mucositis and related problems)

Definition
Abnormal dryness of the mouth due to insufficient secretions.

Causes
- Treatment—radiotherapy can affect the production of saliva from the salivary glands, whilst surgery may remove certain salivary glands.
- Medication, e.g. anti-emetics, diuretics, opioids, some antidepressants.
- Dehydration.

Can cause sensation of food sticking in the mouth as well as increasing the risk of dental caries and gum disease due to the reduction in saliva.

Dietary management
- Encourage adequate fluid intake (8–10 glasses a day), timed to ensure optimum food intake.
- Ensure effective oral care.

- Use of artificial saliva e.g. lozenges, sprays.
- Chewing sugar-free gum or sucking on boiled sweets or ice cubes may help to moisten mouth.
- Softer foods or foods that can be mashed up may be better tolerated.
- Extra sauces, gravy, or butter can be added to moisten meals.
- Sips of fluids with meal. Be warned that excessive fluid intake may lead to early satiety.
- Try very sweet or tart foods and drinks as may stimulate saliva.

Dysphagia

Definition
Difficulty in swallowing food or liquid.

Causes
- Mechanical obstruction—due to site of tumour.
- Extrinsic compression—due to tumour in a lung, bronchus, or from chest wall compressing on the oesophagus.
- Neurological dysfunction—due to surgery or a brain tumour blocking innervation of the swallow reflex.
- Inflammatory—due to side effects of radiotherapy or chemotherapy.
- Oral candidiasis.

Symptoms
- Difficulty in mastication and swallowing.
- Coughing or choking during meals.
- Pain during swallowing.
- Aspiration after swallowing.
- Sensation of food lodged in the throat.

Management
Note: ensure advice is provided by the speech and language therapist to establish if the patient has a safe swallow or is at risk of aspiration.

Dietary management
- Soft foods and foods that can be mashed might be better tolerated.
- Some patients may need to liquidize or even strain their food through a sieve to remove all lumps.
- Milk, cream, white sauces, and condensed soup can be added to foods when liquidizing to moisten the food more and add more calories and protein.
- Extra sauces and gravies can be added to meals.
- Strained baby foods should *not* be used as their nutritional content is low for adults.
- Fluids can aid with swallowing, to 'flush' the food passed the obstruction, but must ensure that this does not affect appetite.
- If required (as advised by the speech and language therapist) thickened fluids can help ensure patient consumes sufficient and thicken to prescribed consistency.

Note: management only acts as a guideline. Specialized advice should be provided by a registered dietitian based on the patient's reported symptoms.

Pain management

Introduction

Pain is not an inevitable symptom of advanced cancer; however it is a common symptom when caring for people with advanced disease. Pain is defined by The International Association for the Study of Pain (IASP) as: 'an unpleasant sensory and emotional experience associated with actual or potential tissue damage or described in terms of such damage'. In other well-known definitions, pain is described as being 'whatever the experiencing person says it is, existing whenever he [she] says it does'[1]. There is much debate about the adequacy of these definitions in terms of the complex multidimensional nature of pain and indeed in terms of whether patients experiencing pain will necessarily report it.

Barriers to effective pain management
- Over- or under-prescribing of analgesia.
- Inappropriate prescribing.
- Lack of a comprehensive assessment.
- Fears about the side effects of drugs.
- Fears about addiction.
- Lack of education in pain management.
- Professional carers' beliefs and values about a person's pain experience.
- Lack of follow-up and reassessment.

Incidence of pain in cancer
- 25% of patients do not experience pain.
- 33% of patients with pain have one pain.
- 33% of patients have two separate pains.
- 33% of patients have three or more pains.

The causes of cancer pain
Pain in patients with cancer may be from many sources. They may have more than one pain, each with a differing cause. Establishing the cause/causes of pain will make it easier to manage.

A person with cancer can have pain related to the following causes:
- The cancer itself:
    - Extension into the soft tissues.
    - Visceral involvement.
    - Bone involvement.
    - Nerve compression or destruction.
    - Raised intracranial pressure.
    - Obstruction, e.g. bowel obstruction.
- Pain related to the cancer treatment, e.g.
    - Radiotherapy skin damage.
    - Chemotherapy-induced mucositis.
- Pain related to the cancer and debility e.g.
    - Lymphoedema.
    - Constipation.

---

1 McCaffery, M (1968). *Nursing practice theories related to cognition, bodily pain and non-environment interactions*. Los Angeles: University of California.

- A concurrent disorder, unrelated to the cancer, e.g.
  - Osteoarthritis.

The perception of pain is determined by

- The patient's mood.
- The patient's morale.
- The meaning of the pain for the individual[2].

Further reading

The International Association for the Study of Pain (IASP). http://www.iasp-pain.org

2 Twycross R G and Lack S (1984). *Therapeutics in Terminal Cancer* London: Churchill Livingstone.

assessment

essing a person's pain requires a number of skills in communication, ch as listening, verbal and written reporting skills, relationship building, and observation. Patients in pain may have more than one pain, each of these needs to be assessed and considered separately. Assessment of pain is an ongoing process that requires systematic updating and re-evaluation of the situation, in other words constant re-assessment.

A narrative approach to pain assessment is often helpful; it keeps the focus on the patient and their experience of pain. This approach focuses the assessment on the person's story and key issues for them related to the experience. A key question using a narrative approach might be 'Would you tell me all about your pain?' A question like this incorporated within a conversation will enable clinical decision-making regarding the appropriate interventions to manage the person's pain (📖 Assessment).

There are many methods of taking a pain history; if a structured and systematic approach to pain assessment is required the following themes and questions may be helpful:
- **Location:** Where is your pain? Is there more than one site? Can you point to the area?
- **Intensity:** How bad is the pain? What number would you give your pain on a scale of 0–10? (0 being no pain and 10 being the worst pain.) Are you able to divert your attention away from the pain? What is the impact of the pain on your activities of daily living?
- **Quality:** What does it feel like? What words would you use to describe your pain?
- **Onset:** What brings on or provokes your pain?
- **Duration:** How long have you had this pain? And how long does it last? Is it constant or does it come and go?
- **Relief:** What relieves or helps your pain?
- **Increase:** Is there anything which increases your pain or makes it worse?
- **Radiation:** Does the pain go anywhere else? Does it move around?
- **Experience:** What are the effects of the pain?
- **Anything else** I need to know about your pain?

Pain assessment tools

Pain assessment tools may be helpful in providing documentary evidence of pain management and to aid communication between the person in pain and the health care professionals. However, assessment tools need to be appropriate to the situation and assess what they purport to assess.

The follow is a selection of pain assessment tools:

Visual analogue scales (VAS)

The VAS is a 10cm line with the anchors or ends marked with 'no pain' and 'worse pain.' This self-reported tool represents the intensity of a person's pain by marking the point on the line which best represents their pain. Some people may find the idea of a line representing their pain as a difficult concept to understand and may not be able to apply this

idea to their pain experience. One criticism of this tool is the difficu.
associated with the VAS, as a person rating their pain as 'worst pain
which then further intensifies. Progression of pain experience may be
more sensitive and more easily understood if the VAS is used vertically,
rather than horizontally. This tool only attempts to assess pain intensity
as opposed to the multi-dimensional aspects of the pain experience.
Photocopying the VAS can change the length of the line, which should be
100mm> If this happens it threatens the reliability and validity of the tool.

No pain .... Worst pain

Verbal rating scale (VRS)

A verbal rating scale is a tool, which uses a series of descriptive words to
represent the intensity of pain, for example:

| None | Mild | Moderate | Severe |

Or

| No Pain | A little pain | A lot of pain | Too much pain |

The verbal rating scale is a simple and quick tool to use however it may
have little resonance for some people in pain if the descriptive words do
not fit with their experience or if a more comprehensive tool is required.

Numerical rating scales (NRS)

The NRS is similar to the VAS but has numbers along the 10cm line to
indicate the intensity of pain.

No pain .....1.....2....3......4.....5......6.....7....8.....9......10......Worst pain

It has some of the same problems as the VAS in that pain may be rated
at 10 and then intensifies further leaving no place on the scale to
acknowledge that increase.

More complex tools aim to capture the multi-dimensional nature of the
pain experience. An example of these is the Brief Pain Inventory
(Fig. 47.1). This multidimensional tool seeks to assess the pain experience
in a more comprehensive way. It attempts to use words to describe the
pain, a body map to locate the pain and questions, which seek to include
the social impact and the physical activity of the person.

Pain diaries

Asking a person in pain to keep a diary of their experiences can be a
helpful way to gain an understanding of how the experience has had an
impact on their life and what interventions have been helpful. Some
people will find this activity positive as it enables them to take a more
active role in managing their pain.

Pain may be assessed differently according to the setting. For example, in
the acute hospital setting there may already be a tool in use and practitioners may be expected to utilize the same tool. Tools need to take
account of the time available for assessment, resources, staff experience,
reliability and validity, and how acceptable they are to the person in pain.

Brief Pain Inventory

Date: __/__/__

Name: _____ _____ _____
          Last   First   Middle Initial

Phone: ( )_____   Sex: ☐ Female ☐ Male

Date of Birth: __/__/__

1) Marital Status (at present)
   1. ☐ Single   3. ☐ Widowed
   2. ☐ Married   4. ☐ Separated/Divorced

2) Education (Circle only the highest grade or degree completed)
   Grade   0   1   2   3   4   5   6   7   8   9
           10   11   12   13   14   15   16   M.A./M.S.
                        Professional degree (please specify) _____

3) Current occupation_____
   (specify titles; if you are not working, tell us your previous occupation)

4) Spouse's Occupation_____

5) Which of the following best describes your current job status?
   ☐ 1. Employed outside the home, full-time
   ☐ 2. Employed outside the home, part-time
   ☐ 3. Homemaker
   ☐ 4. Retired
   ☐ 5. Unemployed
   ☐ 6. Other

6) How long has it been since you first learned your diagnosis? ____ months

7) Have you ever had pain due to your present disease?
   1. ☐ Yes   2. ☐ No   3. ☐ Uncertain

8) When you first received your diagnosis, was pain one of your symptoms?
   1. ☐ Yes   2. ☐ No   3. ☐ Uncertain

9) Have you had surgery in the past month?   1. ☐ Yes   2. ☐ No

10) Throughout our lives, most of us have had pain from time to time (such as minor
    headaches, sprains, and toothaches). Have you had pain other than these everyday
    kinds of pain during the last week?   1. ☐ Yes   2. ☐ No

IF YOU ANSWERED YES TO THE LAST QUESTION, PLEASE GO ON TO QUESTION 11
AND FINISH THIS QUESTIONNAIRE. IF NO, YOU ARE FINISHED WITH THE
QUESTIONNAIRE. THANK YOU.

11) On the diagram, shade in the areas where you feel pain. Put an X on the area that hurts
    the most.

12) Please rate your pain by circling the one number that best describes your pain at its
    worst in the last week.
    0   1   2   3   4   5   6   7   8   9   10
    No   Pain as bad as
    Pain   you can imagine

13) Please rate your pain by circling the one number that best describes your pain at its
    least in the last week.
    0   1   2   3   4   5   6   7   8   9   10
    No   Pain as bad as
    Pain   you can imagine

14) Please rate your pain by circling the one number that best describes your pain on the
    average.
    0   1   2   3   4   5   6   7   8   9   10
    No   Pain as bad as
    Pain   you can imagine

Fig. 47.1 Brief pain inventory. Reproduced with permission from Doyle *et al.* (2005)
The Oxford Textbook of Palliative Medicine, 3rd edn. Oxford: Oxford University Press.

15) Please rate your pain by circling the one number that tells how much pain you have right now.

   0   1   2   3   4   5   6   7   8   9   10
No   Pain as bad as
Pain   you can imagine

16) What kinds of things make your pain feel better (for example, head, medicine, rest)?

_____

17) What kinds of things make your pain worse (for example, walking, standing, lifting)?

_____

18) What treatments or medications are you receiving for your pain?

_____

19) In the last week, how much relief have pain treatments or medications provided? Please circle the one percentage that most shows how much relief you have received.

0% 10%   20%   30% 40% 50% 60%   70%   80%   90% 100%
No   Complete
Relief   Relief

20) If you take pain medication, how many hours does it take before the pain returns?

☐ 1. Pain medication doesn't help at all   ☐ 5. Four hours
☐ 2. One hour   ☐ 6. Five to twelve hours
☐ 3. Two hours   ☐ 7. More than twelve hours
☐ 4. Three hours   ☐ 8. I do not take pain medication

21) Circle the appropriate answer for each item.
I believe my pain is due to:

☐ Yes ☐ No   1. The effects of treatment (for example, medication, surgery, radiation, prosthetic device).

☐ Yes ☐ No   2. My primary disease (meaning the disease currently being treated and evaluated).

☐ Yes ☐ No   3. A medical condition unrelated to primary disease (for example, arthritis).

22) For each of the following words, check yes or no if that adjective applies to your pain.

Aching	☐ Yes	☐ No	Exhausting	☐ Yes	☐ No
Throbbing	☐ Yes	☐ No	Tiring	☐ Yes	☐ No
Shooting	☐ Yes	☐ No	Penetrating	☐ Yes	☐ No
Stabbing	☐ Yes	☐ No	Nagging	☐ Yes	☐ No
Gnawing	☐ Yes	☐ No	Numb	☐ Yes	☐ No
Sharp	☐ Yes	☐ No	Miserable	☐ Yes	☐ No
Tender	☐ Yes	☐ No	Unbearable	☐ Yes	☐ No
Burning	☐ Yes	☐ No			

23) Circle the one number that describes how, during the past week, pain has interfered with your:

A. General Activity

   0   1   2   3   4   5   6   7   8   9   10
Does not   Completely
Interfere   interferes

B. Mood

   0   1   2   3   4   5   6   7   8   9   10
Does not   Completely
Interfere   interferes

C. Walking ability

   0   1   2   3   4   5   6   7   8   9   10
Does not   Completely
Interfere   interferes

D. Normal work (includes both work outside the home and housework)

   0   1   2   3   4   5   6   7   8   9   10
Does not   Completely
Interfere   interferes

E. Relations with other people

   0   1   2   3   4   5   6   7   8   9   10
Does not   Completely
Interfere   interferes

F. Sleep

   0   1   2   3   4   5   6   7   8   9   10
Does not   Completely
Interfere   interferes

G. Enjoyment of life

   0   1   2   3   4   5   6   7   8   9   10
Does not   Completely
Interfere   interferes

Pain Research Group, Department of Neurology, University of Wisconsin-Madison

Fig. 47.1 (Contd.)

Principles of analgesic use

Analgesic drugs should be given
- *Orally* whenever possible.
- *Regularly* in order to prevent pain in advance, rather than trying to alleviate it once it becomes established.
- *Systematically*, starting with mild, to moderate and strong, according to the WHO analgesic ladder[1].

World Health Organization analgesic ladder[1]
- The first step in using the WHO analgesia ladder is to use simple analgesics for example, paracetamol for mild to moderate pain.
- When this is no longer adequate to manage the pain and it persists or increases a 'weak' opioid, such as codeine, should be added.
- If the pain persists or increases when the maximum therapeutic dose has been reached, the next step should be used.
- The third step on the ladder is the use of strong opioids, such as morphine.
- Adjuvant drugs can be used at any point to enhance the analgesic effect.

Often morphine is started at too low a dose. Two tablets of co-codamol 30/500 contains 60mg of codeine, which is already approximately equivalent to oral morphine 5mg every 4 hours. If converting to morphine it will therefore be necessary to use a minimum of morphine 5mg but a starting dose of 10mg 4 hourly may be needed. In older people and those in renal failure a more cautious approach is required, as active morphine metabolites are excreted by the kidney.

When prescribing NSAIDs it is important to check for any history of asthma as this may be exacerbated by NSAIDs, and any history of bleeding or ulceration. This does not exclude use, when NSAIDs are used for prolonged periods or for those people at risk, a gastroprotective drug, for example, lansprazole is usually prescribed.

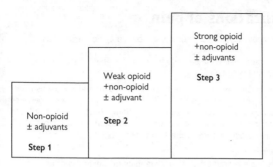

Fig. 47.2 The WHO analgesic ladder[1]

Adjuvant drugs (co-analgesics)

An adjuvant drug refers to an analgesic drug for specific types of pain, drugs that enhance the effect of other analgesics, or drugs that help treat concurrent symptoms. Examples include gabapentin (for neuropathic pain), baclofen (for muscle spasm), midazolam (for anxiety or agitation), and dexamethazone (for nerve root compression), NSAIDs, such as diclofenac (for bone pain). Adjuvant drugs can be added to any step of the analgesic ladder. Commonly more than one adjuvant drug may be required.

1 http://www.who.int/en/

Classifications of pain

There are many ways to classify pain, e.g. pain may be classified as:
- Acute.
- Persistent non-malignant.
- Persistent malignant.

In addition, pain may be classified according to neural mechanism, for example, nociceptive and neuropathic. It is important to distinguish between pain caused by the stimulation of nerve endings (nociceptive pain) and pain caused by nerve dysfunction or compression (neuropathic pain). Patients may have a mixture of the two types.

Neuropathic pain

This usually has a characteristic sharp, stabbing quality and is often partially responsive to treatment with opioids such as morphine. In addition, to the above classifications, it may be helpful to consider pain as opioid- responsive (pain relieved by opioids), semi-responsive (pain partly relieved by opioids), or non-responsive (pain not relieved by opioids).

Concept of total pain

The concept of total pain was introduced by Cicely Saunders in 1964, to describe pain which considered the whole pain experience holistically rather than merely the physical. Total pain encompasses the physical, psychological, social, and spiritual aspects of the experience of pain at the end of life.

Breakthrough pain

Breakthrough pain is that which occurs between regular doses of analgesic drugs. It may or may not be related to activity. The presence of breakthrough pain may suggest that the regular dose of analgesia needs to be increased.

Table 47.1 Nociceptive and neuropathic pain

Pain type	Example	Description
Nociceptive		
Visceral	Liver capsule pain	Sharp
Somatic	Bone pain	Deep aching/gnawing
Muscle spasm	Cramp	Cramp/spasm
Neuropathic		
Peripheral	Neuroma	Burning/stabbing
Central	Spinal cord compression	Numbness/weakness
Mixed	Post-herpetic neuralgia	Cutting/stabbing/shooting/burning

Use of opioid drugs

Morphine is the drug of choice for moderate to severe pain in advanced cancer and is step 3 on the WHO analgesic ladder (see Fig. 47.2).

Starting on morphine

- Start with immediate release tablets or liquid. Adults who are not pain-controlled on regular weak opioids start with 10mg, 4 hourly. 5mg for older people or those with poor renal function.
- Elderly or frail patients start at 2.5–5mg.
- Prescribe a laxative at the same time as commencing morphine.
- Some people will require an anti-emetic if they have a history of nausea or vomiting. These symptoms usually subside within 48 hours of starting morphine. Haloperidol 1.5mg nocte may be helpful.
- Opiate naïve patients (i.e. who are new to morphine) may feel drowsy for the first 2 days after starting morphine but this should not persist for more than a few days.
- When people start morphine for the first time an information booklet is helpful to address any concerns.
- Advise patients to avoid driving for the first week after starting morphine or after any increases in dose.

Titrating the dose of morphine

If the patient is taking 2 or more prn doses in 24 hours, due to break-through pain, increase the regular dose by 30–50%. If the pain is mor-phine-responsive, continue the upward titration of the morphine dose until there is adequate pain relief or intolerable side effects, in which case it may be necessary to consider an alternative.

Morphine preparations

Morphine is available in several immediate- and slow-release preparations.
- Immediate release: oramorph/ sevredol 10mg/5ml, 20mg/ml liquid or tablets (4 hourly).
- Slow-release:
  - 12 hourly: MST and Zomorph® 5, 10, 15, 30, 60, 100, 200mg tablets.
  - 24 hourly: MXL 30, 60, 90, 120, 150, 200mg capsules.
- Rectal morphine, 10, 15, 20, 30mg suppositories.
- Morphine sulphate injection 10, 30, 100mg in 5ml vials.

Converting to slow-release morphine

If a patient's pain is well controlled on oral, immediate-release morphine, converting to slow-release morphine has the benefits of reducing admini-stration to 12 hourly and enabling a more even blood level of the drug. This is done by calculating the total 24-hour dose and dividing by 2. For example: 20mg/4 hourly is 120mg so the slow release dose is MST 60mg 12 hourly. Ensure that a patient taking slow release morphine has access to an immediate release morphine for breakthrough pain.

Calculating breakthrough doses

The breakthrough dose of oral morphine is calculated by dividing the 24 hours dose (180mg) by 6. This would be 20mg in the above example. If the regular, slow release, MST dose is raised, say to 90mg, the breakthrough dose also needs to be increased, resulting in this example in a breakthrough dose of 30mg.

Diamorphine

Diamorphine is commonly used as an injectable strong opioid in a syringe driver. Its advantage over morphine is that it is more soluble in water.

Typically the 24-hour dose is divided by 3 to give the 24-hour S/C dose. For example, 10mg 4 hourly morphine, is 60mg morphine in 24 hours, divided by 3 is 20mg diamorphine in a continuous S/C infusion over 24 hours.

Use of other opioids

In addition to morphine and diamorphine several other strong opioids are available and are used in palliative care including:
- Hydomorphine.
- Oxycodone.
- Fentanyl.
- Alfentanil.
- Methadone.
- Buprenorphine.

Pethidine is rarely used in palliative care due to its short duration of action. The main reasons for using an alternative, strong opioid other than morphine or diamorphine are patient choice, reluctance of the patient to take morphine despite information and explanation, and renal failure. In complex pain situations it may be appropriate to consider alternative opioids, such as fentanyl, in order to reduce the side effect profile and as some pain may respond more effectively to the alternative choice.

Use of syringe drivers in pain control

Syringe drivers are used in palliative care to administer continuous subcutaneous medication when a person is unable to take medication orally. Medication may be given via a syringe driver for pain management and for the management of other symptoms such as agitation. Prior to commencing a syringe driver it is important to discuss its use with the patient and/or family. This may help to allay some of the fear and concern attached to the use of a syringe driver, which may be viewed as a last resort. The advantage of a syringe driver is that it enables the continuous administration of several medications, for multiple symptoms, avoiding the peaks and troughs of oral analgesics.

Indications for use:
• Intractable nausea and/or vomiting.
• Difficulty in swallowing (for example, in the case of head and neck tumours).
• Person too weak to take oral medication.
• Decreased conscious level.

The syringe driver most commonly used in palliative care is the Graseby, MS26, battery operated variety. In acute settings battery pumps may not be used and alternative syringe drivers, such as the Grasby 3200, may be used. The analgesic drug of choice for use in syringe drivers is diamorphine because of its solubility; as a result it can be administered in small volumes of fluid. However, it has been in short supply in some settings, in which case morphine sulphate is used.

The following drugs may be mixed with diamorphine in a syringe driver:
• Cyclizine: anti-emetic
• Haloperidol: anti-emetic/antipsychotic
• Metocloprimide: anti-emetic
• Octreotide: synthetic analogue
• Midazolam: sedative
• Hyoscine butylbromide: anti-muscarinic
• Levomepromazine: anti-emetic/antipsychotic
• Ondansetron: anti-emetic
• Glycopyrronium: anti-muscarinic
• Granisetron: anti-emetic

For more information on drug combinations in syringe drivers see http://palliativedrugs.com

The following drugs are not suitable for subcutaneous use as they cause skin irritation or soreness at the injection site:
• Diazepam.
• Chlorpromazine.
• Prochloperazine.

It is possible to mix two or more drugs in the same syringe for delivery via a syringe driver provided they do not react adversely with each other. Care should be taken when mixing diamorphine and cyclizine in higher concentrations as this can precipitate. The skin site and the driver and tubing need to be checked regularly. Diluting the diamorphine as much as possible before adding the cyclizine can reduce the risk of this happening.

The infusion is given subcutaneously at any suitable site via a 'butterfly needle'. Sites commonly used are the upper arms and the abdomen. The site should be changed if it becomes red, sore, or indurated.

Luer lock connections between the tubing and the syringe provide a safer system. Local guidance relating to the use of syringe drivers are now available in most cancer networks and should be followed, including the procedure for labelling the syringe driver and recommended dilutant.

Non-pharmacological interventions for pain management

The following measures are helpful in the management of pain instead of, or in addition to, pharmacological drugs. They provide an opportunity for nurses in particular to utilize their skills to help and support people in pain.

Transcutanous electrical nerve stimulation (TENS)

TENS is a non-invasive method of pain relief consisting of a small electrical pulse generator, which connects to 2 or 4 electrodes on the skin. The electrical impulse, which is battery powered can be adjusted to deliver a variety of strength, duration, and frequency of impulse. One of the positive aspects of this method is that the person in pain controls the impulse.

TENS is effective in some people however, not everyone will gain relief from this method. Some settings do not endorse nurse administration of TENS and suggest physiotherapists have a key role in the use of this method.

Massage

May be helpful for some people experiencing pain, it is thought to work in a similar way to TENS. Gentle stroking movements of, for example, the hands, feet, or back can be relaxing, provide the comfort of touch and provide an additional analgesic effect. Massage may be particularly effective when there is muscle tension contributing to the pain experience.

Distraction

Distraction therapy, for example, television, radio, reading, music, company, talking, puzzles, etc., is commonly used as a method of pain relief. It enables the person in pain to focus on something other than the pain and is commonly used by people with persistent pain. Often people will have their own ways of managing persistent pain developed over time and may include differing strategies for night and day time. It is important to try to continue these if the person is admitted to hospital.

Relaxation

Relaxation exercises can be taught. One way is to teach the person in pain to systematically tense and then relax all muscles throughout the body, starting from the toes until the muscles of the face are reached. Some people find that relaxation audiotapes are of help and are a guide to this process. Others may find music a source of relaxation and distraction. Visualization provides an opportunity to go outside of one's self to another place as a means of escaping the pain and can be taught as a non-invasive approach to pain management. (Progressive muscle relaxation).

Breathing exercises

These are a helpful strategy to teach a person in pain, particularly while waiting for analgesia to take effect. These may be simply helping a person to slow down their breathing rate by breathing with you or by encouraging the person to extend their exhaled breath by breathing slowly through their mouth. Some people find assistance with breathing exercises useful initially but are then able to utilize this as a strategy themselves.

Comfort measures

Comfort measures, for example, positioning, splinting, heat, and cold are all part of a skilled nurse's repertoire in caring for people in pain. Other useful strategies that contribute to general comfort are:
- Finding a comfortable position in bed or in a chair.
- Using pillows for support.
- The use of pressure-relieving mattresses or aids.
- Fresh bedding, a pleasant outlook in the room or from the window.
- The use of personal effects like family photographs.

Presence—being with the person in pain

Presence and hearing about the person's experience and story can be helpful in itself. If the person along side the patient is confident and sensitive to the experience of pain and is willing and able to be there even when it is distressing to watch, this is usually helpful to the person in pain. Sensitive to the experience means knowing when to talk or be silent, knowing when to use touch, knowing how to 'be' with the person in pain.

Effective communication

Communication with people who are in pain is particularly important. Having information about the pain experiences for example the cause, potential treatments, drug measures, and side effects is usually helpful to people. Having a dialogue with a patient about their experience of pain and understanding their perspective, including the impact of the pain on their quality of life is part of effective communication. However, for some people being able to verbalize their pain is not easy, or is impossible. People with dementia may be unable to verbally report or describe their pain, in which case the nurse has to rely on getting to know the person and being alert to changes in behaviour and body language, which may indicate pain.

Radiotherapy

Radiotherapy has a role in managing pain, particularly bone pain associated with metastatic disease (📖 Metastatic bone disease), and chest pain in lung cancer (📖 Management of non-small cell lung cancer).

Further reading

Dickman, A et al. (2005). *The Syringe Driver: Continuous Subcutaneous Infusions in Palliative Care* 2nd edn Oxford: Oxford University Press.

International Association for the Study of Pain (1986) Classification of chronic pain. Descriptions of chronic pain syndromes and definitions of *pain* terms *Pain* (Supplement 3) S1–S226.

Watson M, Lucas C, Hoy A, Back I (2005) *Oxford Handbook of Palliative Care*. Oxford: Oxford University Press.

Website

📷 www.palliativecare.com/

Symptom management at the end of life

Introduction

Common symptoms at the end of life include:
- Noisy breathing ('death rattle').
- Pain.
- Restlessness.
- Agitation.
- Confusion.
- Breathlessness.
- Weakness.
- Nausea and vomiting.

When managing symptoms at the end of life, it is not usually appropriate to undertake investigations unless they will influence the choice of treatment offered, e.g. to exclude reversible causes.

When it becomes clear that the person is dying, it is important to review the appropriateness of all medication, and any that does not contribute directly to the comfort of the patient may be stopped. For example, analgesia, anti-emetics, anticonvulsants, and anxiolytics may be continued if appropriate via a syringe driver or an alternative route, if the person is unable to take them orally.

A key aspect of end of life care, particularly at home, in the community, is the anticipation of needs and forward planning, having the medication and resources available to respond rapidly as needed, as far as the circumstances allow.

Noisy breathing: 'death rattle'

Death rattle is noisy, rattling breathing that occurs when the dying person is unconscious and close to death, and is unable to cough or clear secretions. It is caused by the collection of secretions in the upper airway, and difficulty in clearing them. Although death rattle can be distressing to family members, it does not need to be, if there is adequate explanation, and management should be tailored to the needs of the patient and family.

Nursing management

It is important to observe the patient for signs of a build-up of secretions, and assess, where possible, the level of distress experienced by the patient. Families need to know the reason for the noisy breathing, options for treatment and to be involved in decision-making. The following measures have a role in prevention and management of death rattle:

- Re-positioning on the patient's side to aid drainage of secretions.
- Frequent mouth care (if the patient is able to tolerate it) is required as the anti-muscarinic drugs will dry the mouth.
- If IV fluids are in progress and the volume of secretions is excessive or causing distress, fluids may be reduced or discontinued to maintain patient comfort (☐ Ethics in cancer care).
- There are several options for drug management of death rattle. Anti-muscarinic drugs may be started at the first sign of noisy breathing, or if the patient is showing signs of distress.
- The following 3 drugs are commonly used in palliative care centres, to treat respiratory secretions at the end of life. There is a lack of evidence regarding the efficacy of one drug over another, and attention should be paid to local protocols.
  - Hyoscine butylbromide (Buscopan®) 20mg stat and 20–60mg/24 hours by SC infusion in a syringe driver.
  - Hyoscine hydrobromide 0.2–0.4mg stat and 0.4–1.2mg/24hrs by SC infusion.
  - Glycopyrronium 0.2–0.4mg stat and 0.6–1.2mg/24 hours by SC infusion in a syringe driver.
- Hyoscine butylbromide has the advantage that it does not precipitate in syringe drivers; however the volume of fluid is larger.
- Suction can be distressing for the patient and is rarely necessary. It can damage the mucosa, may increase the amount of secretions being produced and create a dry mouth. Suction can be used if the above methods do not work, or the if patient is distressed by them.

Further reading

Bennett M, Lucas V, Brennan M, et al. (2002). Using anti-muscarinic drugs in the management of death rattle: evidence-based guidelines for palliative care, *Palliative Medicine* **16**, 369–74.

Wee B L, Coleman, P G, Hillier, R et al. (2006). The sound of death rattle 1: are relatives distressed by hearing this sound? *Palliative Medicine* **20**, 171–5.

Terminal agitation

Terminal agitation is a state of agitation and distress found at the end of life. It can be a very difficult condition for both the patient and their family, and can make the experience of dying a very traumatic event.

There are similarities with acute confusional states, but terminal agitation is associated with the experience of dying, and is not clearly caused by reversible factors (though causes may be multifactorial). The subjective experience of spiritual pain or anguish may be a feature.

It is most important that any reversible causes of agitation at the end of life are identified and treated, for example: anxiety, pain, breathlessness, dehydration, full bladder or rectum, organic brain disease, or the effects of prescribed drugs.

Nursing management

As the patient will usually be acutely distressed by the condition, it is most important to communicate effectively with them and their family, identify their wishes, and respond as fully as possible under the circumstances.

The following are key aspects of management:
- Safety of patient, family, and practitioners.
- Maintain dignity and privacy.
- Communicate effectively.
- Presence of a nurse or family member may reassure the patient.
- Maintain an environment that is free of disruption and distraction.

(See also ⚏ Acute confusional states.)

Terminal sedation

Care needs to be taken giving sedation at the end of life. The expressed needs of the patient and family must be taken into account, as well as the need to maintain the comfort and dignity of the patient (⚏ Ethics in cancer care). The following are options for managing terminal agitation:
- Midazolam 5–10mg stat and 30–60mg/24hr SC infusion in a syringe driver.
- Levomepromazine 25mg stat and 50–100mg/24hr SC infusion in a syringe driver.

If a syringe driver is not available, other benzodiapine or phenothiazine drugs may also be used, in sublingual or rectal routes.

Further reading

Maluso–Bolton M N (2000). Terminal agitation. *Journal of Hospice and Palliative Nursing,* **2**(1), 920.

Psychological reactions to cancer

Introduction

Reactions to cancer

Having cancer is unavoidably distressing. Feelings of distress can be expressed in a number of ways, for example, by crying, seeking reassurance, anger, or hostility. People at any stage of cancer can find it hard to concentrate, make decisions, or take in information. We cannot make assumptions about how an individual will react, or how they will show their distress. Reactions are very individual, and people tend to develop characteristic ways of reacting to painful or stressful events in their lives. This will depend on both personal and social factors.

Personal factors

Some people characteristically react by sharing their feelings with friends or family. Others will keep things to themselves, and not share their feelings, or 'bottle things up'. Neither is right or wrong, and we cannot make assumptions about one way or the other being 'healthy' or 'normal'. People will react in ways that are 'normal' for them.

Social factors

Reactions will also be determined by factors in the social environment. This can include what is expected of gender roles, for example, that men do not cry. Also, roles within families can influence reactions. Individuals may feel that they have to be 'strong' for other family members.

Distress and mood

Distress is only one feature of a person's reaction to illness. Mood (or *affect*) is a term used to describe someone's emotional state, and has a very specific meaning in relation to mental illness, i.e. disorders of mood, including anxiety and depression.

Stress and coping

The concepts of stress and coping are frequently used to understand the reactions of people who are diagnosed with cancer. Stress describes the demands made by the cancer on the individual, and coping describes their efforts to manage these demands. Coping is modified by the appraisal that the individual makes of the stress, i.e. how they appraise their ability to deal with it.

Coping

Individuals develop characteristic ways of coping with stress, and there is some evidence of particular styles that are seen in people with cancer:
- Fatalism.
- Positive avoidance (denial).
- Helplessness–hopelessness.
- Fighting spirit.
- Anxious preoccupation.

Claims have been made that certain coping styles are more effective in dealing with cancer, and may even improve survival (e.g. fighting spirit).

However, the evidence is controversial, and some patients may feel under pressure to adopt a 'positive' attitude to their illness, adding to their existing burden of coping. Coping style itself may not be relied upon as a predictor of the ability to cope.

Poor coping

Certain factors in the patient's history or environment have been identified as significant in limiting their ability to cope, including:

- Lack of social support or social isolation.
- Previous psychiatric history.
- Alcohol or drug abuse.
- History of recent losses.

These factors are useful in identifying the risk of poor coping, enabling support to be targeted at those in greatest need. An inability to cope may show itself as uncontrollable emotions or distress, difficult or disruptive behaviour (e.g. behaviour that upsets family), or excessive alcohol use.

Adjustment and transition

Another way of conceptualizing people's response to cancer is that of adjustment or transition. This is not about response to stress but response to an ongoing and changing situation. Rather than being uniformly stressful, a diagnosis of cancer may bring both positive and negative effects. Alongside the losses experienced by people with cancer, many find an enhanced sense of meaning in their lives, closer relationships and a deepened sense of spirituality. There is the potential for both positive and negative effects of cancer, and the period of adjustment has been described as a 'psychosocial transition'.

Further reading

Barraclough J (1999). *Cancer and Emotion. A Practical Guide to Psycho-oncology* (3rd edn). Chichester: John Wiley & Sons.
Brennan J (2001). Adjustment to cancer—coping or personal transition? *Psycho-oncology* **10**(1), 1–18.

Adjustment, stress reactions, and disorders

Everyone diagnosed with cancer will go through a period of adjustment to the new realities of their situation. In most cases—possibly as many as 50%—they will make positive adjustments with the support of their family, friends, and routine professional care. Most people will have no psychopathology, i.e. no diagnosable mental disorder. As many as 20% of people with cancer will experience a mental disorder. Up to 30% will experience some form of emotional crisis that is severe enough to disrupt their lives for at least a brief period. This can include:

- Rapid mood changes (fear, anger, despair, elation).
- Distress and tearfulness.
- Anxiety and agitation.
- Intrusive thoughts that appear without any conscious control, e.g. thoughts of death, pain, loss of loved ones.
- Attempts to avoid painful or uncomfortable thoughts or feelings associated with the illness.
- Disturbed sleep or nightmares.
- Numbness, disorientation, depersonalization (loss of sense of self), or derealisation (feeling like you are not really there).

These are most likely to be experienced in the initial phases of diagnosis and treatment, but can occur at other traumatic periods of the illness e.g. recurrence or other significant bad news.

Stress reactions

When these features are acute and disabling, but last only a brief period, such as a few hours or a few days, they are called an *acute stress reaction*. They usually resolve spontaneously. If these features persist, for between 2 days to a month, then it is an *acute stress disorder*, and may require treatment. This could involve more active psychological support or short-term use of anxiolytics, such as benzodiazepines. If these features persist beyond 4 weeks, then the patient may be experiencing *post-traumatic stress disorder* (PTSD), a very disabling and distressing condition that can be long-lasting if untreated. PTSD requires referral for specialist psychological treatment (ꀁ Psychological support).

Adjustment disorder

Adjustment disorder is a condition that arises in response to an ongoing situation of change, like the effects of cancer and its treatment. It can manifest itself mainly with the features of anxiety or depression.

Further reading

Brennan J (2004). *Cancer in Context A Practical Guide to Supportive Care*. Oxford: Oxford University Press.

Holland J C (ed) (1998). *Psycho-oncology*. Oxford: Oxford University Press.

Smith M Y, Redd W H, Peyser C, Vogl, D (1999) Post-traumatic stress disorder in cancer: a review. *Psycho-oncology* **8**(6), 521–37.

Supporting the cancer patient through periods of adjustment

The contact a nurse has with a cancer patient will vary considerably, from brief contact in an outpatient department, to more sustained and intensive contact during periods of inpatient care, and this will affect the nature of support that can be offered.

Support existing coping strategies

It is important to establish how a patient normally copes with stressful or demanding situations. This gives the best indication of how they will cope with the demands of the cancer. Ask the patient directly how they normally cope by saying, *'What do you normally do to deal with stress?'* Identify whether usual coping strategies are working. For example, someone who normally copes by working hard will find it more difficult to cope if they are unable to work.

Review alternatives

If usual coping strategies are not working, discuss alternatives. These would need to fit with the individual's current level of functioning, energy and ability. It is best if these are discussed rather than suggested, to enable the patient to review what is possible, or desirable for them. Below are some commonly used coping strategies:

- Distraction: listening to music or watching TV.
- Finding a focus of attention outside of the self: reading, doing puzzles, handiwork.
- Physical activity: walking, gardening.
- Being in company, talking.
- Relaxation, meditation.

Social support structures

Most people derive great benefit from social support, from a sense that they are valued and loved. These supports are usually there when professional support is not. Offering professional support to carers is sometimes the most effective support to the person with cancer.

Provide information and offer choices

Give the patient and their carers, information on support available locally and nationally. This may include health and social services and voluntary and charitable organizations. People are more likely to use a service if they make the choice themselves and they feel it will meet their needs.

Intervene and refer when necessary

If the patient does not appear to be coping, then it may be necessary to intervene, to positively offer support or make a referral to a specialist, e.g. social worker, psycho-oncology, or local support group.

Psychological assessment

All health and social care professionals have a role in psychological assessment. However, many aspects of assessment are specialized, particularly where this involves psychiatric diagnosis. The NICE *Guidance on Supportive and Palliative Care for Adults with Cancer*[1] has provided a 4-level model giving guidance on the appropriate level of assessment for different professional groups (compare with figure in ☐ Psychological support).

Level 1

All health professionals should have the ability to acknowledge psychological distress, and identify the patient's and family's concerns. This requires an awareness of the problems that patients and their families are likely to experience, as outlined in the preceding section, and an ability to elicit concerns.

Level 2

More experienced and specialized nurses, for example, site-specific cancer nurses, can be expected to assess the impact of cancer on patient's daily lives, mood, work and family relationships (including sexual relationships). Some will use specific assessment tools, for example the HADS (☐ Depression).

Level 3

This represents an area of overlap between cancer specialists and mental health specialists who have special training in counselling or psychotherapy models, e.g. cognitive behaviour therapy. They should also have an ability to undertake assessment of some psychopathology, e.g. anxiety, depression, psychosexual problems.

Level 4

This level of psychological assessment can only be undertaken by suitably trained mental health professionals.

1 NICE (2004). *Guidance on Supportive and Palliative Care for Adults with Cancer*. London: Department of Health.

Table 49.1 Levels of psychological assessment (adapted from NICE 2004[1])

Level	Group	Intervention
1	All health care professionals	Recognition of psychological needs
2	Professionals with additional expertise	Screening for psychological distress
3	Trained and accredited professionals	Assessing for distress and some psychopathology
4	Mental health specialists	Diagnosis of psychopathology

Depression

Depression is a persistent low mood that does not respond to events. To the depressed person it is often experienced as a lack of feeling, an emptiness, or loss of meaning in life. Depression differs from sadness in both quality and degree. It is a lack of emotion rather than the presence of sadness. The sad person may be cheered up, but the depressed person's mood does not react. Depression is relatively common in people with cancer, possibly as high as 20%.

Features

Depression is actually a constellation of psychological, physical, and social effects, or symptoms. These include:

Psychological: low mood, poor concentration, loss of interest and pleasure in things. Guilt, remorse and pessimism (depressive cognitions), suicidal ideas.

Physical: loss of energy, fatigue, slowing up, poor sleep and appetite, tension and agitation.

Social: reduced social interaction, withdrawal or social avoidance.

Severity

Not all of these will be found in a depressed person, but the more depressed they are, the more of these will be present. The degree of depression is also significant:

Mild depressive episode: associated with a loss of enjoyment in life, deep dissatisfaction, and loss of purpose.

Moderate depressive episode: associated with more depressive symptoms, some severe, more likely to experience sleep disturbance and fatigue, tension and irritability.

Severe depressive episode: likely to be distressed and agitated or physically and mentally slowed up (psychomotor retardation), with depressive cognitions and suicidal ideas. Social and occupational functioning is severely disrupted.

Assessment

The diagnosis of depression is a specialist mental health activity. However, all health and social care professionals can undertake assessment for depression. Some of the features usually used to diagnose cancer are present in many people who are physically ill, and cannot therefore be relied on for diagnostic purposes. These include fatigue, sleep, and appetite disturbance. Other factors that affect psychological assessment include:

• Weakness and exhaustion.
• Nutritional deficiency.
• Cognitive impairment.
• Pain.
• Drugs such as opiates, corticosteroids, benzodiazepines.

It is therefore important to identify treatable causes of distress, and focus assessment on psychological and social features that are clearly diagnostic of depression.

Key diagnostic features of depression

The primary diagnostic feature of depression is persistent, unvarying mood of at least 2 weeks duration.

In addition, the following features confirm the diagnosis:
- Fearful, depressed, or worried appearance.
- Reduced interest and enjoyment of life, social withdrawal.
- Depressive thoughts e.g. guilt, remorse, and pessimism.

Assessment strategies

The best way to assess for depression is to engage the patient directly in conversation. In this way, the nurse can both observe the patient's behaviour, and gain direct information about how the patient is feeling. In observing the patient, note the following signs of depression:
- Avoidance of eye contact.
- A lack of rapport or emotional warmth.
- Speech lacks spontaneity, is monotonous or monosyllabic.

The most useful single question to ask is *'Do you feel depressed?'*. If the answer is yes, then it is useful to identify whether any of the above features are also present.

Carers are a very good source of information. They can say whether the patient's current mood and behaviour are normal for them, or unusual.

Hospital Anxiety and Depression Scale (HADS)

The Hospital Anxiety and Depression Scale (HADS)[1] has been developed specifically to detect depression and anxiety in the physically ill, focusing on the psychological and social manifestations of depression and anxiety. It is quick and easy to use, and it can provide a useful score to underpin a verbal assessment. It gives a score for both anxiety and depression on a scale of 0–21. 8–10 is a borderline score, and scores of 11–21 are clinically significant.

Treat the depression

When depression is present, the patient should be offered treatment. Mild to moderate depression may be treated by non-specialist medical staff, such as GPs. However, severe depression requires a specialist mental health referral.

---

1 Zigmond A S and Snaith R P (1983). The hospital anxiety and depression scale. *Acta Psychiatrica Scandinavica*, **67**, 361–70.

Suicide and suicidal ideas

Suicidal ideas are common in people with depression and in people who have been diagnosed with cancer. This may take two forms:

- Considering suicide as a future option if life becomes unbearable because of pain or lack of dignity. This can be greatly helped by giving the patient and carers information about palliative care options in advanced disease.
- The presence of passive suicidal ideas, that is, wishing to be dead, but not wishing to actively do anything about it. This can occur at difficult stages of illness and treatment, and is usually transitory.

Suicide is not a common event. Approximately 3000 people commit suicide in the UK every year. Suicidal ideas should always be taken seriously. Most people who have suicidal ideas tell someone about them. Although suicidal ideas are not themselves treatable, people experiencing them can be offered support to reduce the risk of acting on them. Suicidal ideas are associated with depression, and depression is treatable.

It is also important to recognize those at increased risk of suicide. The following factors increase the risk of suicide:

- Male gender.
- Older age.
- Mental illness (e.g. depression, schizophrenia).
- Alcohol or drug dependence.
- History of previous self-harm.
- Physical illness—especially with chronic pain.
- Socially isolated.

Nursing management

If patients express suicidal ideas, they should always be taken seriously. It is wrong to believe that someone telling you about suicidal ideas means that they are less likely to do it. Most people who do commit suicide have confided their intentions in someone. Let the patient know that you take their feelings seriously. It is important to make a distinction between passive suicidal ideas (see above) and active suicidal ideas, i.e. when the patient has active intention or plans to kill themselves.

- Spend time with the patient, establishing what their current intentions are.
- Alert your colleagues to what you know of the patient's suicidal ideas, and discuss this as a team.
- Inform senior colleagues who have clinical and managerial responsibility, e.g. senior medical and nursing staff.
- If there is any suspicion that the patient has active suicidal ideas they are likely to act on, then involve a psychiatric colleague urgently.
- It may be necessary to observe the patient closely until the psychiatrist or other mental health specialist arrives.

Active suicidal ideas and active suicidal intention should be shared immediately with colleagues and lead to a referral to a psychiatric colleague.

Treatment of depression

It is very important to treat depression. Depression involves considerable suffering for both the patient and their carers. It is also associated with an increased risk of suicide. Depressed patients are less likely to cooperate with and make progress in their treatment.

Drug treatments

Most episodes of depression will respond to the use of antidepressant medication. Two main groups of antidepressants are in use:
- *Tricyclic antidepressants:* these include amitriptylline, imipramine, and dothiepin. These are effective treatments for depression, but they are not generally recommended for physically ill people as they can have a range of side effects, including dry mouth, blurred vision, and constipation. Tricyclics are not advised for use in suicidal patients as they are cardiotoxic in overdose.
- *Selective serotonin reuptake inhibitors (SSRIs):* these drugs are also effective for depression, but are associated with less side effects, and are therefore used more commonly with the physically ill. Examples are citalopram and fluvoxamine. Fluoxetine can cause agitation, so should be used with caution. Side effects of SSRIs include nausea, vomiting, and headaches. There is a discontinuation syndrome associated with SSRIs that causes insomnia, fatigue, and agitation. It is advisable to reduce the dose gradually, giving it on alternate days, to prevent this. SSRIs should be used with caution or avoided in any patients with hepatic or renal impairment, or who are taking anticoagulants or NSAIDs. Venlafaxine is a related antidepressant that is also used in the physically ill.

Psychological treatments

Some mild to moderate depressive episodes can be helped by psychological means alone, and many depressive episodes will be helped by a combination of medication and psychological treatment.

Cognitive behavioural therapy (CBT)

This is the preferred psychological treatment for depression. There is evidence that negative thought patterns perpetuate a depressed person's pessimistic view of the world, and that helping them to change these patterns overcomes their depressive world-view. CBT is best carried out by a specialist mental health professional trained in its use. Other cognitive behavioural techniques, including problem solving, and a form of CBT designed for use with people with cancer called *adjuvant psychological therapy*, can be used by cancer care professionals with additional training.

Support of the depressed patient

Alongside specific treatments for depression, effective nursing care can help the patient to make a full recovery. Depression can generate cycles of pessimism and hopelessness, which the nurse can help to counteract.

- Respect the patient and acknowledge how they feel, but demonstrate confidence that things can get better.
- Be careful not to collude with and confirm the patient's depressive view of the world. Show empathy with the person, (e.g. *'you must be feeling very low at the moment'*), not the mood (e.g. *'yes, life is awful isn't it?'*).
- Actively engage the patient. This shows them that they are worth getting to know, and counters any loss of self-esteem. Depressed patients will often withdraw from social contact, and the depression may be missed if efforts are not made to engage with them.
- Be aware of the danger of suicide or self-harming activity. Depression is a high risk factor for suicide.
- Be aware of the danger of self-neglect. Help the patient to maintain adequate standards of hygiene and appearance as deterioration undermines self-confidence and morale.
- Get to know the social situation. Support family and friends who will find the situation hard to deal with. Identify factors that will perpetuate or prolong the depression, e.g. relationship or financial problems.
- Encourage physical activity which promotes physical well-being and prevents further deterioration.
- Encourage a return to normal activities as soon as possible.
- Refer on for mental health assessment and treatment when necessary.

Further reading

Endicott J (1984). Measurement of depression in out-patients with cancer. *Cancer* **53**, 2243–48.

Lloyd-Williams, M (1999). The assessment of depression in palliative care patients. *European Journal of Palliative Care* **6**(5), 150–3.

Massie M J, Popkin M (1998). Depressive disorders. In: Holland JC (ed) *Psycho-oncology*. Oxford: Oxford University Press.

Moorey S, Greer S (2002). *Cognitive Behaviour Therapy for People with Cancer* (2nd edn). Oxford: Oxford University Press.

Anxiety

Unlike depression, anxiety is a universal and ever present human experience. It is helpful to educate patients about its effects, so that they can distinguish them from other effects of illness and treatment.

Features

The following are common features of anxiety:

Psychological: fearfulness, apprehension, uncertainty, poor concentration, worrying thoughts, a sense of impending doom.

Physical: tachycardia, hyperventilation, sweating, tremor, frequency of micturition, diarrhoea.

Anxiety is associated with the following behaviour: agitation, seeking reassurance, restlessness, pacing.

Anxiety as a problem

Anxiety can become a problem because of:
- The degree or intensity of the anxiety.
- The duration of the anxiety.
- The nature or effects of the anxiety.

Anxiety can have the following effects, which will impair quality of life and make treating the cancer more difficult:
- Difficulty concentrating.
- Loss of patience or irritability.
- Difficulty taking in information.
- Difficulty making decisions.
- Pain may become more difficult to tolerate.
- Loss of appetite, nausea.
- Sexual dysfunction.
- Sleep disturbance.
- Fatigue.

Panic attacks

These are intense, acute attacks or episodes of severe anxiety, characterized by:
- Chest pain, palpitations, and shortness of breath.
- Intense apprehension or fear, a sense of impending catastrophe.
- Fear of losing control or going mad, or that death is imminent.
- Feelings of depersonalization or derealisation.

Anxiety in cancer care

Aside from the anxieties of everyday life, having a diagnosis of cancer can provoke specific anxieties for patients and their families. As disease status changes, and the patient progresses through treatment, new situations present new challenges. Particular situations that can provoke anxiety include:

- Going for hospital appointments and waiting for the results of investigations. Test results can have major implications for the patient's future, and many patients report the period leading up to this as a particularly anxious time.
- Periods of uncertainty about prognosis or treatment outcome. The period after the end of treatment can be a particularly unsettling time for cancer patients.
- Prior to and during painful investigative procedures.
- Prior to surgery or other treatments, especially if they are new to the patient.
- Prior to discharge after a long period of hospitalization.
- Situations of vulnerability, e.g. being undressed in the presence of staff.
- Any other change in the patient's circumstances which is perceived as threatening.

Physical causes of anxiety

Organic
- Endocrine disorders e.g. hyperthyroidism hypoglycaemia
- Cardiovascular disorders e.g. congestive cardiac failure, arrhythmias
- Respiratory disorders e.g. chronic obstructive pulmonary disease
- Metabolic conditions e.g. hypoxia, encephalitis
- Neurological conditions e.g. delirium

Drugs
- Corticosteroids, bronchodilators
- Drug and alcohol withdrawal

Anxiety management

Anxiety management is a series of techniques that can be taught to patients as general strategies for coping, or for dealing with anxiety and stressful situations during treatment.

General anxiety management strategies

Relaxation training

Progressive muscle relaxation (PMR) teaches us to recognize the different feeling of relaxed and tense muscles. PMR usually involves lying or sitting in a calm, comfortable setting and progressively tightening and relaxing groups of muscles, from the head down or the feet up. PMR can be taught to individuals or groups and there are numerous tapes patients can practise with at home (see box below).

Time management and goal planning

Using time purposefully enhances the feeling of being in control and reduces opportunities for dwelling on problems. Achieving modest goals can help during periods of adjustment by giving a sense of satisfaction and enhancing self-esteem. Setting unrealistic targets has the opposite effect. You can encourage patients to work with their carers to plan targets to be achieved each day.

Exercise and rest

Regular exercise, within the limits imposed by the disease, helps to relieve muscular tension and promote a sense of well-being. Good sleep hygiene gives a sense of refreshment and relieves fatigue. Patients who are tense and anxious should avoid or restrict the use of stimulants like coffee, which increase tension and impair sleep.

Progressive muscle relaxation

This can be taught to people who are experiencing anxiety or going through a stressful time, as a preventative measure for dealing with anxiety. It can be practised by the person on their own or with others. 20 minutes a day is a good routine. Audiotapes and CDs are available that take people through the exercises:

- Find a quiet place and make yourself comfortable, removing shoes and loosening clothing, sitting or lying down.
- Focus on the breathing, breathing in through the nose and out through the mouth. Imagine tension leaving the body with the out breath. Try to relax as much as possible before the exercise.
- Focus on a muscle group, first breathing in and tensing, then holding for a few seconds, then relaxing the muscles and breathing out. Relax before next stage.
- Go through the following muscle groups: hands, arms, neck and shoulders, face and forehead, chest and back, abdominal muscles, buttocks, legs, feet. At each stage, tense the muscles as tightly as possible, then release. Focus on the muscle group alone, try to keep the rest of the body relaxed.

Progress to visualization or stay relaxed and get up slowly.

Anxiety first aid
Managing hyperventilation
Hyperventilation (over-breathing or rapid shallow breathing) is a common effect of anxiety, which worsens and extends the episode of anxiety. Managing hyperventilation involves breathing slowly and deeply, by focusing on the breathing. It helps to breathe from the diaphragm rather than the ribs; a hand can be placed on the stomach, to observe the rise and fall of the diaphragm. It is helpful to demonstrate this to the anxious person. In an emergency, the hands can be cupped over the mouth and nose to restrict the passage of oxygen. The use of bags over the mouth can be dangerous, and detracts from the patient's sense of gaining control through their own effort.

Managing panic attacks
Panic attacks are often precipitated by a thought or feeling. Panic then reinforces whatever fear precipitated the attack. The combination of chest pain, shortness of breath, and tacchycardia, with the psychological experience of fear and impending doom can be very distressing. The following steps can be taught:
- Slow deep breathing.
- Identify any precipitants.
- Understand the process of panic.

Distraction
It can help for the patient to distract themselves from anxious thoughts by finding an external focus for their attention, e.g. by talking to someone, listening to music, or reading a book.

Visualization
This can be developed during relaxation training, visualizing a peaceful or relaxing place that the patient associates with well-being and contentment.

Pharmacological treatment of anxiety

Pharmacological treatment of anxiety should be approached with caution. There are three main reasons for this:
- The most commonly used drugs can develop dependency.
- Reliance on drugs can reduce the patient's sense of personal control.
- All drugs have side effects which may cause additional problems for the patient.

For these reasons, anxiety management techniques are recommended in the first place for treating anxiety. However, anxiolytic drugs do have a place in the short-term management of anxiety, particularly during acutely distressing or unpleasant medical procedures and in end of life care. Benzodiazepines are the main group of anxiolytic drugs in use e.g. diazepam, lorazepam. Midazolam can be used in situations where rapid seation is necessary. Problems associated with this group are excessive drowsiness and respiratory depression. Because they can also lead to disinhibition, they should not be given to people who have suicidal ideas.

The other group of anxiolytic drugs in common use are the beta-blockers, e.g. propranolol, which are particularly useful for controlling palpitations. Antidepressants, such as the SSRIs, e.g. citalopram, can be used for longer-term management of anxiety, particularly if associated with depression.

Assessment and support of the anxious patient

An assessment of anxiety should involve the following:
- How severe and incapacitating is the anxiety and how long does it last?
- What effect does the anxiety have on the patient's health and quality of life?
- Is there a trigger to the anxiety? Identifying what starts off or triggers anxiety will help the patient find alternative ways of responding to their concerns.
- What physical effects is the patient experiencing? This will help the patient distinguish the effects of anxiety from other effects of illness and treatment.
- Are there background factors which maintain the anxiety? This could include any ongoing worries or questions the patient needs to be answered.
- How does the patient normally deal with anxiety? This provides an opportunity for the patient to review the effectiveness of their anxiety management and consider alternatives.

In addition to anxiety management and treatment strategies, the way that care is delivered can minimize anxiety for the patient and aid their coping. Anxiety can be minimized by:
- Helping the patient feel in control.
- Involving the patient and their carers in decision-making and offering choices, in a manner and at a pace that is acceptable to the patient.
- Providing clear information, based on the patient's view of their information needs.

It is also important to provide reassurance by dealing effectively with treatable causes of anxiety, and by demonstrating a professional understanding of anxiety and its management. An important element in the management of anxiety is *containment*, that is, demonstrating calmness and confidence in managing the anxiety in the face of the patient's uncertainty and apprehension.

Further reading

Stark D P H, House A (2000). Anxiety in cancer patients. *British Journal of Cancer*, **83**(10), 1261–7.

Other psychological problems encountered in people with cancer

Acute confusional states

Acute confusion or delirium is an acute organic brain syndrome, characterized by problems with level of consciousness, attention, and memory. Acute confusion may be transient and reversible. Key features are a clouding of consciousness, and difficulty registering or making sense of new information. Clouding of consciousness ranges from reduced awareness of the environment or drowsiness, to stupor and coma.

Presentation

It is more common in terminal illness, and in older people, particularly when they have been removed from a familiar environment. 'Sundown syndrome' describes a worsening of symptoms towards the evening. The following are common:

- Clouding of consciousness—reduced awareness of the environment.
- Impaired attention and memory—especially recent events.
- Disorientation in time, place, or person.
- Impaired abstract thinking and comprehension.
- Perceptual distortions—illusions or hallucinations.
- Transient delusions—usually paranoid.
- Disturbed cycle of sleeping and waking, nightmares
- Emotional disturbance—depression, anxiety, fear, irritability, euphoria, apathy, perplexity
- Psychomotor disturbance—agitation, restless, or under-activity.

Patients commonly appear perplexed or apathetic, and sometimes distressed, anxious, or fearful. Misunderstandings, related to poor orientation, or different interpretations of external events may lead to fear and suspicion, or paranoid behaviour.

The presentation is similar to chronic confusional states, or dementia, but unlike acute confusion, these conditions are not associated with clouding of consciousness, and are irreversible.

Causes

There are a number of physical or physiological causes of confusion:

- Prescribed drugs—opioids, corticosteroids, psychotropic drugs.
- Drug withdrawal—e.g. benzodiazepines or opioids, alcohol.
- Infection—respiratory or urinary infection, septicaemia, encephalitis, or meningitis.
- Brain pathology—primary or secondary tumour.
- Metabolic—dehydration, electrolyte disturbance, hypoxia, hypercalcaemia, organ failure.
- Endocrine disorders—hypoglycaemia, myxoedema, thyrotoxicosis.
- Trauma—head injury, subdural haematoma.
- Severe pain.
- Hearing and sight defects.

Nursing management of acute confusion

Assessment

Identify and treat the cause and any contributory factors (e.g. sensory deprivation). Many of the psychological symptoms associated with confusional states are caused by difficulties in processing new information.

Manage confused thoughts

Aim to keep all communication clear, brief, and to the point. Avoid over-taxing the patient's short attention span. Ask only one question at a time.

Encourage correct orientation

Aid orientation by the use of cues such as mealtimes or visiting times. Make the environment as familiar as possible, using the patient's own possessions. Ensure that the patient's hearing aid or glasses are being worn.

Prevent and respond to distress

Listen to the patient's worries or concerns, which may be expressed indirectly. Use touch to calm the patient, if this proves helpful. Reduce all invasive or painful interventions to a minimum.

Respond to hallucinations and delusions

Try to offer explanations rather than reassurance. Acknowledge distress and concern when faced with delusional ideas.

Safety issues

Individual nursing care, on a one-to-one basis, will usually keep the confused patient safe. Avoid the use of physical restraint, which undermines the nurse–patient relationship.

Medication

This may be helpful in ensuring a good night's sleep, or in calming an extremely distressed patient. The choice of medication will relate to the specific problem, e.g. analgesics for pain, benzodiaepines for anxiety, haloperidol for delirium. Any medication should be kept to the minimum effective dose. Sedating the patient may further impair their consciousness and worsen their confusional state.

Psychoses and their management

Psychoses are disorders of thought, feeling, and perception, that lead to difficulties relating to both the internal world of self, and to the world at large. Psychotic states may be mild and transient, in response to a clear precipitant, or enduring and disabling, e.g. schizophrenia.

The presentation of acute psychosis can be similar to that of acute confusional states, but disturbance in the level of consciousness is rare. Psychotic disorders differ from confusional states in that they are usually functional rather than organic, i.e. there is no clear physical cause.

Psychotic episodes are rarely encountered in the cancer care setting, but they are distressing and difficult to manage when they are. There are two main ways they will be encountered:
- People with existing psychotic illness who develop cancer.
- Acute psychotic reactions in someone with cancer.

Presentation
- The person's attention and concentration may be impaired.
- Thought disorders: the person may believe that their thoughts are being controlled, inserted or removed by others.
- Hallucinations: auditory hallucinations are the most common, but visual, olfactory, and tactile hallucinations are also possible.
- Delusions: incongruous beliefs that are frequently persecutory.
- Mood: may be blunted or incongruous.
- Behaviour: may be paranoid or suspicious, impulsive, or unpredictable.
- Appearance: clothing may appear bizarre, or the individual may neglect their appearance.

Nursing management
Get expert mental health advice and support
The management of psychosis can be very complex and unpredictable. If the patient is already known to a mental health team, it may be possible to arrange support from professionals, such as mental health nurses, who already know the patient.

Establish a relationship
The experience of psychosis is usually very distressing to patients, relatives and staff alike. Some nurses may withdraw rather than engage with the patient, but this is likely to alienate the patient and their family. Openness, consistency, and genuine concern on the nurse's part will promote therapeutic rapport.

Maintain safety
Some patients may be at increased risk of suicide and self-harm when psychotic. Safety measures should include nursing individuals in observation areas, preferably on the ground floor. Agitation and threatening behaviour are possible (📖 Violence and aggression).

Medication

Medication is essential in controlling the distressing and disab. toms of psychosis. Anti-psychotic medication such as major tranq. are prescribed to calm agitation, reduce thought disorders and perce abnormalities. These drugs have difficult side effects, and these shoula monitored.

...e and aggression

...s of violence and aggression have been increasingly reported in ... care situations. These are not especially associated with the cancer ...e setting, but they may occur. There are a number of reasons why ...eople may become aggressive or violent:

- Anger or frustration.
- Fear or confusion.
- Delusional misinterpretation or intoxication.
- Loss of control or disinhibition.
- Previous history of violence.
- Limited ability to interpret the environment e.g. learning disabilities.

Assessment
An assessment should establish whether the violent or aggressive behaviour is the result of real and understandable factors in the environment, such as anger or frustration, that are amenable to reason. If the behaviour is the result of an altered mental state, e.g. delirium, psychosis, drugs, or alcohol, they will respond to treatment.

Principles of anger management
- Respond to the person, not the behaviour, as far as possible.
- Maintain your professional composure and priorities.
- Put limits on unacceptable behaviour.
- Ensure a safe environment.
- Defuse the situation by acting calmly and showing concern.
- Acknowledge how the person feels.
- Seek reasons for the behaviour.
- Problem-solve—help the person identify their problems and find solutions.

Principles of dealing with violence
- It is always better to prevent or defuse potentially violent situations than to deal with actual violence.
- Familiarize yourself with the local policy for violent incidents, and know who to call on for assistance.
- Maintain communication, and be clear about the action you are taking.
- Relocate vulnerable people to a safer environment.
- Always act within your own area of confidence.
- Review the incident with the staff concerned, to defuse feelings and learn for the future (debriefing).

Legal and professional framework for action
Most interventions carried out with confused, or potentially violent patients in hospital are done under Common Law. That is, rights and responsibilities that have been established by previous decisions in law courts.

Action is carried out under the following principles:
- *Necessity*: staff may need to restrain or treat a patient who is
  to himself or others without their consent, in an emergency.
- *Duty of care*: staff have a duty to provide care to those who need
  Failure to do so may result in negligence.
- *Capacity*: the patient's ability to make informed decisions on whether
  or not to accept treatment.

...l misuse

- ...ol is part of the British and European way of life. Used
  ...derately, it has no harmful effects and may bring positive health
  ...enefits, e.g. protection against heart disease.
- Excessive alcohol use is associated with cardiovascular, digestive,
  neurological, psychological, and social problems, with cancers of the
  head and neck, oesophagus, stomach, pancreas, colon, and breast.
- The incidence of alcohol-related deaths in the UK may be as high as
  20,000 per annum, with as many as 25% resulting from accidents.

Alcohol units

Alcohol units are the accepted measurement of alcohol consumption in
the UK: one unit represents 8g of ethanol. Table 50.1 below shows the
units in standard measures of alcohol.

Sensible drinking

The recommended limits of sensible drinking in the UK are:
- Men: 21 units of alcohol per week, or 3–4 units per day.
- Women: 14 units of alcohol per week, or 2–3 units per day.

27% of men and 15% of women regularly drink in excess of these
recommended limits in England.

Hazardous drinking

This is defined as the regular consumption of:
- More than 5 units of alcohol per day by men.
- More than 3 units of alcohol per day by women.

Binge drinking

This is defined as drinking more than half the recommended weekly
number of alcohol units in one session, i.e. 10 units for men, 7 units for
women.

Harmful drinking

This is defined as a pattern of heavy drinking that results in damage to
physical or mental health.

Alcohol dependence

This is physical dependence on alcohol, with altered behaviour that is
associated with the increased emphasis on alcohol within the person's
life. This can result in financial and work problems, damaged relationships, a range of health problems, and accidents. It may manifest as:
- The strong or overpowering desire to drink alcohol.
- Symptoms of withdrawal, including tremor, nausea, vomiting,
  perspiration, seizures. These can start within 3–6 hours of the last
  drink, and may last 5–7 days.
- Delirium tremens: this is a very dangerous condition that occurs in
  approximately 5% of people withdrawing from alcohol. It often
  presents with confusion and agitation, hallucinations (often tactile), and
  paranoia. Its onset is within 24–48 hours of the last drink.

Table 50.1 Alcohol units in standard drinks measures

Beer, lager cider	Average strength 3–4% alcohol by volume	Half pint Pint	ʒ
Strong beer, lager, cider	5% alcohol by volume	Pint	3 unr
		Bottle (500ml)	3 units
Wine	Average strength 12% alcohol by volume (wine ranges 8–14%)	Small glass (125ml)	1 unit
		Bottle (750ml)	9 units
Fortified wine, e.g. sherry, port	20% alcohol by volume	Standard pub measure (50ml)	1 unit
		Bottle (750ml)	15 units
Spirits, e.g. whisky, brandy, vodka, gin	40% alcohol by volume	Standard pub measure (35ml)	1.5 units
		Bottle (750 ml)	30 units

Website

www.alcoholconcern.org.uk/servlets/home

management of people who
alcohol dependent

A patient who is alcohol dependent may present with a number of problems in the cancer care setting. The person's use of alcohol may cause additional health problems, may interact unfavourably with treatment, e.g. medication, or may make it hard for them to cooperate consistently with treatment, or to attend appointments. The disruption of relationships and finances can lead to ongoing problems within the family structure. The resulting loss of trust and confidence can also make it very difficult to offer support to the patient and their family. People who are alcohol dependent are at greater risk of depression, suicide, and attempted suicide.

Assessment

Dependence is likely to be present in men who consistently drink more than 50 units a week, and in women who drink more than 35 units a week.

According to ICD-10[1] criteria, alcohol dependence is diagnosed if three or more of the following have been present during the previous year:
- A strong desire or compulsion to drink.
- Difficulty controlling drinking.
- Physical withdrawal state, drinking to relieve withdrawal.
- Increased tolerance of alcohol, drinking more to achieve the same effect.
- Neglect of other interests, more time spent getting drink, or recovering from its effects.
- Persisting with drinking, despite the harmful effects of alcohol.

Principles of intervention

Do an alcohol assessment. Key questions are:
- *How much do you drink?*
- *How often do you drink?*

Alcohol assessment should be undertaken prior to surgery in patients where alcohol abuse is suspected. This should be considered in cancers known to be associated with alcohol abuse, e.g. cancers of the head and neck. If undetected, complications due to alcohol withdrawal can occur after surgery. Refer to local guidelines where these are available.

Drinkers are not always honest or accurate about their consumption. Get information from the family where possible.

Intervene at any stage of problem drinking. Provide information on the health risks associated with drinking, what constitutes sensible drinking, and how to cut down.

1 ICD-10. http://www.3.who.int/icd/currentversion/fr_icd.htm

Many well-motivated people can reduce their drinking with information and informal support from their family and from alcohol support groups. Professional support is targeted on the alcohol dependent.

Detoxification

Detoxification is the planned withdrawal of alcohol from dependent individuals, under professional supervision. It is usually done at the patient's home, or via an outpatient clinic. It can be done in hospital with specialist intensive support. The recommended drug for withdrawal is chlordiazepoxide, which dampens withdrawal symptoms, lowers the risk of convulsions, and is less likely to be misused than other benzodiazepines.

Website

www.alcoholconcern.org.uk/servlets/home

Chapter 51

Altered body image

⌐troduction

Altered Body Image is a term used to describe a state of disturbance when the person's changed body image does not enable the person to experience their usual sense of self, or it inhibits their ability to engage in social interaction. This can be experienced as a profound sense of dissatisfaction or distress, affecting the individual's personal and social identity.

Changes in physical appearance are very common in people with cancer, and can include:
- Hair loss during chemotherapy.
- Skin reactions during radiotherapy.
- Weight loss or weight gain.
- Effects of corticosteroids.
- Effects of surgery e.g. mastectomy, colostomy.

Some cancers are associated with particular disturbances of body appearance and function; these include cancers of the head and neck that lead to visibly altered appearance, and disturbance of speech, eating and breathing. Changes in body image also have psychological and social elements. Our body image is part of our self-image, how we think about ourselves as a person, and this is also part of our perception of our self worth, or self esteem. Price's model[1] of body image is widely used within nursing to understand altered body image. It has 3 components:
- Body reality (the way our body really is).
- Body ideal (the way we want our body to look and function).
- Body presentation (the way we dress, pose, move, act).

These components exist in a state of balance that usually give us a sense of satisfactory body image. If one of them changes, we will compensate. For example, if our body reality changes as a result of treatment so that it is less like our body ideal, we may alter our body presentation to compensate for this. This might involve wearing a wig to compensate for hair loss, or using make-up to mask the effects of surgery.

1 Price B (1990). *Body Image, Nursing Concepts and Care.* London:Prentice Hall.

Assessment and support

Assessment

Assessment is necessary at times when disruption to body image is suspected, particularly following major treatments. Assessment of body image should include the following:

- The person's perception of their body image.
- Their attitude to treatment.
- Their need for information.
- Their coping strategies.
- Their social support.
- Expectations of what can be achieved cosmetically.

Support

Supporting the patient with altered body image is based on achieving the best cosmetic and functional outcome, dealing with specific problems (e.g. eating problems after head and neck surgery), supporting social interactions, and enabling optimum adjustment to the new body reality.

Preparation

- Preparing the patient in advance for the effects of treatment.
- Discussion of likely effects on lifestyle and self-image.
- Providing information and help with decision-making with treatment options.
- Providing photographs or other images of how appearance may change after treatment (📖 Breast reconstruction).

Cosmetics and prosthetics

- Discussing options for any further cosmetic treatment.
- Discussing prosthetics options and their impact on lifestyle.
- Giving practical advice regarding wearing wigs and other prosthetics.
- Support when looking at scars for the first time.
- Advice on realistic expectations for cosmetic surgery and the best timing of this in relation to cancer treatment.
- Look Good Feel Better groups (📖 Hair loss (alopecia)).

Social support

- Supporting coping strategies (📖 Psychological reactions to cancer).
- Mobilizing social support, including any specialist support groups.
- Talking to and meeting other patients—patients are often happy to discuss the results of their surgery.
- Advise on how partners and children may cope i.e. hugging children after mastectomy.
- Advice for partners on what to expect and how to deal with anticipated problems.

Some people develop phobic elements, e.g. avoiding looking at a mastectomy scar. This may impact on the patient's ability to notice changes that would suggest the possibility of recurrence. They may benefit from referral for specialist mental health intervention[2].

2 Newell R (1991). Body image disturbance: cognitive-behavioural formulation and intervention, *Journal of Advanced Nursing*, **16**, 1400–5.

Chapter 52

Sexual health and canc

uction

...r is associated with a number of sexual problems. Some of these are
. ect physical result of the cancer or its treatment (see Table 52.1):

Disfigurement or loss of sexual organs through surgery (e.g. breasts,
testes, gynaecological surgery).
- Nerve damage after pelvic surgery affecting sexual response and
function.
- Disfigurement or loss of sensation to other areas of the body, such as
the hand, tongue, face, or mouth.
- Personality changes or loss of inhibition resulting from brain
involvement or surgery.
- Side effects of chemotherapy or radiotherapy (e.g. vaginal dryness).
- Infertility, or early menopause through surgery or chemotherapy.
- Impotence or loss of sexual response as a consequence of medication
(e.g. some anti-depressants, anti-hypertensives, anti-convulsants, and
anti-emetics).

Other sexual problems are more indirect effects of illness or treatment:
- Feeling unattractive or lost personal sense of sexuality because of
altered body image, or loss of control of bodily functions.
- Loss of intimacy because of pain, disability, or fatigue.
- Impotence in the man or loss of sexual response in the woman for
psychological reasons.

Sexual health is defined by the WHO[1] as:
- A capacity to enjoy and control sexual and reproductive behaviour in
accordance with a social and personal ethic.
- Freedom from fear, shame, guilt, false beliefs, and other psychological
factors inhibiting sexual response and impairing sexual relationships.
- Freedom from organic disorders, diseases, and deficiencies that
interfere with sexual and reproductive functions.

Our sexual health is part of our general health, at all stages of the life
span. The Royal College of Nursing[2] describes sexuality and sexual health
as 'an appropriate and legitimate area of nursing activity'. Research also
shows that patients want nurses to provide information and initiate
conversations about sexuality.

Human sexuality is complex and is unique to each individual. It is
composed of:
- Physical factors that define biological sex.
- Psychological factors that contribute towards personal gender identity.
- Social and cultural factors that influence sexual behaviour.

Our sexuality affects many areas of our lives, and the effects of cancer on
sexuality can include: disruptions to sexual response and sexual
behaviour, body and self image, emotional life and intimate relationships,
and the ability to reproduce.

---

1 World Health Organization (1986). *Concepts for Sexual Health*. EUR/ICP/MCH 521. Copenhagen: WHO.
2 Royal College of Nursing (2000). *Sexuality and Sexual Health in Nursing Practice*. London: Royal College of Nursing.

Table 52.1 Treatment-related sexual problems

Problem	Treatment caused by	Management options
• Vaginal dryness, thinning, and loss of elasticity.	• Chemotherapy. • Pelvic radiotherapy and treatment-induced menopause. • Bone marrow transplant—graft-versus-host disease.	• Use of hydrating creams, lubricant gels, and oestrogen-based pessaries and creams.
• Vaginal infections, e.g. thrush.	• Chemotherapy.	• Antifungal agents.
• Narrowing, scarring of vagina.	• Pelvic radiotherapy (external and internal). • Bone marrow transplant—graft-versus-host disease.	• Use of vaginal dilators. • Finger stimulation can be done alone, or as a couple.
• Pain on intercourse.	• Chemotherapy. • Radiotherapy. • Surgery to pelvic area.	• Analgesia + general strategies for overcoming sexual difficulties (below). • Different positions are helpful. E.g. woman on top, so able to control the depth/angle of penetration.
• Irregular or absence of periods.	• Chemotherapy.	• Periods usually return—caution, pregnancy can occur in the absence of periods.
• Signs of early menopause, e.g. hot flushes, irritability.	• Chemotherapy. • Hormonal therapy. • Pelvic radiotherapy.	• Hormone replacement therapy if not hormone dependant tumour.
• Reduced testosterone in men.	• Chemotherapy.	• Usually recovers, or testosterone replacement therapy an option.
• Infertility.	• Chemotherapy. • Pelvic radiotherapy. • Surgery.	• Sperm banking for men.
• Erectile dysfunction in men.	• Bone marrow transplant—graft-versus-host disease. • Hormonal therapy. • Pelvic radiotherapy. • Surgery.	• Use of medications that improve blood flow to penis, e.g. sildenafil, also use of vacuum devices or injections (into the penis).
• Loss of desire. Inability to achieve orgasm.	• Any treatment + fatigue, pain, altered body image.	• Thorough physical and psychological assessment. • Treatment of any physical causes or overcoming sexual difficulties. • Refer to psychosexual therapist.

Assessment and communication about sexual health

Communication

Communication about sexuality is frequently a problem, either because of embarrassment on the part of the patient or nurse, or because sexuality may not be seen to be relevant to cancer or its treatment.

In order to communicate on the subject of sexuality, the nurse should:
• Understand the role of sexuality in personal identity and health.
• Have a willingness to discuss sexuality with patients and significant others.
• Give the patient and their partner permission to share information about their sexual health.
• Have an understanding of common sexual problems associated with cancer.

Assessment

When assessing the sexual health of an individual, or of a couple, be careful not to make assumptions about their needs on the basis of age or any other personal factors. A person's sexuality is unique to them. There are models designed specifically to assess sexuality, including the PLISSIT[1] model, and the BETTER[2] model. They follow similar stages that can be summarized:
• Let the patient know it is acceptable to talk about sexuality, and provide a safe environment to do so.
• Talk about sexuality as an element of health and quality of life, encompassing physical and emotional intimacy.
• Provide information about the sexual problems associated with cancer and its treatments as part of informed consent.
• Attempt to address any problems that are raised, within the limits of your own knowledge and competence.
• Find sources of additional support, expert advice or treatment, and refer on as necessary, e.g. psychosexual counselling.

The Ex-PLISSIT[3] model further emphasizes the importance of developing a climate of permission-giving, providing privacy and visible acknowledgement of individuals as sexual beings, for example, providing literature for gay men, lesbians, and bisexuals. The different stages of the Ex-PLISSIT model do not necessarily follow in a neat order. It is necessary to review and evaluate after an intervention, for example, asking if written literature was useful, and if it raised any issues for the patient or their partner. This may lead to further questions or to a more personal level of disclosure by the patient.

---

1 Annon, J (1971). The PLISSIT Model: a proposed conceptual scheme for the behavioural treatment of sexual problems, *Journal of Sex Education and Therapy* **2**, 1–15.
2 Mick J A, Hughes M, Cohen M Z (2004). Using the BETTER model to assess sexuality, *Clinical Journal of Oncology Nursing*, **8**(1), 84–6.
3 Davis S, Taylor B (2006). From PLISSIT to Ex-PLISSIT, In Davis S (Ed.) *Rehabilitation: The Use of Theories and Models in Practice*, Oxford: Elsevier Ltd.

Creating an inclusive environment

It is important not to make assumptions about other people's sexuality, or to demonstrate assumptions through the use of language. For example, the question 'Are you married?' assumes a heterosexual orientation, and might make it difficult for someone who is not heterosexual to respond. Phrase questions about sexuality as openly as possible, combining them with an awareness that sexuality is an issue, for example, 'Having cancer and going through treatment can have an impact on people's sex lives. Do you have any questions you would like to ask?' Having leaflets available for patients, that deal with a range of sexual problems, and different sexualities, is another way of demonstrating an inclusive environment (see, for example, CancerBACKUP website[4])

General strategies for overcoming sexual difficulties for patients and their partners

- Make time for intimacy, create a comfortable and relaxed environment
- Explore other ways of being intimate.
- Explore different positions, and options for mutual pleasure and sexual satisfaction.
- Avoid the pressure of lovemaking when tired, uncomfortable, or in pain.
- Acknowledge differences in sexual desire between partners and try to work with these.

4 ⊞ Cancer BACKUP: www.cancerbackup.org.uk/Resourcessupport/Relationshipscommunication/
Sexuality

Skin and mucosal alterations

Hair loss (alopecia)

Hair loss can be a distressing side effect of cancer treatment; it impacts on body image and feelings of attractiveness, creates anxiety and causes a visual reminder of the disease and treatment. Alopecia is not a major side effect for most people, but a small group of patients will become extremely distressed by it.

Causes

Chemotherapy and radiotherapy damage cells that are dividing. Since most scalp follicles are in a state of rapid growth, patients are susceptible to hair loss during treatment. Alopecia can be a localized effect of radiotherapy, with scalp hair most susceptible. About half the patients who experience scalp alopecia will also lose other body hair, e.g. pubic, facial, or axillary hair. Many chemotherapy agents can cause alopecia. Drugs that generally cause severe alopecia include cyclophosphamide, ifosphamide anthracyclines, vinca alkaloids, and taxanes.

Prognosis

Hair loss generally begins 7–10 days after chemotherapy commences. Many patients get scalp sensitivity during hair loss. Hair will re-grow about 4–6 weeks after treatment finishes in virtually all cases. New hair often changes colour and texture—it may be coarser, curlier, greyer, or thinner.

Hair lost due to radiotherapy will start to regrow about 8–9 weeks after treatment. Regrowth tends to be slower and the texture may be finer. If the radiotherapy dose is particularly high, it can be possible for hair not to re-grow.

Nursing support

It is important to prepare patients for their hair loss. As prevention of hair loss is often not possible, the emphasis should be on psychological support and measures to minimize the impact on the person's appearance (📖 Altered body image).

Assessing and understanding the person's sense of loss, or the level of importance the individual and their family attach to their hair loss, allows appropriate support to be planned. This support will include listening to and valuing the individual's concerns, considering methods to minimize hair loss, informing them about options such as wigs, hats, and turbans and offering practical advice on scalp and hair protection.

Those facing hair loss are often more concerned about the reaction of their friends and family than their own actual loss of hair.

Key areas to cover with patients
- Why hair loss occurs.
- When it will begin and end, and the degree of hair loss, including areas other than the scalp.
- How the hair will fall out—quickly or over time—and any changes in the hair afterwards.

- Scalp cooling options—including potential risks and benefits.
- Other symptoms or complaints associated with hair loss—such as scalp sensitivity.
- Potential psychosocial impact.
- How to cope with hair loss—including information on wigs, hats, turbans etc.
- Scalp care and eye care—if eyelashes are lost.

Minimizing hair loss
- Advice is often given on minimizing hair loss—this includes cutting it short, reducing washing and shampooing, avoiding hair manipulation, dyes and perms, use of wide-toothed combs, or soft hairbrushes.
- These measures may enable individuals to gain some sense of control in managing their hair loss, but there is little evidence to suggest that they actually reduce hair loss.
- Careful shaving of the head once hair loss is severe, will allow an even re-growth when it returns.

Wigs and other head coverings
- Wigs are available free of charge on the NHS to anyone facing the prospect of treatment-related alopecia. They can also be bought privately.
- Wigs should be professionally fitted, and should be selected before the patient has lost their hair in order to match the colour, style, and hair texture. Otherwise a photo and a snip of hair can be used to choose an appropriate wig. Some patients find wigs feel strange, uncomfortable or hot, others may not be satisfied with the final look.
- Most cancer centres also offer a range of headscarves and turbans. Hats and caps can also hide alopecia effectively.

Scalp and face protection
- Patients should wear a head covering to protect themselves from the sun, wind, and cold. A high factor sun cream should also be applied if any sun exposure is expected.
- If eyebrows and eyelashes have been lost, then sunglasses, wide brimmed hats and false eyelashes can all protect the eyes from injury.

Look Good... Feel Better

A number of centres in the UK are now offering the 'Look Good... Feel Better' programme, where women can have a makeover by a professional beautician. They also receive advice on how to look and feel their best throughout cancer treatment. www.lookgoodfeelbetter.org

Scalp cooling (scalp hypothermia)

- The most common attempt to reduce hair loss has been scalp cooling. This causes vasoconstriction of the scalp, reduction in the uptake of drugs in the hair follicles, and therefore reduces hair loss.
- Because scalp cooling has to be maintained throughout the period that cytotoxic drugs are circulating, it is generally only used for regimens of short duration (<2 hours).
- Cooling commences shortly before chemotherapy administration (normally 15–20 minutes), and is generally maintained after treatment for a period of time based on the drug's plasma half-life.
- Effectiveness of scalp cooling varies, but in general, around 50% of patients in anthracycline and taxane based regimens should have a good to excellent response with scalp hypothermia.

Methods of scalp cooling

The two methods are:
- Refrigerated gel filled caps: these require changing regularly throughout the treatment.
- Cooling machines: these attach to caps similar to the above, and maintain them at a constant temperature throughout treatment. They are less time-consuming for nursing staff.

Caps need to be close fitting, and in some centres the hair is wet before treatment to increase cold conductivity.

Side effects include headache, dizziness, nausea and vomiting, a heavy feeling on the head, and transient light-headedness following cap removal.

Scalp metastases

- Concern has been raised that scalp cooling may increase the risk of scalp metastases. In the case of solid tumours this risk is extremely low, and there is no strong evidence to suggest that scalp cooling increases this risk. Further studies are required to clarify this issue.
- Scalp cooling should not be given in cases where scalp skin metastases exist, or in haematological malignancies where the risk of scalp metastases is highest e.g. lymphoma or leukaemia.
- Nurses should discuss the risk of scalp metastases with individuals having scalp cooling, to enable informed choice.

Further reading

Massey C S (2004). A multicentre study to determine the efficacy and patient acceptability of the Paxman Scalp Cooler to prevent hair loss in patients receiving chemotherapy. *European Journal of Oncology Nursing*, **8**(2), 121–130.

Oral mucositis and related problems

Oral mucositis (OM) is a major problem for patients receiving cancer chemotherapy and radiotherapy. The oral mucosa is made up of rapidly dividing squamous epithelial cells. With a life span of approximately one week, they are extremely prone to damage from chemotherapy or radiotherapy. The impact of OM is severe, including pain, infection, altered taste, decreased nutritional intake, dehydration, diarrhoea, bleeding, and altered body image. In extreme cases airway obstruction can occur.

Definitions

The terms OM and stomatitis are often used interchangeably. Strictly speaking, OM is the inflammation of oral mucosa due to chemotherapy or radiotherapy treatments. This process may also occur anywhere in the gut and is covered by the general term 'mucositis'. Stomatitis is any inflammation of the oral and oropharyngeal mucous membrane and includes infections of oral tissue.

Causes and risk factors

- 80% patients having radiotherapy for head and neck cancers get OM.
- Radiotherapy causes mucosal atrophy and fibrosis of the salivary glands, causing not only OM but xerostomia (reduced saliva). Radiotherapy damage can be long term.
- Chemotherapy causes reduced renewal, atrophy, and ulceration of the oral mucosa. As patients become neutropaenic, superimposed infections cause further ulceration, damage, and inflammatory response.
- Up to 40% of patients receiving chemotherapy have mucositis (higher rates in haematological malignancies). Drugs most frequently used are:
  - Anthracycline antibiotics e.g. doxorubicin.
  - Taxanes e.g. paclitaxel.
  - Antimetabolites e.g. methotrexate, 5-FU, raltitrexed.
- Other risk factors for OM include:
  - Previous radiotherapy.
  - Poor oral hygiene.
  - Dental cavities.
  - Improperly fitting denture.
  - Gingival disease.
  - Nutritional deficiency.
  - Smoking and alcohol consumption.
  - Oxygen therapy.

Prevention of mucositis

Practices for preventing and treating OM are many and varied. There is little convincing evidence for one particular unified approach.

Oral care protocols

A UK systematic review[1] and recent guidelines from the Multinational Association of Supportive Cancer Care (MASCC) and the International Society for Oral Oncology (ISOO)[2] both suggest that there is limited evidence of benefit from pharmacological intervention. Key recommendations include:

- Oral care protocols and education of both staff and patients.
- Use of a soft toothbrush.
- Radiotherapy induced OM:
  - Use of midline radiation blocks, 3 dimensional radiotherapy.
  - Benzydamine mouthwash (anti-inflammatory and antibacterial properties).
- Chemotherapy induced OM:
  - 30 min cryotherapy (sucking ice-chips) for bolus 5FU.
- In high dose and stem cell transplant settings, palfermin (Kepivance®), a keratinocyte growth factor has recently been shown to reduce the duration and severity of oral mucositis.

Treatment of oral mucositis

There is some limited evidence that both granulocyte colony stimulating factor and allopurinol mouthwash can reduce the duration of mucositis[1].

Management of mucositis

The following advice is based on the best currently available evidence[2]. Due to the limits of this evidence, if a specific treatment is not working for a patient, it is important to be flexible in your management approach, and to consider some of the many alternative treatments that are available.

Oral care protocol

A systematic oral care protocol should be used to carry out the management of OM. It should include the following elements:

- Assessment and monitoring.
- Managing the process and symptoms.
  - Maintaining integrity of the oral mucosa.
  - Preventing secondary infections.
  - Providing pain relief—maintain comfort.
  - Ensuring adequate nutritional intake.
- Patient education.

1 Worthington H V, Clarkson J E, Eden O B (2004). Interventions for treating oral mucositis for patients with cancer receiving treatment. *The Cochrane Database of Systematic reviews*, Issue 2.
2 Rubenstein E B, Peterson D E, Schubert M (2004). Clinical Practice Guidelines for the Prevention and Treatment of Cancer Therapy–Induced Oral and Gastrointestinal Mucositis. *Cancer* **100**(9) S2026–46.

Assessment

Regular assessment is essential. The oral cavity should be assessed daily. A consistent assessment method or tool should be used, such as the WHO grading system, Table 53.1 or the Oral Assessment Guide[3]. Equipment required for effective assessment includes a pen torch and a tongue depressor.

Routine dental procedures should be carried out prior to treatment, if possible, including treatment of underlying dental problems. This is not always possible due to risk of infection or haemorrhage; it may need to be delayed until after some or all cancer treatment.

3 Eilers J et al. (1988). Development, testing and application of the oral assessment guide. *Oncology Nursing Forum*, **15**(3), 325–30.

Table 53.1 World Health Organization assessment scale for oral mucositis

Mucositis grade					
Scale	0	1	2	3	4
WHO oral Toxicity scale	None	Soreness and erythema	Erythema, ulcers, patient can swallow solid diet	Ulcers, extensive erythema, patient cannot swallow solid diet	Mucositis to extent that alimentation is not possible

Oral mucositis: managing the process and symptoms

Maintain the integrity of oral mucosa by the following measures

Oral hygiene

- Maintaining excellent oral hygiene is important in managing mucositis and preventing superimposed infections. Patients should be encouraged to brush with a softheaded toothbrush and toothpaste after each meal and before bed.
- If wearing dentures, they should be removed from the mouth and brushed after meals and before bed. The oral cavity should also be rinsed clean on each occasion.
- The frequency of oral hygiene should be increased to 2-hourly or even hourly for those with severe mucositis—or at high risk of developing it—and also for those on oxygen therapy.
- If patients are unable to tolerate a toothbrush, foam swabs can be used instead.
- For patients with low saliva, regular water, ice chips, nebulized saline, and saliva replacement products can be tried.
- Lips should be moisturized with lubricants such as paraffin gel and aqueous cream.
- If there is bleeding in the mouth, full blood counts and clotting checks may be required, and replacement blood products given as necessary. Tranexamic acid, as a mouthwash can be used.

Mouthwashes

- There is little evidence that one mouthwash is better than another; the main benefit may be from the mechanical impact of swilling. Commercial mouthwashes should not be used as they contain alcohol and other astringents, causing oral irritation.
- Chlorhexidine based mouthwashes (e.g. Corsodyl®)
  - These can reduce plaque and oral bacteria, and are often recommended for patients with haematological cancers, where infection risks are highest. There is no evidence that they are effective in managing OM.
  - They can cause burning and stinging due to their alcohol content. Some patients find that diluting it in half with water can reduce the irritation.
  - Therefore *chlorhexidine should not be used* to manage OM outside of the high dose chemotherapy setting.
- For standard dose chemotherapy, normal saline or water may be as effective as any mouthwash; these are not irritants so provide a safer option.
- Benzydamine (Difflam®) mouthwash is recommended for patients receiving radiotherapy for head and neck cancers due to its anti-inflammatory and cleansing properties.

Prevention of secondary infections

Regular assessment is essential. Swab suspected areas and administer anti-viral/anti-fungal treatment if indicated (📖 Candidiasis).

Pain relief

A range of preparations can be used to reduce pain and inflammation:
- Benzydamine (Difflam®) mouthwash—a local anaesthetic mouthwash
- Protective gels/coating agents—can be used to ease the pain of mouth ulceration, though again the evidence for their effectiveness is limited. Orabase is applied directly to mouth lesions and can include a steroid to reduce inflammation (adcortyl in orabase). Gelclair is mixed with water and used as a mouthwash.
- Sucralfate—an antacid preparation which can coat ulcers and may reduce discomfort.
- Aspirin gargles—can be used as an anti-inflammatory analgesic. Patients on some chemotherapy regimens will be advised not to swallow aspirin due to the increased risk of bleeding.
- Many patients will require opioids to manage pain.
  - Regular oral morphine is the first choice, however, a continuous infusion may be required.
  - Patient controlled analgesia is recommended, as there is evidence that patients use lower overall doses of opioid for a similar benefit.

Maintenance of nutrition

- Food should be tender. Moist sauces and soft, bland foods might help. Foods that irritate the mouth or throat should be avoided.
- If unable to tolerate food, nutritional support such as high calorie drinks, NG feeding may be required (📖 Nutritional support).
- IV fluids will also be required for patients unable to tolerate sufficient fluid orally.

Patient education

Nurses need to be involved in teaching and subsequently reinforcing optimal oral hygiene practices, including proper brushing, flossing, and mouth rinsing. Nurses should also educate patients about the risk of infection and the signs and symptoms that they need to report to their GP or clinic.

Patients should be educated about pain relief measures and on avoiding alcohol and tobacco, to minimize oral complications.

Nursing support

- OM can have a major impact on a patient's quality of life. It often occurs in combination with other side effects of treatment. Accurate information, effective assessment and speedy management are all essential to try to reduce the impact of severe mucositis.
- Consider methods to ease communication difficulties when patients are unable to talk. Asking closed questions that require simple yes or no answers may be most appropriate at times.
- Do not underestimate the severity of pain, and ensure the most effective analgesia is administered. Patients may have anxieties about using opioids, and might need support and education about the safety and effectiveness of their use in these circumstances.

Oesophagitis

Patients with treatment-induced mucositis are also at risk of oesophagitis. Presenting symptoms are dysphagia, painful swallowing, and epigastric pain. Continuous pain indicates progressing oesophagitis. Oesophagitis pain can be extremely distressing, causing severe discomfort every time the person swallows.

Particular risk factors include:
- Radiation to the oesophagus.
- Oesophageal cancer, high dose chemotherapy, total body irradiation.
- Concurrent chemo-radiotherapy.
- Ulcer disease, alcohol, and tobacco use.

In immuno-suppressed patient, an infective cause must be considered. *Candida* is the most common cause, though herpes simplex can also cause oesophagitis.

Management
- Amifostine can be used to reduce oesophagitis induced by combined chemo-irradiation in patients with NSCLC.
- Nursing management is symptom relief and supportive care. Humidifying the bedroom air can help, particularly at night.

Pain management
- NSAIDs should be administered if not contraindicated.
- Sucralfate solution can relieve some discomfort.
- No smoking and avoid irritants.
- For severe pain, opioids should be used (📖 Oral mucositis management).
- Anaesthetic sprays can help throat discomfort, but there is a risk of reducing the gag reflex, so they should be used with caution.

Nutritional support
- Advise moist foods, such as sauces and gravies and cold foods such as jellies, fruit nectars.
- No citrus juices or hot and spicy food.

(See 📖 Nutritional support for further advice).

Oral care in advanced cancer

- Most problems in advanced cancer are due to reduced saliva production and poor oral hygiene leading to xerostomia (dry mouth) and candidiasis.
- Other problems include mucositis, altered taste, and hyper-salivation (drooling).
- A dry and dirty mouth should be cleaned as usual by oral hygiene.
- Chewing pineapple can also cleanse the mouth.

Xerostomia (dry mouth)

This can impact on speech, chewing, and swallowing. Common causes include: radiotherapy, oxygen, anxiety, dehydration, candidiasis, antimuscarincs, antidepressants, and opioids.

Management

Ensure reversible causes are treated. Offer regular water, ice chips, nebulized saline, and saliva replacement products, particularly before meals.

Saliva stimulants, such as pilocarpine can also be effective, but are better for non-radiation induced xerostomia (📖 Nutritional support).

Candidiasis

Oral thrush is extremely common, both in immuno-suppressed patients, and those with advanced cancer. Accurate and regular assessment of the oral cavity is essential to establish diagnosis and early management.

Presenting features

- Dry mouth, loss of taste.
- Smooth red tongue.
- White plaques on tongue or mucous membranes.
- Soreness.
- Dysphagia.

Management

- Take swabs (not usual in palliative care setting).
- Treat with oral fluconazole or ketoconazole. Nystatin suspension or pastilles 6 hourly can be used topically.

Note: nystatin has reduced activity if combined with chlorhexidine. Do not administer nystatin until at least 30 minutes after chlorhexidine mouthwash.

Hypersalivation

This is not common in the cancer setting. Hyoscine or a range of antimuscarinic drugs can be used to reduce production of saliva.

Further reading

Clarkson J E, Worthington H V, Eden OB (2003). Interventions for preventing oral mucositis for patients with cancer receiving treatment. *The Cochrane Database of Systematic reviews*, Issue 3.

alignant wounds

.hese are caused by local extension or tumour embolization into the epithelium. They can be extremely distressing, as they are a visual reminder of the disease, and can produce odour, discharge, bleeding, pain, and infection. All of these can impact on body image and quality of life.

If appropriate, surgical removal, with or without radiotherapy, can reduce pain, drainage, and odour, and provide infection control. This may be contraindicated in widespread disease. If healing is not possible and the prognosis is generally poor, then the principle of management is symptom control.

The nurse's role is crucial in the management of malignant wounds. Flexibility, creativity, and patience are all required, since the potential success of any approach may be limited. There is often a need to systematically try a range of approaches to achieve optimum management. Psychological support throughout is essential for what can be an embarrassing and traumatic symptom.

> The overall aim of treatment for malignant wounds is to reduce the impact on quality of life and to optimize comfort. Specific management of each the following is required:
> - Control of odour
> - Pain
> - Bleeding
> - Infection
> - Cosmesis
> - Comfort
> - Wound exudate
> - Psychological impacts

It is essential to involve the patient and their family in planning care. They need to have realistic expectations of the likely outcomes of any treatment and support.

General principles of wound management

There are a variety of different products that can be used to dress malignant wounds e.g. alginates, hydrocolloids, foams, and charcoals. (See Table 53.2).

General guidelines are

- Limit frequency of dressing changes if possible. High absorbency dressings and extra pads can help.
- Use non-stick dressings to reduce trauma to the wound.
- Barrier creams should be used to protect surrounding skin.
- Use of quick acting analgesia or relaxation techniques during the dressing procedure may make it more bearable for the patient.
- If the wound is bleeding, adrenaline soaked dressings or Kaltostat® can be useful.
- Metronidazole, systemically or topically, can be helpful in managing odour in the short term. Long-term use can cause an increase in number of aerobic bacteria. Charcoal dressings and deodorizers may also be useful. Other options include regular baths, showering the area clean, and using perfumes.

Table 53.2 Wound products

Type	Indications	Examples
Alginates	Extremely absorbent. Useful for bleeding wounds and infected wounds with moderate to high levels of exudate.	Kaltostat®, Sorbsan®
Hydrocolloids	Used with light to moderate exudate.	Comfeel®, Granu-flex®, Tegasorb®
Foams	Useful for superficial exuding wounds, and also for placing in cavities.	Allevyn® (cavity), lyofoam
Charcoal	Excellent absorbent deodorizer. Useful as a secondary dressing if odour is a problem	Clinisorb®, Kaltocarb®, Lyofoam-C®

Note: contact a wound specialist for advice on the latest products, and on any wounds that are particularly difficult to manage.

Further reading

Twycross R, Wilcock A (2001). *Symptom Management in Advanced Cancer*, 3rd edn. Oxford: Oxford Radcliffe Medical Press.

Watson M S, Lucas C F, Hoy A M, Black I N (2005). *Oxford Handbook of Palliative Care*. Oxford: Oxford University Press.

Lymphoedema

Lymphoedema is an accumulation of lymphatic fluid within interstitial tissues. The accumulation and stagnation of plasma proteins in the fluid causes local inflammation and fibrotic skin changes. This leads to skin folds filled with fluid, which distort the limb or other affected area. This can become very severe, making the limb or affected area grossly distorted, increasing in both size and weight. Lymphorrhoea is the leakage of fluid from damaged skin.

It is a progressive, chronic, and extremely distressing condition that is frequently disabling. Most commonly affecting the limbs, it can also affect the trunk, head, and neck. It is associated with profound disturbance of physical, psychological, and social functioning.

Lymphoedema is a common problem in breast cancer, cancers of the head and neck, and in advanced pelvic disease e.g. prostate and bladder cancer.

Causes
In cancer, it is mostly caused by damage to lymph nodes and vessels, either by treatments for cancer or by the disease itself.
- Fibrosis resulting from surgery and radiotherapy are the most common treatment-related causes, e.g. axillary clearance or axillary radiotherapy for breast cancer.
- Up to 40% of patients having axillary surgery combined with radiotherapy develop lymphoedema.

Other potential causes include:
- Local malignant disease.
- Blockage of lymphatic vessels.
- Inflammatory processes.
- Trauma.
- Infection.
- Invasive procedures such as venepuncture.

Problems associated with lymphoedema
Altered body image: the dramatic changes in body appearance and function are associated with a high level of body image disturbance.

Fatigue, exhaustion: these can be caused by the weight of lymphoedematous limbs, lack of exercise or underlying pathological processes.

Sexual problems: many people will feel themselves unattractive or lose interest in sex because of tiredness, pain, or discomfort.

Disability and loss of mobility: limbs may be heavy as well as distorted, and this can seriously limit activity.

Social isolation and reduction of pleasurable activities: loss of function combined with unease at body changes can lead to social isolation, involving a loss of friendships or other supportive activities, in some cases associated with depression.

Pain and discomfort: lymphoedema itself does not usually
but underlying infective or inflammatory processes may. It is .
associated with discomfort, and loss of or altered sensations
affected part.

Infection: this can be a problem in damaged tissue.

Treatments
Treatments are not generally curative, but aim to improve drainage,
reduce capillary filtration, and prevent complications.

Massage: manual lymphatic drainage (MLD) is a gentle, rhythmic form of
massage used to promote movement of lymph from affected areas into
the lymphatic drainage system. Simple lymphatic drainage is an alternative, simplfied version that patients or their carers can perform.

Compression: this is the most common treatment for lymphoedema. It
involves:
- *Low-stretch bandages.* These are worn 24 hours a day, being replaced
  regularly.
- *Compression garments*, including stockings and sleeves, usually
  removed at night.

Compression should not be used in patients with thrombosis, SVCO or
where the area is infected.

Exercise: gentle exercise promotes lymphatic drainage. Activity should be
tailored to fit with normal activity as far as possible.

Nursing management
In many areas, specialist lymphoedema units and nurses are available to
deal with this problem. It is also very important to work together with
allied health professionals in the multidisciplinary management of lymphoedema. The following are essential elements of the nursing care of
lymphoedema:
- *Hygiene and skin care.* This guards against infection, skin dryness, and
  cracking.
- *Education and information.* The condition can be very distressing and
  frightening, so patients and their families need accurate information on
  the condition. This is empowering and promotes self-care.
- *Avoidance of trauma.* Damage to the skin must be minimized. Potential
  trauma includes venepuncture, sunburn, and accidents. Post-
  mastectomy, women should not have blood tests or chemotherapy
  drugs administered into the arm on the same side as their surgery.
- *Support.* Professional support should aim to assist with changes to
  self-image. There are also patient support groups that can be accessed
  directly (see website).

Website
⊞ Lymphoedema Support Network: www.lymphoedema.org/lsn/

Section 8

Oncological emergencies

Oncological emergen

...axis

...as is a severe systemic allergic reaction with multi-system ...ment. Onset is normally immediate, but there can be a delay of ...

...s caused by the immunologically induced release of chemical mediators (histamine, kinins, prostaglandins, and platelet activating factors), from mast cells and basophils. This leads to smooth muscle contraction, vascular permeability, vasodilation, cardiovascular stimulation, and gastric acid secretion.

Common causes of anaphylaxis

Medical products: antibiotics (especially penicillins), blood products, aspirin, NSAIDs, chemotherapy agents (see box opposite), vaccines

Non-medical: insect stings, latex, peanuts, shellfish, strawberries

Clinical features

- *Respiratory system*: swelling of the lips, tongue, pharynx, and epiglottis may lead to complete upper airway obstruction. Lower airway involvement may develop with dyspnoea, wheeze, stridor, chest tightness, and hypoxia.
- *Skin*: flushing, erythema, pruritis, urticaria.
- *Cardiovascular*: tachycardia, hypotension, arrhythmias, ECG changes, ischaemic chest pains.
- *GI tract*: nausea, vomiting, diarrhoea, abdominal cramps.

Assessment

It is essential to diagnose anaphylaxis early, and not to mistake it for other episodes, such as vaso-vagal (fainting) or panic attacks.

Allergic reactions in oncology

These guidelines are for the management of acute anaphylaxis. In oncology many allergic reactions are milder in nature and may be treated successfully with IV steroids and antihistamines, without the need to use adrenaline. Careful monitoring is required to observe for potential progression to acute anaphylaxis.

Treatment

- Discontinue administration of suspected allergen e.g. drug, blood product. If there are any signs of respiratory distress or circulatory collapse call the emergency (crash) team immediately.
- Secure airway: if there is severe upper airway oedema, the patient may require emergency tracheal intubation and ventilation.
- Give immediate 100% oxygen: if bronchoconstriction give salbutamol 5mg nebulized with oxygen.

- Administer IM adrenaline/epinephrine: 1:1000 0.3–0.5m, every 5–15 minutes if no improvement.
- Give IV fluids to restore BP: lie patient flat unless respiratory worsens.
- Maintain continuous monitoring of cardiovascular and respiratory s
- Antihistamines (H1 blockers: chlorphenamine 10–20mg IV and H2 blockers ranitidine 50mg) can be given as second line treatment.

Note on adrenaline: patients on beta-blockers may not respond to adrenaline or can get severe hypertension. Patients on tricyclic antidepressants are at higher risk of cardiac arrhythmias.

Nursing care

- *Anxiety:* patients and their families may be extremely fearful during and after an episode of anaphylaxis, and will require a lot of emotional support. If a chemotherapy agent causes anaphylaxis it could have implications for their future treatment. This will need to be sensitively explored with the patient.
- *Observation:* if anaphylaxis occurs as an out patient, then ensure the patient is admitted and observed for 24 hours (relapses can occur in first 24 hour period).
- *Drug reactions:* ensure these are properly reported and recorded in the patient's notes.

Chemotherapy agents with high risk of anaphylaxis

- Alemtuzamab
- Asparaginase
- Carboplatin
- Cisplatin
- Dacarbazine
- Docetaxel
- Liposomal Doxorubcin
- Etoposide
- Paclitaxel
- Rituximab
- Trastuzamab

Prevention of anaphylaxis due to chemotherapy

- Monoclonal antibodies: premedication of analgesic and antihistamine.
- Taxanes: premedication with corticosteroid, antihistamine, and H2-receptor antagonist (major reactions still around 1–3%)

Note: for prevention of blood product reactions see 📖 Blood product support.

Further reading

Ferns T, Chojnacka I (2003). The causes of anaphylaxis and its management in adults. *British Journal of Nursing,* **12**(17), 1006–12.
Gobel H (2005). Chemotherapy-induced hypersensitivity reactions. *Oncology Nursing Forum,* **32** (5), 1027–35.

ated intravascular

ation (DIC)

the abnormal generation of thrombin over a sustained period of
causing generalized intravascular coagulation, leading to
onsumption of platelets and clotting factors. DIC can be chronic or
acute. In the cancer setting the most common causes are sepsis,
leukaemias, and adenocarcinomas.

Note: acute pro-myelocytic leukaemia (AML M3) is virtually always
associated with some level of DIC at diagnosis.

Presenting signs and symptoms

- Most common is bleeding, which can be widespread.
- Purpura, ecchymosis (purple marks or skin discoloration), and
  petechiae (red pinprick marks). There are often multiple sites e.g. skin,
  gums, nose, lungs, venepuncture, and central line sites.
- Blood in urine and stools.
- Can cause uncontrollable haemorrhage leading to shock and death.

Important note: Chronic DIC may be sub-clinical, whereas acute DIC
develops over a few hours and is a true oncological emergency.

Diagnosis

By clinical presentation and blood tests showing decreased platelets and
fibrinogen plus increased clotting times (see Table 54.1).

Management

- Treat underlying cause.
- Support patient with blood products if bleeding, or if the deletion of
  clotting factors is well established.

There is no clear evidence as to the most effective approach.

Commonly used blood products

- Fresh frozen plasma: 2–4 units if clotting times are prolonged (there
  is some controversy as to how helpful FFP is)
- Platelets: 10 units for platelet counts <50 x 10^9/L.
- Cryoprecipitate: keep fibrinogen >1g/L (8 units).

Heparin can be used (mainly in chronic DIC) to inhibit excess thrombin
and halt the process of clotting (clotting cascade). Clinical trials do not
show clear benefits and there is a possible increased risk of bleeding.

Nursing management

- *Assessment for signs and symptoms of bleeding:* this must be from head
  to toe and extremely thorough; include all pressure areas, back,
  mouth, vision changes (retinal bleeding), sputum, nose bleeds, line
  sites, urine, stool.
- *Regular administration of blood products:* and regular review of blood
  counts (📖 Blood product support).

- *Bleeding*:
  - *Line sites/oozing venepuncture sites:* apply pressure (5–1υ minimum) and change dressings regularly.
  - *Nose bleeds:* instruct the patient to sit up and pinch the soft ρ the nose for 10–15min. The nurse may have to do this for the patient.
- *Vital signs measurements:* P, BP (cuff may cause extensive bruising), RR. Look for signs of shock (due to blood loss) and respiratory distress (due to pulmonary oedema). Accurate fluid balance and CVP. Chest pain could signal cardiac tamponade, requiring immediate medical intervention.
- *Fear/anxiety:* the symptoms of DIC can be extremely distressing. Careful explanation of the cause, all the treatments, their goals and side effects is required. Calm and efficient care, despite the potential emergency, can help to reassure the patient (📖 Anxiety management).

Table 54.1 Laboratory markers

Test	Finding
Platelet count	Decreased
Prothrombin time	Prolonged
Activated partial thromboplastin time	Prolonged
Thrombin time	Prolonged
Fibrinogen	Decreased

Further reading

Gobel H (1999). Disseminated Intravascular Coagulation. *Seminars in Oncology Nursing*, **15**(3), 174–182.

Levi M and Ten Cate H (1999). Disseminated Intravascular Coagulation *New England Journal of Medicine*, **341**(8) 586–592.

...ncy induced hypercalcaemia

- ...e most common oncological emergency associated with
  ...r. It occurs in 10% of patients with cancer, in most cases with
  ...anced disease.
- ...t is most commonly seen in breast, multiple myeloma, and lung cancer.
  Also in head and neck cancer, lymphomas, leukaemias, renal, and
  prostate cancer. It can be seen in any cancer.
- It can occur with or without bone metastases, though in 80% of cases
  patients do have skeletal disease.
- Overall prognosis is poor. The median survival is 3–4 months, with
  80% mortality in one year.

Normal calcium homeostasis

- 99% of calcium (Ca) is in bones (with phosphorous). 1% in
  serum—half freely ionized; half bound to protein.
- Calcium has a role in: bone formation, muscle (cardiac) contractility,
  clotting, and nerve impulse transmission.
- Normal homeostasis is controlled by parathyroid hormone (PTH),
  vitamin D, calcitonin, and renal excretion.
- If serum calcium is low, PTH stimulates bone resorption and renal
  resorption. It also stimulates gut absorption of calcium via vitamin D.

Calcitonin antagonizes PTH, and is released if serum calcium is high. It
is only short-acting.

Causes of hypercalcaemia

There are two possible mechanisms (not mutually exclusive):
- Local bone metastases directly stimulate osteoclast activity (causing
  breakdown of bone structure) and release humoral hypercalcaemia
  factors.
- Some tumours (e.g. renal, head and neck, lung, haematological) release
  systemic parathyroid hormone related protein (PTHrP) and other
  cytokines, which stimulate osteoclast activity.

In both cases, increased bone resorption releases calcium into the
bloodstream. Renal excretion of calcium may also be reduced.

Note: PTHrP has the same effect as PTH (see upper box opposite), but
without any feedback loop so it continues to act regardless of Ca level.

Presenting signs and symptoms

(See also lower box opposite for early detection.)
- Mental status: irritability, lethargy, depression, confusion, psychoses.
- Cardio-vascular: ECG changes, bradycardia, atrial arrythmias.
- Gastro-intestinal: anorexia, nausea and vomiting, constipation, ileus.
- Musculo-skeletal: fatigue, weakness, bone pain.
- Renal: thirst, polyuria, dehydration, renal failure.

Diagnosis

- Blood test for corrected calcium.
- Normal calcium 2.12–2.65mmols/L. If >3mmol/L then start t...
  and symptoms. Untreated levels of >4mmol/L can cause death
  few days.

Corrected calcium

Since calcium is bound to albumin, ionized calcium levels vary depending on the albumin level, i.e. patients with a low albumin level have higher levels of ionized calcium.

Corrected calcium (m/mols) = measured calcium + $0.02 \times (40\text{-albumin}[g/L])$

Early detection

Hypercalcaemia can easily be overlooked. Early symptoms include thirst, decreased appetite, nausea, frequent voiding of urine, increased fatigue, constipation, lethargy, and personality changes. These symptoms are non-specific, and may have many other causes.

It is important to consider who is at risk and assess individuals for potential signs/symptoms.

Patient/family education

This is important to support a quick response to possible symptoms. Teaching should include:
- Early symptoms (see above).
- Maintenance of mobility and adequate hydration.
- The need for early assessment and treatment.

Management

If the patient is asymptomatic, then treatment is not normally required. Continue to monitor calcium levels and give advice on early signs and symptoms of hypercalcaemia, including reduction of exacerbating factors. Patients should be encouraged to maintain adequate hydration with oral fluids.

The key principles of management are:

Treat the malignancy: radiotherapy, chemotherapy, or surgery should be used as appropriate. If the disease is refractory—or at an advanced stage—then palliation is the main aim.

Remove any exacerbating causes: e.g. drugs such as vitamins A and D, thiazide diuretics. Immobility may require extra analgesia, mobility equipment, physiotherapy, and occupational therapy input.

Note: there is no need to reduce oral dietary calcium, as absorption will already below.

........ately if the individual is symptomatic. 2–3 litres of normal
.... day will reduce calcium levels, but rarely back to normal. Loop
.....s such as frusemide 20–40mg can be used to assist in maintaining
...... balance once the patient is rehydrated. Maintain electrolyte-
.....onitoring check for hypokalaemia and hyponatraemia.

Bisphosphonate infusion

Bisphosphonates inhibit osteoclast activity, and reduce bone resorption.
They take 48 hours to work effectively. They are given after initial
rehydration therapy.

Drug management of hypercalcaemia

Pamidronate and sodium clodronate are effective in about 70–80% of
cases. The effects last for about 2–3 weeks. Zoledronic acid is more
expensive, but infusion times are shorter, and it may be effective for up
to 6 weeks.
- Pamidronate: 30-90mg IV I over 2–4 hr
- Zoledronic acid: 4mg IVI over 15 min
- Sodium clodronate: 1.5g IVI over 4 hr
- Ibandronic acid: 2–4 mg IVI over 1–2 hr

Bisphosphonates can cause transient fever and bone pains (manage
with paracetamol) and also a risk of hypocalcaemia.

Many patients maintain normal calcium through monthly treatment
with bisphosphonates (Ⅲ Metastatic bone disease).

Oral ibandronic acid is increasingly used in palliative settings as
maintenance therapy.

Steroids: only used in haematological malignancies to reduce osteoclast
activity.

Nursing management of hypercalcaemia

Patients may be extremely dehydrated, drowsy and confused, nauseated,
vomiting, and in pain. They can require intensive nursing support in
managing their symptoms, maintaining their safety, and monitoring their
response to medical treatment.

Nursing assessment

- Manage fluid balance, accurate monitoring of input and output. Patient
  may not be mobile for weighing.
- Monitor all vital signs, (P, BP, RR) including neurological and cardiovascular status, signs and symptoms of fluid overload and renal failure.
  Monitor for response to treatment i.e. reduced blood calcium levels,
  improved consciousness levels, reduction in fatigue, lethargy, and
  GI symptoms.

Renal and GI
- Assist with fluid input.
- Assess nausea, anti-emetics, assist with drinking, administration, and management of IVI.
- Check for oliguria, anuria,
- Assess for constipation and manage as appropriate (📖 Constipation).

Neurological

Patient may be confused or have altered consciousness levels. This can be extremely distressing for the patient and their family (📖 Acute confusional states).

- Assist patient with activities of daily living.
- Assist in orientating to time and place.
- Reassure that as calcium levels improve, confusion and consciousness levels should return to normal.

Musculoskeletal

Mobility can prevent exacerbation of hypercalcaemia. Encourage walking and weight bearing exercise unless contraindicated due to risk of pathological fractures. Analgesia may need assessment and review to enable mobilization. Patient may need nursing assistance with mobility. Equipment, physiotherapy, and OT can all be helpful in encouraging and maintaining independence.

Hypercalcaemia in the terminal phase

In some cases a decision not to treat the hypercalcaemia may be taken if the patient is close to death. A full assessment needs to be carried out, considering the patient's symptoms and also their recent response to hypercalcaemia treatment. This requires sensitive management; relatives may be expecting continuing treatment of hypercalcaemia if this has happened in the past. Management is aimed at palliation of the other symptoms such as pain and confusion.

Further reading

Heatley S (2004). Metastatic bone disease and tumour-induced hypercalcaemia: treatment options. *International Journal of Palliative Nursing*, **10**(1), 41–6.

McDonnell Keenan A K (2005). Hpercalcemia. In Yarbro C H, Frogge M H, Goodman M (eds) (2005). *Cancer Nursing, Principles and practice*. 6th edn pp.791–807. Massachusetts: Jones and Bartlett.

Spinal cord compression (SCC)

- SCC occurs in about 5% of cancer patients. Most commonly in breast, lung, and prostate cancer and multiple myeloma.
- 10% of patients with spinal metastases develop SCC.
- Sites of SCC: 70% thoracic, 20% lumbosacral, 10% cervical:
  - Different sites can produce different motor neurone signs.
  - Multiple points of compression can occur, producing confusing neurological signs.

Pathology

- *Extrinsic:* vertebral body tumour invading epidural space, vertebral collapse.
- *Intrinsic:* intradural/intramedullary metastases.

Diagnosis

- Medical history—presenting signs and symptoms.
- Neurological examination.
- MRI is the gold standard—assesses soft tissue as well as bone. Assess for meningeal metastases and multiple areas of compression.

Diagnostic delay

- Delay in the diagnosis of SCC can be devastating in term of quality of life.
- It is very important to have a high index of suspicion in patients with spinal metastases, or those with known advanced breast, prostate or lung cancer.
- Nurses need to educate patients about what SCC is, what the risks are, and the common signs and symptoms. They need to know why they must inform professionals of signs such as back pain, difficulties in passing urine, or leg weakness.

Management

Depends in part on prognostic factors:

- Patient's performance status. Will they cope with surgery or radiotherapy?
- Is there a potential to reverse the compression? If there is severe dysfunction, then the chance of improvement is poor.
- Tumour histology. Haematological malignancies tend to respond best.
- Has the patient a very short prognosis?
- Does the patient want emergency treatment?

Nurses have an important role in supporting the patient and their family with these decisions, clarifying the risks and benefits of different treatment strategies.

Treatment

Steroids

Immediate treatment is given with high-dose dexamethasone, particularly if rapidly progressing myelopathy. Lower doses can be started if there is stable, slow progress.

Radiotherapy

This is the standard treatment unless there is an unstable spine or vertebral collapse. If the patient has severe back pain, radiotherapy can often be effective even if there is no improvement in neurological status. Opioids and non-steroidal anti-inflammatory drugs are also used for pain relief. In lymphoma, chemotherapy should be considered.

Surgery

Options are vertebral body resection or laminectomy. Can be used if there is extensive vertebral collapse, or if the tumour is radiotherapy resistant. The best results are achieved when the tumour is anterior to the spine. Surgery is also used where the diagnosis is uncertain or there is a single lesion that might be totally removed. Good performance status patients with a single site of compression may do better with decompressive surgery combined with radiotherapy.

Mortality rates from surgery can be high in patients with metastatic cancer. Careful patient selection is essential.

Table 54.2 Presenting symptoms

Back pain (>90% of cases)	Weakness	Sensory loss	Autonomic dysfunction (late findings)
• Often described as band-like. • Localized or radiating. • Usually intense, progressive and persistent. Often neuropathic in nature.	• Unsteady gait, ataxia.	• Numbness and tingling.	• Urinary hesitancy, retention, incontinence. • Constipation, incontinence.

Late presentation with profound weakness or loss of sphincter control suggests poor prognosis and little chance of reversing the compression and therefore the symptoms.

Prognosis

Approximately 70% of patients ambulant prior to treatment will regain full function. Around 30% of these will survive for one year. Only 5% of those who were paraplegic will regain function. Those who remain paraplegic generally have a life expectancy of only a few weeks.

Nursing management

Assessment and early detection

Pain assessment is crucial. Knowing the early signs of SCC and educating patients and their families about these can prevent a late diagnosis (see Table 54.2).

Rehabilitation

For patients with SCC, nursing care and goals will depend on the degree of neurological deficit. Realistic goals need to be set in collaboration with the patient and the family.

These need to include the preferred place of care, so that the involvement of community or hospice services can be arranged early on.

Early involvement of physiotherapists, occupational therapists, and the palliative care team are essential to maximize the patient's rehabilitation and to enable them to maintain as much independence as possible (📖 Rehabilitation).

Symptom management

Patients with severe neurological deficits will require full nursing care. Assessment of their skin condition, regular turning, the use of low-pressure mattresses and maintaining adequate nutrition, are all essential to prevent skin breakdown and pressure sores. Bowel or bladder programmes will need to be started.

Education for patients and their family is required about physical care, mobility, injury prevention due to sensory deficits, risks of chest and urinary infection, and management of bowel and bladder care.

Facing the last months of life as a paraplegic can have a huge impact on quality of life. Referral to a specialist palliative care team is essential.

Further reading

Bucholtz JD (1999). Metastatic epidural spinal cord compression. *Seminars in Oncology Nursing*, **15** (3), 150–9.

Watson MS, Lucas CF, Hoy AM, Black IN (2005). *Oxford Handbook of Palliative Care*. Oxford: Oxford University Press.

Superior vena cava obstruction (SVCO)

This occurs when the SVC is obstructed by extrinsic compression (in about 80% of cases), tumour invasion, or thrombosis. It results in impaired drainage of the head, neck and upper extremities.

Causes

- 97% are caused by cancer, of which 75% are bronchus, particularly SCLC.
- 15% are caused by lymphoma.
- SVCO can also be caused by thrombus formation from a central line.

Clinical features

- Dyspnoea: the most common feature, caused by tracheal or bronchial compression.
- Face, neck, and arm oedema: often worse in the morning and when bending down.
- Cough, headaches, hoarseness, facial erythema, or superficial vein distension of the upper torso.

There is usually a gradual onset (not a true emergency), but rapid onset can cause severe, life-threatening symptoms such as respiratory distress and stridor. The prognosis is generally dependent on the type of cancer and the stage of the disease.

Diagnosis

Unless it is a life-threatening emergency, it is important to establish an accurate diagnosis of SVCO and the cause. Over 50% of cases present without a known diagnosis of malignancy.
- *CT scan:* ideally with contrast. Establish patency of the SVC and external or internal compression.
- *Venogram:* if there is no obvious external cause and /or if stent placement or thrombolysis is considered.
- *Tissue samples:* for definitive diagnosis (if unknown).

Treatment

Radiotherapy, chemotherapy, and surgical stenting provide the main treatment options for SVCO.
- *Stenting:* insertion of metal stent via femoral vein. This is the first choice in an emergency, as it provides immediate relief. It can also be used when radiotherapy or chemotherapy are no longer options. It should be considered as part of initial therapy in NSCLC. If a clot is suspected to be exacerbating SVCO, thrombolysis can be combined with stenting.

Note: if a clot from a central line is causing SVCO, then removing the line normally resolves the obstruction.
- *Chemotherapy:* used for chemo-sensitive tumours, such as SCLC and lymphoma, as it provides systemic treatment of disease as well. Symptom relief in 7–10 days.

- *Radiotherapy:* used for NSCLC and also when there is poor performance status or relapse post chemotherapy in SCLC or lymphoma. Symptom relief in 3–4 days.
- *Steroids:* dexamethasone 8–16mg PO/IV. There is a lack of evidence for the use of steroids, but they can reduce radiotherapy-induced oedema, and they have an anti-tumour effect in lymphoma.

Nursing

It is important to be aware of those most at risk of developing SVCO; e.g. people with SCLC. Being aware of early signs such as increasing shortness of breath, tightness or fullness of the neck, arms, and chest can allow SVCO to be treated before it becomes an emergency.

Management

This involves the assessment and support of respiratory, cardiac, and neurological systems. Emotional and psychosocial support is important where there is breathlessness and recent diagnosis or poor prognosis. (📖 Breathlessness).

Observations

- Observe for signs of worsening SVCO such as increasing anxiety, respiratory distress, decreased O_2 saturation, stridor, or hoarseness.
- Also look for signs of blurred vision and mental status changes—these are signs of cerebral oedema.
- Vital signs monitoring—frequent respiratory, cardiac, neurological assessment. Venepuncture, BP and IVs are contraindicated in upper extremities.
- Fluid balance monitoring—over-hydration could exacerbate symptoms.

Interventions

- Maintain the patent's airway.
- Support O_2 perfusion. O_2 therapy can temporarily relieve dyspnoea, restrict activity assisting with activities of daily living, maintain patient in a supported upright position.
- Anxiety management. Aim to reduce anxiety and feeling of drowning or suffocating (📖 Anxiety management).

Further reading

Haapoja I S and Blendowski C (1999). Superior vena cava syndrome. *Seminars in Oncology Nursing*, **15**(3), 183–9.

Rowell N P and Gleeson F V (2001). Steroids, radiotherapy, chemotherapy and stents for superior vena caval obstruction in carcinoma of the bronchus. *Cochrane library*, Issue 1, Oxford: Update Software.

Syndrome of inappropriate antidiuretic hormone (SIADH)

This is a paraneoplastic syndrome, caused by unregulated release of ectopic antidiuretic hormone (ADH) by the tumour.

High levels of ADH leads to water being conserved in the kidney and concentrated urine. This causes plasma hypo-osmolarity and hyponatraemia ('water intoxication'). Plasma volume moves into the cells in an attempt to equalize the osmotic gradient. This leads to intracellular oedema; cerebral oedema leads to reduced neural function and eventually death.

Physiology

ADH, also known as arginine vasopressin (AVP) is produced by the hypothalamus and has a role in maintaining accurate fluid balance. It conserves levels of fluid in the body by reducing the output of urine. It is regulated by plasma volume and osmolarity (the concentration of solutes in blood). Dehydration, vomiting, diarrhoea, or bleeding would all decrease the volume of extracellular fluid, increase plasma osmolarity, and stimulate ADH production and release.

Incidence

- Common in SCLC. Rare but also found in head and neck, oesophageal and haematological cancers.
- Non-ectopic causes include:
  - Infection, COPD.
  - Chemotherapy agents (vinca alkaloids, cyclophosphamide, ifosfamide, cisplatin, docetaxel).
  - Other drugs: tricyclic antidepressants, carbamazapine, morphine.

Presentation

- Most patients present with a slowly developing asymptomatic hyponatraemia. If hyponatraemia develops rapidly the symptoms are more severe, as the brain does not have time to effect compensatory mechanisms against cerebral oedema.
- At sodium levels below 125mmol/L common symptoms are nausea, anorexia, fatigue, weakness, and muscle cramps.
- As hyponatraemia worsens symptoms include confusion, lethargy, and psychotic behaviour eventually leading to seizures and death.

Diagnosis

Hyponatraemia is common in advanced cancer due to several causes including cardiac and hepatic failure, diuretics and hyperglycaemia. To diagnose SIADH:
- There is a need to exclude all non-entopic causes.
- The following criteria are essential:
  - Decreased plasma osmolarity, normal plasma volume.
  - Serum sodium < 130mmol/L.
  - Concentrated urine and high urinary sodium.

Management
The key is successful treatment of the cause, e.g. the malignancy, and stabilization of the patient, by correcting hyponatraemia.

Chronic/asymptomatic hyponatraemia
Fluid restriction to 500–1000ml/24h is generally sufficient. It takes several days to correct sodium levels.

Oral medication
Demeclocycline can be used. It inhibits the action of ADH on the renal tubules. Renal function must be monitored closely due to the risk of acute renal failure.

Severe/symptomatic hyponatraemia
- This is a true emergency, with a mortality of >5%.
- Management involves conservative measures as above. If these fail and the patient deteriorates, administration of IV hypertonic saline (3%) may be tried. This requires meticulous monitoring (1–2-hourly) of electrolytes, since correcting hyponatraemia too quickly can cause cerebral dehydration and neurological damage. Best carried out in a high-dependency/intensive care setting.

Nursing management
- Meticulous fluid balance monitoring including fluid balance chart, signs of fluid overload or dryness.
- Weight, lying/standing blood pressure.
- Urine measurement; volume, osmolarity.
- Educate patients on the need for fluid restriction and support with the impact of this.
- Support with oral care, managing thirst.
- For management of confused patient, see 📖 Acute confusional states.

Chemotherapy treatment and SIADH

Patients may present with SIADH as part of their initial diagnosis. They may require treatment with chemotherapy regimens that need high levels of hydration, e.g. cisplatin or cyclophosphamide.
- If they have hyponatraemia, treatment should go ahead since treating the cancer will effectively reduce the SIADH. Balancing the hydration needs for chemotherapy and management of the hyponatraemia will require meticulous monitoring.

Tumour lysis syndrome

This is an oncological emergency caused by tumour cell breakdown releasing cellular contents—uric acid, phosphorous and potassium—into the bloodstream.

Tumour lysis syndrome (TLS) is most commonly seen during aggressive treatment of large, rapidly dividing tumours, e.g. high-grade lymphoma, acute leukaemia, and chronic myeloid leukaemia in blast crisis. It is rare in solid tumours, although it has been recorded in small cell lung cancer and metastatic breast cancer.

Risk factors

Patients at increased risk are those with pre-existing renal impairment, high uric acid or electrolyte levels, and dehydration before treatment.

Timing

The syndrome generally starts within 48 hours of treatment commencing, but can last 5–7 days.

Presenting signs and symptoms

- *Acute renal failure:* due to uric acid blocking distal tubules.
- *Cardiac arrhythmia:* due to raised potassium and phosphorus (which also causes lower blood calcium).
- *Gastrointestinal and neurological effects:* due to raised potassium and phosphorus.

Common clinical manifestations of tumour lysis syndrome

Renal effects	Cardiovascular effects	GI effects	Neuromuscular effects
• Decreased urine output	• Hypertension	• Nausea and vomiting	• Muscle weakness
• Increased urea and creatinine	• Tachycardia	• Diarrhoea	• Muscle cramps, twitching
• Flank pain	• ECG changes	• Anorexia	• Parasthaesia
• Acute renal failure	• Ventricular tachycardia	• Intestinal colic	• Tetany
	• Cardiac arrest		• Confusion, delirium

Management strategy

Education

- Nurses need to educate patients about what TLS is and the common signs and symptoms. Patients need to know why it is essential to immediately report any of the signs or symptoms of TLS.
- Explain the importance of maintaining a good fluid intake (>3L) and output of urine.

Prevention of renal failure and electrolyte imbalance

- Nursing assessment and patient monitoring for risk factors and signs of TLS (see table above).
- Pharmacological treatment.
  - Allopurinol: 300mg before and during chemotherapy. This inhibits the enzyme xanthine oxidase, and blocks the conversion of nucleic acids into uric acid. It does not affect pre-existing uric acid, therefore takes 1–3 days to start reducing uric acid levels. A small proportion of patients have severe allergic reactions.
  - Rasburicase (IV) converts uric acid into allantoin. It decreases uric acid levels far quicker then allopurinol. It can be used for patients with a haematological malignancy and a high tumour burden at risk of high volume cell lysis. It is currently far more expensive than allopurinol.
- Aggressive hydration and diuresis: IV fluids, loop diuretics.
- Alkalization of urine with IV sodium bicarbonate is sometimes used to increase solubility of uric acid (keep above pH 6 or 7). This is controversial. Use cautiously as alkalization can cause calcium phosphate precipitation, increasing problem with hypocalcaemia.
- Electrolyte monitoring: urea, creatinine, and electrolytes.

Treatment of established TLS

- High potassium (>5mmol/L)—use calcium gluconate and loop diuretics, e.g. frusemide 40mg bd.
- High phosphate levels (>1.45mmol/L)—use aluminium containing antacids, every 4–6 hours (may need laxatives due to constipating effect).
- High uric acid levels. Consider switching from allopurinol to rasburicase. Continue other preventative methods as above.
- Some patients require intensive nursing support of any symptoms, e.g. nausea and vomiting, diarrhoea, muscle cramps, flank pain, and confusion.
- If electrolyte imbalance continues to worsen (e.g. potassium>6mmol/L) haemodialysis may be required.

Further reading

Gobel B H (2002). Management of Tumour Lysis Syndrome: prevention and treatment. *Seminars in Oncology Nursing*, **18**(3), S12–16.

Lydon J (2005). Tumor lysis syndrome. In Yarbro C H, Frogge M H, Goodman M (eds) *Cancer Nursing, Principles and practice.* 6th edn pp.946–958. Massachusetts: Jones and Bartlett.

For detailed information on Rasburicase got to: UK Medicines Information Pharmacists Group at: www.ukmi.nhs.uk/NewMaterial/html/docs/rasburicase.pdf

Useful websites

There are a number of extremely useful websites where up-to-date, evidence-based information, and options for information and support are available. We have included a range of websites with a broad focus on many aspects of cancer and also some more specialized websites.

Websites with Information on many aspects of cancer

Cancer Backup: www.cancerbackup.org.uk/Home
Cancer information charity, with up-to-date cancer information, practical advice and support for cancer patients, their families, and carers.

Department of Health: www.dh.gov.uk
UK government's health department website—includes a lot of key cancer policy documents.

Macmillan Cancer Support:
www.macmillan.org.uk/home.aspx
Leading national organization promoting the needs of people with cancer, campaigning for better services and funding research.

National Cancer Institute: www.cancer.gov/
Excellent American website covering evidence-based summaries of cancer treatment and side-effect management.

National Cancer Research Institue:
www.ncri.org.uk/
Promotes research into all aspects of cancer.

National Electronic Library for Health: www.nelh.nhs.uk/
Gateway to a large number of excellent evidence-based electronic resources.

National Library for health: Cancer section:
www.library.nhs.uk/cancer/

National Institute for Health and Clinical Excellence: www.nice.org.uk
Up-to-date information on latest clinical treatment recommendations.

Oncology Nursing Society: www.ons.org/
Website of the main Cancer nursing organization in America. Excellent breadth of information and link for a range of other sites.

Scotland's Health on the web (NHS Scotland):
www.show.scot.nhs.uk/publicationsindex.htm

World Health Organization: www.who.int/topics/cancer/en/
An excellent site for exploring a broad world perspective of cancer management and prevention.

More specialized websites

Adjuvant! Online: www.adjuvantonline.com/
Provides information to help health professionals and patients with early cancer discuss the risks and benefits of getting additional therapy (adjuvant therapy: usually chemotherapy, hormone therapy, or both) after surgery.

British Association of Head and Neck Oncology Nurses (BAHNON): www.bahnon.org.uk
Provides guidelines and protocols for health professionals.

British Association for Parenteral and Enteral Nutrition: www.bapen.org.uk/

British Columbia Cancer Agency website: www.bccancer.bc.ca/default.htm
Provides in-depth information on cancer management guidelines and treatment protocols.

British Committee for Standards in Haematology (BCSH) website: www.bcshguidelines.com/
Provides guidelines for management of haematological disorders and also blood product administration guidelines.

Cancer Black Care: www.cancerblackcare.org/
Cancer support service for the black and minority ethnic community.

CancerQuest: http://cancerquest.org/
Excellent interactive cancer biology website, which assumes no previous knowledge of the subject.

Cancer Research UK Website: http://info.cancerresearchuk.org/cancerstats/
Excellent resource for UK cancer statistical information.

Central Office for Research Ethics Committees: www.corec.org.uk
Useful website to explore a number of issues related to cancer research, including drug trials.

Changing Faces: www.changingfaces.org.uk
Changing Faces is a national charity based in the UK that supports and represents people who have disfigurements of the face or body from any cause.

Cochrane Collaboration: www.cochrane.org/
Provides up-to-date, accurate information about the effects of healthcare by producing and disseminating systematic reviews of healthcare interventions.

DIPEx: www.dipex.org
DIPEx provides access to a wide variety of personal experiences of health and illness, of use to patients, families, and professionals.

Lymphoedema Support Network: www.lymphoedema.org/lsn/

Maggie's Cancer Caring Centres www.maggiescentres.org.uk/
National charity with regional centres dedicated to support for people adjusting to living with cancer.

National AIDS Manual (NAM) excellent website with up-to date treatment news: www.aidsmap.com/

National Council for Palliative Care:
www.ncpc.org.uk/palliative_care.html

National Extravasation Information Service:
www.extravasation.org.uk/home.html

NHS Cancer Screening Programmes: www.cancerscreening.nhs.uk/

Palliativecare.com: www.palliativecare.com
Offers resources and information on Palliative Care Specialty and Palliative care.

Prostate Cancer Charity:
www.prostate-cancer.org.uk/info/publications.asp

Scottish Intercollegiate Guidelines Network
www.sign.ac.uk/guidelines/
Provides clinical guidelines for different cancer treatments in Scotland. Similar role in Scotland that NICE has in England and Wales.

Society of Radiographers: www.sor.org/
Provides information about the role of radiographers, including some guidelines on managing adverse effects of radiotherapy.

Teen Info on Cancer www.click4tic.org.uk/Home
Information, advice, and support for teenagers with cancer.

Index